The Role of Healthy Eating and Physical Activity in Longevity

The Role of Healthy Eating and Physical Activity in Longevity

Guest Editor

Bartłomiej Konrad Sołtysik

MDPI

Basel • Beijing • Wuhan • Barcelona • Belgrade • Novi Sad • Cluj • Manchester

Guest Editor
Bartłomiej Konrad Sołtysik
Department of Geriatrics
Medical University of Lodz
Łódź
Poland

Editorial Office
MDPI AG
Grosspeteranlage 5
4052 Basel, Switzerland

This is a reprint of the Special Issue, published open access by the journal *Nutrients* (ISSN 2072-6643), freely accessible at: https://www.mdpi.com/journal/nutrients/special_issues/1F7RB29KUJ.

For citation purposes, cite each article independently as indicated on the article page online and as indicated below:

Lastname, A.A.; Lastname, B.B. Article Title. *Journal Name* **Year**, *Volume Number*, Page Range.

ISBN 978-3-7258-7248-0 (Hbk)
ISBN 978-3-7258-7249-7 (PDF)
https://doi.org/10.3390/books978-3-7258-7249-7

Contents

About the Editor

Bartłomiej Konrad Sołtysik

Bartłomiej Konrad Sołtysik is an academic physician and researcher at the Medical University of Lodz, Poland, where he works at the Department and Clinic of Geriatrics. His academic work focuses on healthy aging, geriatric medicine, nutrition, and lifestyle determinants of health in older adults. He is involved in teaching medical students and supervising graduate research, as well as conducting clinical and epidemiological studies related to aging, cardiometabolic risk, and functional status in older populations. Dr. Sołtysik has authored numerous peer-reviewed publications in international scientific journals in the fields of geriatrics, nutrition, and aging research.

nutrients

MDPI

Editorial

From Lifespan to Healthspan: Integrating Nutrition and Physical Activity in Healthy Ageing

Bartłomiej K. Sołtysik

Department of Geriatrics and Internal Medicine, Healthy Ageing Research Centre (HARC), Medical University of Lodz, Pomorska Street 251, 92-213 Lodz, Poland; bartlomiej.soltysik@umed.lodz.pl

Population ageing is no longer a future scenario but a present reality, reshaping not only the epidemiology of chronic disease but also the fundamental goals of medicine and public health [1]. As life expectancy continues to increase, the central challenge is no longer how to live longer, but how to live longer while preserving physical function, independence, and quality of life [2]. In this context, lifestyle-related factors, particularly diet and physical activity, stand out as among the most accessible and most powerful determinants [3]. Yet, despite decades of accumulating evidence, the burden attributable to modifiable lifestyle risks remains strikingly high, with dietary factors still ranking among the leading contributors to global morbidity and mortality [1].

Importantly, the biological and behavioural processes that shape ageing trajectories begin long before old age itself. Patterns of physical inactivity, suboptimal diet quality, and psychosocial stress tend to cluster early in adult life and may silently shape long-term metabolic, cardiovascular, and functional risk. Recent large-scale observational data in young adults compellingly illustrate how these lifestyles components coexist and reinforce one another, while also revealing that the majority of individuals are aware of the need for change but struggle to translate this awareness into sustained behavioural improvement (contribution 1). This life-course perspective provides a natural conceptual frame for the present Special Issue, which brings together contributions spanning molecular mechanisms, clinical studies, and population-level observations.

A recurring theme emerging from this Special Issue is that the relationship between nutrition, physical activity, and ageing is not merely additive, but fundamentally synergistic. Diet shapes metabolic and inflammatory tone, while movement modifies body composition, mitochondrial function, insulin sensitivity, and resilience to physiological stress [4]. Collectively, these processes determine vulnerability to frailty, sarcopenia, disability, and cardiometabolic disease [5]. Several contributions highlight, from different angles, that muscle health in ageing is not simply a matter of preserving mass, but of maintaining metabolic quality and functional efficiency. Interventions such as medium-chain triglyceride supplementation appear capable of shifting skeletal muscle substrate utilization and improving muscle quality without necessarily increasing muscle size, thereby offering a plausible mechanistic explanation for previously observed benefits in gait stability and balance in older adults (contribution 2). Simultaneously, observational data in older populations reinforce the central role of adequate protein intake in maintaining muscle mass, while also suggesting that the nutritional determinants of muscle health may be more complex and more strongly modulated by lifestyle factors in women than in men (contribution 3). Complementing this perspective, evidence synthesized on nitrate-rich beetroot supplementation suggests that nutritional modulation of vascular and muscular energetics can translate into meaningful improvements in physical performance, particularly in non-elite or ageing populations, even if cognitive benefits remain less consistent (contribution 4).

Beyond the musculoskeletal system, the contributions in this Issue also converge on the importance of low-grade inflammation, oxidative stress, and metabolic resilience as core features of biological ageing. Even in apparently healthy older adults, inflammatory and vascular risk markers are frequently elevated, reflecting the well-described phenomenon of "inflammaging" [6]. Notably, targeted, polyphenol-rich nutritional interventions appear capable of attenuating this low-grade inflammatory burden and improving vascular parameters over relatively short timeframes, supporting the concept that diet can modulate ageing-related pathophysiology even before disease becomes clinically apparent (contribution 5). At the other end of the age spectrum, data in physically active adolescents show that antioxidant status and redox balance are influenced more by habitual dietary patterns and nutrient timing than by single bouts of exercise. This illustrates the complexity and context-dependence of redox regulation and cautions against overly simplistic interpretations of antioxidant supplementation or acute exercise effects (contribution 6). By acting together, these findings reinforce the view that nutrition acts not merely as fuel, but as a regulator of inflammatory tone and stress adaptation capacity.

Several contributions also extend the discussion from functional outcomes to more fundamental mechanisms of ageing. Experimental evidence from animal models indicates that dietary interventions can influence genomic stability, DNA repair capacity, and mitochondrial function processes that occupy a central position in contemporary theories of ageing biology [7]. While caloric- and dietary restriction remain the most robust experimental strategies in this field, a broader spectrum of nutritional and metabolic interventions is now being explored, converging on the idea that metabolic–genomic crosstalk represents a critical interface between lifestyle and the biology of ageing (contribution 7) [8]. At the same time, the translational dimension of these insights should not be underestimated. The example of the Mediterranean diet in chronic inflammatory diseases shows that even the most biologically plausible and evidence-supported dietary patterns require careful adaptation to clinical context, patient preferences, and long-term feasibility in order to achieve durable benefits in real-world settings (contribution 8).

As a whole, the contributions assembled in this Special Issue offer a coherent and nuanced picture of how diet and physical activity shape ageing trajectories from early adulthood to old age and from molecular mechanisms to functional outcomes. A consistent message is that healthy longevity is not the product of any single intervention, nutrient, or training modality, but rather is the result of sustained, integrated lifestyle strategies that act on interconnected metabolic, inflammatory, vascular, and musculoskeletal pathways. Perhaps most importantly, these studies collectively remind us that the prevention of frailty, disability, and loss of independence cannot be postponed until old age itself, but must begin much earlier, through long-term investment in dietary quality and habitual physical activity [9]. Future research should therefore focus not only on refining mechanistic understanding, but also on developing scalable, pragmatic, and behaviourally informed approaches capable of delivering meaningful and lasting gains in healthspan at the population level.

Conflicts of Interest: The author declares no conflict of interest.

List of Contributions:

1. Lucini, D.; Luconi, E.; Giovanelli, L.; Marano, G.; Bernardelli, G.; Guidetti, R.; Morello, E.; Cribellati, S.; Brambilla, M.M.; Biganzoli, E.M. Assessing Lifestyle in a Large Cohort of Undergraduate Students: Significance of Stress, Exercise and Nutrition. *Nutrients* **2024**, *16*, 4339. https://doi.org/10.3390/nu16244339.

2. Mutoh, T.; Kataoka, H.; Tatewaki, Y.; Taki, Y. Medium-Chain Triglyceride Dietary Supplements Reduce Glucose Metabolism of Gait-Related Skeletal Muscle in Older Adults: A Longitudinal ^{18}F-FDG PET/CT Analysis. *Nutrients* **2025**, *17*, 1707. https://doi.org/10.3390/nu17101707.
3. Sołtysik, B.K.; Balicki, P.; Kowalczyk, K.; Lutostańska, A.; Dmuchowska, J.; Pigłowska, M.; Kostka, T. Dietary and Physical Activity Correlates of Muscle Mass in 60–65-Year-Old Seniors: A Gender-Specific Analysis. *Nutrients* **2025**, *17*, 1930. https://doi.org/10.3390/nu17111930.
4. Nowak, A.; Szymańska, A.; Kwaśniewska, M.; Kochan, E.; Lipert, A. Beetroot Juice Supplementation as a Healthy Aging Strategy Through Improving Physical Performance and Cognitive Functions: A Systematic Review. *Nutrients* **2025**, *17*, 3954. https://doi.org/10.3390/nu17243954.
5. Farhat, G.; Malla, J.; Vadher, J.; Al-Dujaili, E.A.S. Effects of Pomegranate Extract on Inflammatory Markers and Cardiometabolic Risk Factors in Adults Aged 55–70 Years: A Randomised Controlled Parallel Trial. *Nutrients* **2025**, *17*, 1235. https://doi.org/10.3390/nu17071235.
6. Gawron-Skarbek, A.; Wróblewski, A.M.; Chrzczanowicz, J.; Nowak, D.; Kostka, T. Salivary Total Antioxidant Capacity of Sportive Adolescents—The Effect of Antioxidant Vitamin Intake with Usual Diet and Physical Exercises. *Nutrients* **2025**, *17*, 3610. https://doi.org/10.3390/nu17223610.
7. van Galen, I.; Hoeijmakers, J.H.J.; Vermeij, W.P. The Use of Nutritional Interventions to Enhance Genomic Stability in Mice and Delay Aging. *Nutrients* **2026**, *18*, 246. https://doi.org/10.3390/nu18020246.
8. Naik, R.G.; Purcell, S.A.; Gold, S.L.; Christiansen, V.; D'aloisio, L.D.; Raman, M.; Haskey, N. From Evidence to Practice: A Narrative Framework for Integrating the Mediterranean Diet into Inflammatory Bowel Disease Management. *Nutrients* **2025**, *17*, 470. https://doi.org/10.3390/nu17030470.

References

1. GBD 2019 Risk Factors Collaborators. Global burden of 87 risk factors in 204 countries and territories, 1990–2019: A systematic analysis for the Global Burden of Disease Study 2019. *Lancet* **2020**, *396*, 1223–1249. [CrossRef] [PubMed]
2. Kirkland, J.L.; Stout, M.B.; Sierra, F. Resilience in Aging Mice. *J. Gerontol. A Biol. Sci. Med. Sci.* **2016**, *71*, 1407–1414. [CrossRef]
3. Willett, W.; Rockström, J.; Loken, B.; Springmann, M.; Lang, T.; Vermeulen, S.; Garnett, T.; Tilman, D.; DeClerck, F.; Wood, A.; et al. Food in the Anthropocene: The EAT-Lancet Commission on healthy diets from sustainable food systems. *Lancet* **2019**, *393*, 447–492. [CrossRef]
4. Bull, F.C.; Al-Ansari, S.S.; Biddle, S.; Borodulin, K.; Buman, M.P.; Cardon, G.; Carty, C.; Chaput, J.P.; Chastin, S.; Chou, R.; et al. World Health Organization 2020 guidelines on physical activity and sedentary behaviour. *Br. J. Sports Med.* **2020**, *54*, 1451–1462. [CrossRef] [PubMed]
5. Cruz-Jentoft, A.J.; Bahat, G.; Bauer, J.; Boirie, Y.; Bruyère, O.; Cederholm, T.; Cooper, C.; Landi, F.; Rolland, Y.; Sayer, A.A.; et al. Sarcopenia: Revised European consensus on definition and diagnosis. *Age Ageing* **2019**, *48*, 16–31. [CrossRef] [PubMed]
6. Franceschi, C.; Capri, M.; Monti, D.; Giunta, S.; Olivieri, F.; Sevini, F.; Panourgia, M.P.; Invidia, L.; Celani, L.; Scurti, M.; et al. Inflammaging and anti-inflammaging: A systemic perspective on aging and longevity emerged from studies in humans. *Mech. Ageing Dev.* **2007**, *128*, 92–105. [CrossRef] [PubMed]
7. López-Otín, C.; Blasco, M.A.; Partridge, L.; Serrano, M.; Kroemer, G. Hallmarks of aging: An expanding universe. *Cell* **2023**, *186*, 243–278. [CrossRef] [PubMed]
8. Fontana, L.; Partridge, L. Promoting health and longevity through diet: From model organisms to humans. *Cell* **2015**, *161*, 106–118. [CrossRef] [PubMed]
9. Fielding, R.A.; Guralnik, J.M.; King, A.C.; Pahor, M.; McDermott, M.M.; Tudor-Locke, C.; Manini, T.M.; Glynn, N.W.; Marsh, A.P.; Axtell, R.S.; et al. Dose of physical activity, physical functioning and disability risk in mobility-limited older adults: Results from the LIFE study randomized trial. *PLoS ONE* **2017**, *12*, e0182155. [CrossRef] [PubMed]

https://doi.org/10.3390/nu18030528

nutrients

MDPI

Article

Salivary Total Antioxidant Capacity of Sportive Adolescents—The Effect of Antioxidant Vitamin Intake with Usual Diet and Physical Exercises

Anna Gawron-Skarbek [1,*], Adam Marek Wróblewski [2,*], Jacek Chrzczanowicz [3], Dariusz Nowak [4] and Tomasz Kostka [1]

1 Department of Geriatrics, Medical University of Lodz, 92-213 Lodz, Poland; tomasz.kostka@umed.lodz.pl
2 Department of Medical Biochemistry, Medical University of Lodz, 92-215 Lodz, Poland
3 Cardiac Rehabilitation Centre, Copernicus Memorial Hospital, 93-438 Lodz, Poland; jacekchrz@interia.pl
4 Department of Clinical Physiology, Medical University of Lodz, 92-215 Lodz, Poland; dariusz.nowak@umed.lodz.pl
* Correspondence: anna.gawron@umed.lodz.pl (A.G.-S.); adam.wroblewski@umed.lodz.pl (A.M.W.)

Abstract: Background: The body requires effective antioxidant defense mechanisms to counter the effect of oxidative stress. The aim of the study was to evaluate the postprandial effect of antioxidative vitamin (C, E and β-carotene) consumption during breakfast and of aerobic exercise on salivary total antioxidant capacity (TAC). **Methods:** Fifty-one healthy male adolescents were examined (13–18 years; 15.4 ± 1.6). Dietary interviews including vitamin C, E, and β-carotene intake were performed twice, once on the examination day and again the day before. Salivary TAC was assessed using the DPPH method (2.2-diphenyl-1-picryl-hydrazyl) and expressed as % of free radical reduction. Saliva samples were assayed at three subsequent time-points: fasting (DPPH 1), after a meal—breakfast—(DPPH 2), and after aerobic exercise training (DPPH 3). **Results:** DPPH 2 was higher than DPPH 1 (16.8 ± 7.5 vs. 14.9 ± 7.2% of reduction; $p = 0.03$), and no differences were noted between DPPH 2 and DPPH 3 (16.8 ± 7.5 vs. 16.3 ± 6.5%; $p > 0.05$), nor between DPPH 1 and DPPH 3. Subjects with higher BMI demonstrated higher values of DPPH at all time-points of the study ($p < 0.05$). In turn, neither the DPPH values nor the changes in DPPH were related to weekly exercise-related energy expenditure ($p > 0.05$). No singular DPPH index was associated with the level of vitamin E or β-carotene intake with meals on the day before the study; however, DPPH 1 (rho = −0.38; $p < 0.01$) and DPPH 2 (rho = −0.45; $p < 0.001$) negatively correlated with vitamin C intake on the day before examination. **Conclusions:** In physically active adolescents, daily vitamin C consumption decreased salivary TAC, and the consumption of antioxidant nutrients/vitamins as part of a regular breakfast directly enhanced the antioxidant capacity of saliva; nevertheless, subsequent physical exercise had no detectable impact.

Keywords: total antioxidant capacity; saliva; DPPH; exercise; vitamin C; vitamin E; beta-carotene; young athletes

1. Introduction

Homeostasis between pro- and antioxidant compounds is maintained by the continual activity of a range of processes. The human body has a complex antioxidative defense system comprising three main lines of defense: free radical scavengers, antioxidant enzymes (e.g., glutathione peroxidase, superoxide dismutase and catalase), and the Fenton reaction system, which enables chelation of free metal ions. Free radical scavengers neutralize free radicals to become more stable radicals themselves. Moreover, vitamin C can regenerate oxidized antioxidant molecules [1].

The antioxidant defense system is affected by a number of factors, including physical effort [2], diet [3,4], smoking [5,6], health status/diseases [7,8], and applied pharmacotherapy. However, there is little concrete data regarding the influence of physical exercise on the antioxidant barrier and, as such, no formula aimed at improving antioxidant capacity currently exists [9–12]. Therefore, it is unclear whether enhancing antioxidant status would be more desirable for the body than maintaining the balance between oxidative stress and antioxidant potential.

Antioxidant capacity can be assessed by different methods, which achieve different results. Such methods include measuring the concentration or activity of singular antioxidants in body fluids (blood plasma/serum, saliva, urine, tears) or in cells/tissues, or by assessing Total Antioxidant Capacity/Status (TAC/TAS) [13–15]. Although TAC evaluation methods have certain limitations, e.g., sensitivity to only a defined group of antioxidants [16,17], this approach is widely used in experimental and clinical studies [15]. Recently, a promising new method for assessing TAC has been developed that could be useful in clinical studies. This method measures the total activity of circulating low-molecular-weight nonenzymatic antioxidants based on the ability of deproteinized body fluids (e.g., plasma, serum, and saliva) to decompose a 2.2-diphenyl-1-picryl-hydrazyl (DPPH) radical.

Human saliva is a mixture of gingival crevicular fluid (GCF), with a similar composition to plasma/serum, and it is the first line of defense against oxidative stress [14,18]. It includes a large number of organic and inorganic compounds which can be used as indicators of health status. As such, and due to its availability and noninvasive mode of collection, saliva could be used in diagnoses of pathological conditions/diseases in the oral cavity, as well as some systemic disorders [19]. For instance, salivary TAC is also known to be influenced by oral health status [20,21].

In the available literature there are no studies assessing simultaneously the impact of dietary antioxidants and exercise on salivary TAC in adolescents. Filling this gap of knowledge would enable better insight into planning these two basic non-pharmacologic behaviors in young people. Therefore, the aim of the study was to (1) evaluate the postprandial effect of consuming antioxidative vitamins (C, E, and β-carotene) as part of the typical breakfast, (2) measure the effect of aerobic exercise on salivary TAC, and (3) assess the relationship between the regular daily intake of antioxidative vitamins and the TAC of saliva in a group of healthy, young, physically active boys.

2. Materials and Methods

2.1. Subjects

The study included 83 healthy, physically active students in the Kazimierz Górski memorial sports school in Lodz (Poland). All were residents of the school dormitory, and were receiving their meals in the school canteen. The age range was 13–18 years, and the participants' training experience $\geq$1 year; Physical Activity Level = 2.2 ÷ 2.4 [22]. Of these, 27 students were excluded from the study due to the following various reasons: absence from school, physical injury, lack of time in the second and/or in the third stage of the study, mild infection, or laboratory difficulties with saliva testing (i.e., presence of precipitates in the sample). Complete data was therefore collected from 56 adolescents. As only five female participants with complete data were enrolled, they were excluded from the study. Finally, 51 male students were included in the analysis (15.4 $\pm$ 1.6 years).

The whole study group was free from inflammation, chronic diseases (any medicaments were applied), and physical injury. The subjects were not overweight, obese (according to the BMI percentile chart for boys at age of 5 to 19 years), nor had an addiction history (tobacco, alcohol, and drugs). All students were provided with meals on a daily basis in the school canteen (institutional food). None used any special diet. The study protocol was approved by the local ethics committee (RNN/15/15/KE/L) and informed consent was obtained from parents or legal guardians.

2.2. Protocol and Measures

The examinations took place in the school. The laboratory measurements were performed in the Department of Clinical Physiology, Medical University of Lodz, and the dietary intake was analyzed in the Department of Hygiene and Health Promotion, Medical University of Lodz. The students were asked to report to the school hall, after overnight fasting, between 7:00 and 7:45 a.m. They were also asked not to brush their teeth before sample collection, just to slightly gargle the oral cavity with water (time window between tooth cleaning and saliva collection was ±10 h).

An unstimulated saliva sample was given by each student and reading pH 1 was assayed immediately. Following this, the subjects were interviewed for demographic and behavioral features related to dietary habits, physical activity, oral hygiene, smoking, and drug use; the data was collected using a questionnaire designed for the study based on WHO CINDI recommendations [23]. Anthropometric and blood pressure measurements were performed, and a 24 h dietary recall from the day before an examination was obtained from each individual.

Next, the subjects consumed their breakfast at the school canteen. A second saliva sample was then collected within an hour, before their usual exercise training, and reading pH 2 was tested. Then the dietary intake from breakfast was recorded and the students went to their training. Each of the respondents, both the day before and on the day of the study, could eat what the kitchen offered in any amount according to their usual preferences.

After aerobic exercise (physical activity intervention) the third saliva sample was collected and pH 3 was recorded. A single training unit lasted 1.5 h and consisted of three parts: a warm-up (±20 min, including jogging, jumping, stretching, and activities reflecting the type of movements/actions during the sport events), a main training session with discipline-specific exercises (±60 min), and a cool down (±15 min, including stretching of muscle groups loaded during a training session). Exercise training was the same for all the participants.

2.2.1. Anthropometric and Blood Pressure Data

Height and weight were measured and Body Mass Index (BMI; $kg\cdot m^{-2}$) was calculated [24]. Waist and hip circumference measurements were taken, and Waist-to-Hip Ratio (WHR) was computed as an index of visceral obesity. An electronic manometer with oscillometric technique (UA-767PC) was used to measure systolic (SBP) and diastolic blood pressure (DBP), and heart rate (HR) at rest [25].

2.2.2. Energy Expenditure

The exercise-related energy expenditure ($kcal\cdot week^{-1}$) was calculated based on the time (hours and minutes) scheduled for recreational/sports physical activities. The calculation was performed according to Fox et al. [26].

2.2.3. Nutritional Assessment

Dietary recall was supported using an album of photographs of food products and dishes from the National Food and Nutrition Institute (NFNI) in Warsaw [27]. The Diet

5.0 software (license No: 52/PD/2013), also designed by the NFNI, was used to assess nutrient, vitamin, mineral, and energy intake in the daily food rations (DFR) [22,28].

2.2.4. Salivary TAC and pH

Before the unstimulated saliva samples (±5 mL) were secured [29], pH assays were performed with test paper (Whatman, Maidstone, UK). In the laboratory, the samples were centrifuged to separate all debris (10,000 rpm, 10 min, 4 °C). The supernatant was stored at −80 °C until the experiment, but not longer than 30 days.

Salivary TAC was assessed using the spectrophotometric (Ultrospec III with Spectro-Kinetics software—LKB Biochrom Pharmacia, Cambridge, UK) DPPH test, as described previously [15,30,31]. The analysis comprised samples of saliva collected at three subsequent time-points: fasting (DPPH 1), after a meal—usually breakfast—(DPPH 2), and after aerobic exercise intervention (DPPH 3). For singular DPPH determination, 25 μL of deproteinized saliva was added to 975 μL of DPPH reagent mixture. To enhance the data reliability, all individual results were calculated as a mean, from three separate experiments (expressed as % of DPPH reduction). The measurement procedures were performed by a qualified laboratory technician who was blinded to the participant qualification criteria and the time-point of the analyzed samples.

2.3. Statistical Analysis

Data were verified for the normality of distribution using the Shapiro–Wilk test, and homogeneity of variance using Levene's test. Variables that did not meet the assumption of normality were analyzed with non-parametric statistical tests. DPPH and pH values between the three time-points were compared using the T-test for dependent samples and the Wilcoxon matched-pairs test. The results for continuous variables were presented as mean ± SD and median (Q1–Q3). The Spearman rank correlation with 95% confidence intervals (CI) was used to determine the relationships between the selected numerical variables. Effect sizes based on Cohen's d were calculated. An effect size of 0.2 to <0.5 and ≥0.5 to <0.8 has been suggested to represent a small and medium effect, respectively, while an effect size ≥ 0.8 represents a large effect. The level of statistical significance was set at $p < 0.05$. Statistica version 13 was used (StatSoft Polska Sp. z o. o., Kraków, Poland).

3. Results

3.1. General Characteristics

Detailed demographic, anthropometric resting blood pressure and energy expenditure data are presented in Table 1. The entire study group was within the normal BMI range and did not have high blood pressure.

Table 1. Baseline characteristics of the study group.

Parameter	Mean ± SD Median (Q1–Q3)
Age [years]	15.4 ± 1.6 16.0 (14.0–17.0)
Height [m]	1.76 ± 0.1 1.76 (1.69–1.82)
Body Mass [kg]	66.8 ± 12.4 68.0 (60.0–76.0)
Body Mass Index [kg·m^{-2}]	21.4 ± 2.2 21.9 (20.2–22.9)
Waist Circumference [cm]	72.2 ± 5.6 72.0 (70.0–75.0)

Table 1. *Cont.*

Parameter	Mean ± SD Median (Q1–Q3)
Hip Circumference [cm]	89.5 ± 8.2 90.0 (82.0–95.0)
Waist-to-Hip Ratio	0.81 ± 0.05 0.81 (0.78–0.83)
Systolic Blood Pressure [mmHg]	124.6 ± 12.8 124.0 (116.0–131.0)
Diastolic Blood Pressure [mmHg]	68.6 ± 9.8 68.0 (62.0–75.0)
Heart Rate [beats per minute]	68.6 ± 9.8 68.0 (62.0–75.0)
Exercise-related Energy Expenditure [kcal·week^{-1}]	7000 ± 1804 6300 (6000–8400)

3.2. Nutrient Intake

Table 2 presents data regarding energy and the consumption of various DFR nutrients with meals on the day before the study and with the breakfast on the day of the study; Table 3 presents the intake of the antioxidant vitamins C, E, and β-carotene.

Table 2. Dietary characteristics of the study group based on a 24 h dietary recall and from the breakfast on a study day.

Parameter	24 h Mean ± SD Median (Q1–Q3)	Breakfast Mean ± SD Median (Q1–Q3)
Total energy [kcal·d^{-1}]	3008 ± 880 3106 (2317–3434)	756 ± 588 610 (554–720)
Proteins [g]	104.4 ± 32.0 103.5 (86.1–124.6)	22.1 ± 9.8 20.6 (16.4–25.6)
Animal proteins [g]	61.4 ± 25.4 60.6 (44.4–78.1)	11.2 ± 7.8 10.6 (6.2–13.6)
Plant proteins [g]	42.6 ± 11.1 42.5 (35.8–48.4)	11.0 ± 3.7 10.2 (9.7–12.4)
Carbohydrates [g]	453.9 ± 136.0 456.5 (380.7–522.2)	92.2 ± 31.9 78.8 (74.4–114.6)
Absorbable carbohydrates [g]	429.6 ± 131.9 437.8 (360.6–495.0)	88.6 ± 31.1 73.4 (71.1–110.3)
Sucrose [g]	111.3 ± 62.9 105.8 (79.8–132.9)	11.0 ± 7.9 7.9 (6.4–13.5)
Fiber [g]	24.4 ± 7.9 23.5 (18.4–29.5)	3.7 ± 2.2 2.7 (2.2–4.3)
Fats [g]	95.0 ± 39.9 96.1 (67.3–115.8)	34.8 ± 62.4 22.3 (18.2–27.6)
Saturated fatty acids [g]	40.7 ± 17.4 40.6 (27.8–50.7)	19.4 ± 39.4 12.3 (8.9–16.4)
Monounsaturated fatty acids [g]	36.6 ± 17.9 34.0 (24.1–45.2)	10.7 ± 17.8 7.5 (5.3–8.4)
Polyunsaturated fatty acids [g]	11.1 ± 4.9 10.8 (7.2–12.8)	2.6 ± 3.7 1.8 (1.6–2.2)
Cholesterol [mg]	322.8 ± 137.7 298.1 (241.3–362.3)	102.9 ± 185.2 68.6 (44.2–88.8)

Table 3. Vitamin C, vitamin E, and β-carotene intake with daily food rations on the day before the study, based on a 24 h dietary recall, and with breakfast on the day of the study, in a group of adolescents.

Parameter	24 h Mean ± SD Median (Q1–Q3)	Breakfast Mean ± SD Median (Q1–Q3)
Vitamin C [mg]	100.5 ± 99.2 69.0 (39.8–113.4)	6.3 ± 7.6 2.5 (0.0–10.2)
Vitamin E [mg]	8.8 ± 4.2 8.0 (6.2–10.3)	2.1 ± 3.7 1.3 (1.1–1.7)
β-carotene [μg]	4757 ± 5968 3355 (1283–5658)	192 ± 298 111 (76–192)

3.3. Analyses of DPPH Changes and Selected Correlates

A significant difference was observed between DPPH 1 and DPPH 2, i.e., the DPPH values increased after eating a meal (potential antioxidant effect of vitamin C, E, and β-carotene intake): 14.9 ± 7.2%; 95% CI = 12.8–16.9% vs. 16.8 ± 7.5%; 95% CI = 14.7–18.9%; $p = 0.03$. However, the level of DPPH was not affected by exercise (DPPH 1 vs. DPPH 3: 14.9 ± 7.2%; 95% CI = 12.8–16.9% vs. 16.3 ± 6.5%; 95% CI = 14.4–18.1; $p > 0.05$) (Figure 1).

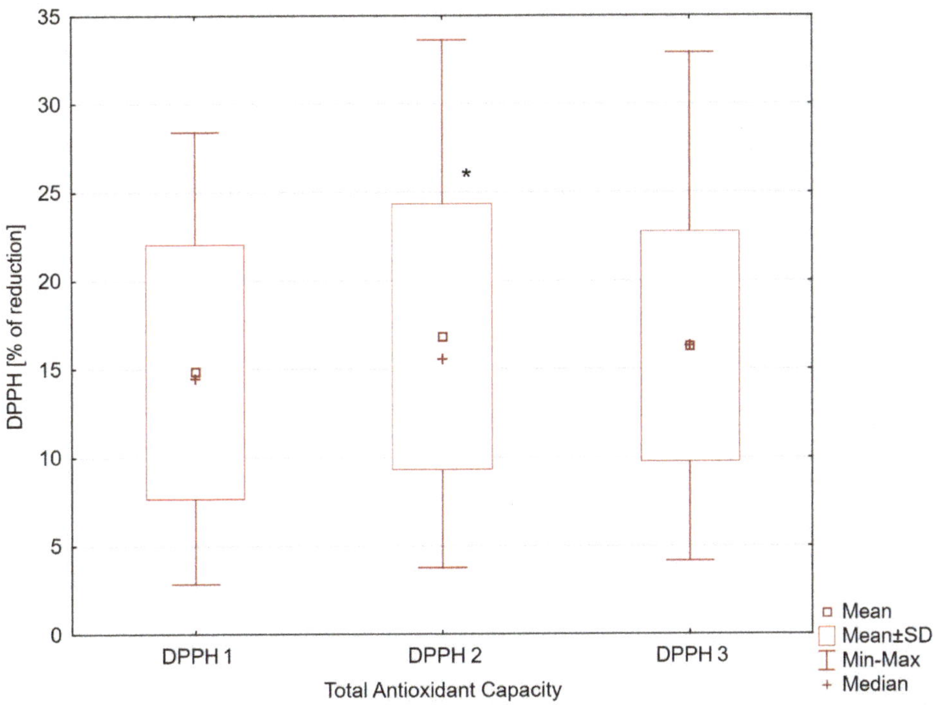

Figure 1. Salivary DPPH values: fasting (DPPH 1), after dietary intake (DPPH 2), and after aerobic exercise intervention (DPPH 3) in group of male adolescents. *—$p < 0.05$.

Higher DPPH 1 (rho = 0.31; 95% CI = 0.03–0.54; $p = 0.03$), DPPH 2 (rho = 0.36; 95% CI = 0.09–0.59; $p = 0.01$), and DPPH 3 (rho = 0.31; 95% CI = 0.03–0.55; $p = 0.03$) were noted in subjects with higher BMI values (Figure 2a,b; small effect size). In turn, neither the

DPPH values nor the changes in DPPH (neither ΔDPPH 3–DPPH 1, nor ΔDPPH 3–DPPH 2) were associated with exercise-related energy expenditure ($p > 0.05$).

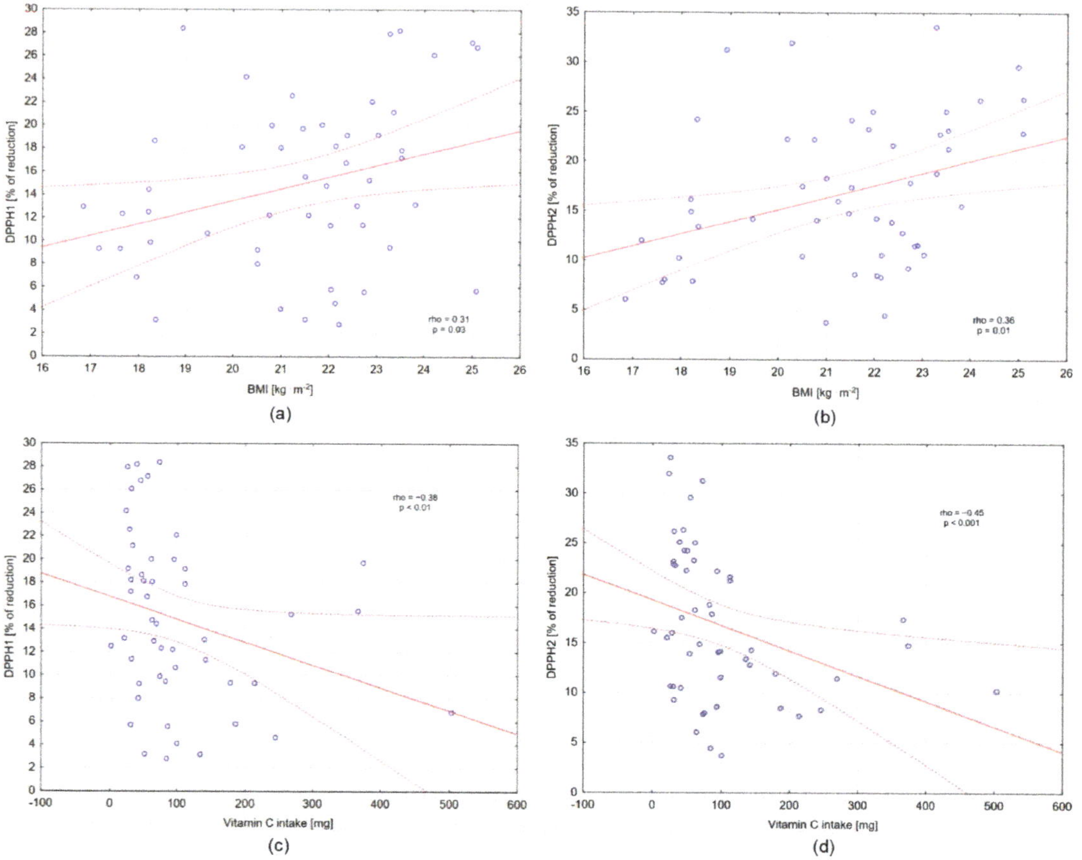

Figure 2. Correlations between DPPH and BMI (**a**,**b**), and between DPPH and vitamin C intake on day before the examination (**c**,**d**).

No singular DPPH index was associated with the level of vitamin E or β-carotene intake with meals on the day before the study; however, DPPH 1 (rho = −0.38; 95% CI = −0.60–−0.11; $p < 0.01$) and DPPH 2 (rho = −0.45; 95% CI = −0.65–−0.19; $p < 0.001$) negatively correlated with vitamin C intake (Figure 2c,d; small effect size). Individuals with higher vitamin C intake demonstrated lower fasting and postprandial salivary TAC. Vitamin C consumed with meals the day prior to the study had no effect on DPPH 3.

Meanwhile, the level of vitamins C, E, and β-carotene consumed with breakfast on the day of the examination was not related to either DPPH 2 or DPPH 3, nor to a change in DPPH (ΔDPPH 2–DPPH 1).

4. Discussion

Few reports have examined the antioxidant capacity of saliva in adolescents, especially interventional studies [32]. As such, the present study is one of the few to use saliva to determine the effect of physical activity and the amount of antioxidant vitamins consumed with a meal (not as supplements) on TAC (DPPH) levels. It was observed that salivary TAC of the studied active male adolescents significantly increased after breakfast, which could be related to the consumption of antioxidant vitamins contained in a meal. We may suppose that the observed postprandial increase in TAC could be related also to non-vitamin components of meals—to the polyphenols contained, for example, in tea, fruit, and vegetables—or perhaps also to the sources of fructose (fruit), or purine rings (meat), as substrates for future uric acid synthesis. In contrast, the aerobic exercise intervention had no influence on salivary TAC, as indicated by DPPH testing, in a relatively short period after the intervention.

These results are partially consistent with those of a previous study in a group of older adults, which showed that, unlike supplementation, higher habitual dietary intake of vitamin C corresponds to lower salivary TAC when measured via FRAS (Ferric Reducing Ability of Saliva), but neither vitamin C, E, nor β-carotene affected salivary TAC when assessed via DPPH [33]. A recent systematic review suggested that increased dietary antioxidant intake is more closely linked to enhanced salivary TAC in different age groups [34,35]. Kamodyová et al. report that a high single intake of a 250 mg dose of vitamin C augmented salivary TAC and ferric reducing antioxidant power (FRAP) in healthy subjects (n = 19) [36]. Although the intake of vitamins C, E, and β-carotene with meals was not as high in the current study, the effect on salivary TAC was still present.

The studied adolescents did not consume a vitamin-rich diet, but it seems that this was enough to improve the antioxidant capacity of saliva. It should be noticed that some data variability, as the intake of vitamin C, vitamin E, and β-carotene had a high variability among participants, could be related to the differentiated dietary preferences of youth—some of them did not like vegetables or fruits, and others quite the opposite. Interestingly, our findings indicate negative correlations between the level of vitamin C intake from a 24 h interview and either DPPH 1 or DPPH 2 in the study group. Adolescents whose daily vitamin C intake was higher the day before the study showed lower fasting and postprandial antioxidant capacity of saliva on the next day. However, this relationship was no longer identified after exercise. This could mean that although the postprandial antioxidant effect in saliva occurs, it may be short-lived, and that after a longer break from the meal, the antioxidant effect in saliva is counterbalanced by habitual vitamin C intake. It may be the case that this is intended to increase the level of antioxidant defense in the oral cavity in saliva. Several existing studies indicate pro-oxidative properties of vitamin C at low concentrations ("second face" of vitamin C), especially in the presence of interlocutory metal ions (Fe and Cu), which may putatively attenuate the antioxidant defense system [37–40]. Interestingly, the bioavailability of vitamin C/ascorbic acid is dose-dependent, i.e., higher absorption is observed at lower doses, and it is actively transported through cell membranes.

The amount of serum vitamin C can be modified in relation to dietary supply by active vitamin C transporters (SVCT1 and SVCT2) [41]. Hence, the vitamin C level in saliva could be influenced by its absorption with previous meals, thus determining the level of salivary TAC.

It seems that salivary TAC may be vulnerable to antioxidant intake in a time-dependent and antioxidant-specific manner. Recent (breakfast) intake may increase TAC while more remote (the day before) intake may be related to lower TAC, but only in relation to vitamin C intake and not to vitamin E or β-carotene intake. However, considering the contradictory results of previous research, which suggests an indirect relationship between antioxidant vitamin intake and TAC, and the possible contribution of other factors, further analyses are required to better understand the nature of the free radical scavenging mechanisms used in the body.

On the other hand, the meta-analysis of 22 studies indicated an increase in salivary TAC despite the oxidative stress linked to dental caries, implying the existence of a compensatory mechanism activated when necessary [20]. Another meta-analysis showed attenuated TAC in plasma, serum, and GCF in periodontitis; however, salivary TAC was unchanged [21]. Thus, further research should focus on a comprehensive assessment of the body's oxidative status (e.g., plasma, GCF, and cellular oxidative status of adjacent tissues) to identify the potential antioxidative reservoir utilized to counterbalance salivary oxidative stress on demand.

The following certain factors may have a significant influence on the effect of physical exercise on saliva TAC level: the time of sample measurement (in our case, immediately after the end of training), the type of exercises (aerobic or anaerobic), and its duration and intensity. In the present study, no significant increase in salivary TAC was observed after aerobic exercise, which may indicate that the physically active adolescent boys have more advanced adaptive capacities for physical effort than typical adolescents, at least in saliva. This higher level of exercise tolerance may have resulted from their everyday sporting school activities; however, exercise-related energy expenditure was not found to influence TAC/DPPH index in saliva.

Grzesiak-Gasek et al. report an increase in salivary TAC in thirty young (13–16 years) swimmers after swimming training, which they attribute to an adaptive mechanism or a defensive reaction to increased oxidative stress induced by physical exercise. After resting, salivary TAC level decreased but remained higher than at rest [42]. Also, González et al. [2] indicate increased TAC in healthy subjects immediately after aerobic exercise (after 10,000 m race) and a decrease in the salivary marker of oxidative stress (lipid hydroperoxide).

In contrast to our present research, Mahdivand et al. report a decrease in TAC (assessed by FRAP) both immediately after and 24 h after a single session of combined strength and endurance training in a group of 20 male athletes [43]. In turn, Deminice et al. [44] note that salivary uric acid, a main endogenous antioxidant, increased post-acute resistance training and that salivary uric acid correlated with blood serum acid. Further studies are needed to assess TAC simultaneously in saliva and other fluids, such as blood plasma, to confirm the presence of systemic antioxidative mechanism homeostasis among well-trained adolescents.

However, due to the small number of similar studies, it is difficult to relate our present results to the wider literature. Nevertheless, Pani et al. [45] reported a significantly lower reduction in salivary TAC in dental students engaging in high levels of exercise compared to their counterparts from a low-exercise group, during examination week. This supports the theory that more physically active people have better adaptation mechanisms. They conclude that regular exercises may protect against the oxidative stress associated with academic stress. Additionally, Munther et al. also confirm that total salivary antioxidant activity was higher in men who exercised compared to those who did not, regardless of smoking [46].

In contrast, taekwondo athletes were found to have a markedly suppressed salivary antioxidant capacity immediately after a training session, though it quickly returned to pre-exercise values [10], regardless of whether green tea or water was consumed by subjects. Similarly, exhaustive aerobic exercise was found to induce oxidative stress in the saliva of young girls, which affected TAC levels (DPPH) [47]. Furthermore, Babaei et al. observed that acute physical exercise contributed to a decrease in salivary vitamin C concentration in sedentary men, which may have impacted antioxidant capacity [48]. These examples illustrate the complex relationship between physical exercise and salivary TAC according to type of physical activity (aerobic/anaerobic), its intensity, or one's level of proficiency in sport. A systematic review, by Alves et al., of the effects of physical exercise and its accompanying changes in salivary oxidative stress/antioxidant capacities also concluded that the wide heterogeneity of study methodology leads to divergent data [49].

An interesting additional observation was the identification of positive correlations between DPPH 1, DPPH 2, and DPPH 3, and BMI. At each salivary TAC measurement time-point, a higher antioxidant capacity of saliva indicated a better, but not impaired, nutritional status, as assessed by BMI. Unfortunately, few papers describe the relationship between salivary TAC and nutritional status in young subjects with normal weight (no overweight/obesity); however, a study of salivary TAC in a group of thirty-year-old participants by Safabakhsh et al. did not identify significant differences between the obese and normal-weighted individuals [50]. On the other hand, Gunjalli et al. reported higher salivary TAC in overweight and obese 6- to 12-year-old children in India compared to their slim counterparts. The authors note that these children belong to a high socioeconomic class and attribute the outcome to a diet rich in phytonutrients and antioxidants [51]. Also, Zalewska et al. report that overweight and obese adolescents (aged 11–18) demonstrate stronger antioxidant barrier in saliva (higher TAC) and higher concentrations of individual antioxidants, such as uric acid or enzymes, superoxide dismutase, catalase, and peroxidase, compared to controls [52]. Based on these findings and our present results, it can be assumed that a poorer nutritional status, but not being underweight, may translate into the weaker antioxidant capabilities of saliva; however, this hypothesis requires additional research, ideally in groups without any accompanying health problems.

The study does have some limitations. For example, it would have benefited from a larger sample size. In addition, regarding recruitment, the subjects were included based on the typical time period that boys enter puberty in Poland; this is currently believed to be around 13–14 years of age. However, no assessment of the stage of the development of each participant was made, which could influence the level of the antioxidant adaptive mechanisms of saliva. The puberty period may affect the antioxidative activity of saliva [8] but, for example, in the study by Esenlik et al. [53], on patients with fixed orthodontic appliances, no difference was found regarding the antioxidant status of saliva between the pubertal and postpubertal groups. Future studies should assess the potential impact of the stage of puberty on salivary antioxidant status. Due to the small number of girls who agreed to participate in the project (i.e., five participants), the study included only male individuals, which weakens the possibility of extrapolating the results to the entire population. Further research should be aimed at female athletes and adolescents in other sports disciplines to permit further generalization. Furthermore, the DPPH method itself is limited in that it omits protein antioxidants (enzymes, albumins, and glutathione) which might also affect the final results; in addition, it cannot be excluded that the DPPH effect was local rather than systemic, and greater changes in saliva could occur later in the oral cavity rather than in the circulation (in blood plasma).

Nevertheless, the study also has a number of strengths. The subject selection allowed the formation of a homogeneous group consisting of healthy, sportive young male adolescents with similar anthropometric and dietary characteristics: all subjects were engaged in a similar lifestyle and ate meals served by the same canteen. In addition, the group was not subject to possible confounding factors, i.e., no participants smoked, or were overweight or obese. Our results also provide an opportunity to identify some nutritional shortcomings in the diet of young athletes fed by the mass catering system. Still, further studies are needed to confirm these findings and to shed more light on the habitual antioxidant vitamin intake- and physical exercise-related modulation of salivary TAC.

5. Conclusions

In conclusion, in physically active adolescents, daily vitamin C consumption decreased salivary TAC, and the consumption of antioxidant nutrients/vitamins as part of a regular breakfast directly enhanced the antioxidant capacity of saliva. In addition, subsequent physical exercise had no detectable impact; however, the potential systemic impact of physical training cannot be excluded. Despite limited evidence, salivary TAC seems to be a promising index for assessing biochemical changes in the body caused by behavior-dependent factors.

Author Contributions: Conceptualization, A.G.-S., J.C. and T.K.; methodology, A.G.-S., J.C. and D.N.; software, A.G.-S., J.C., A.M.W. and D.N.; validation, A.G.-S., J.C. and A.M.W.; formal analysis, A.G.-S., A.M.W. and J.C.; investigation, A.G.-S. and A.M.W.; resources, A.G.-S., J.C. and D.N.; data curation, A.G.-S., J.C. and A.M.W.; writing—original draft preparation, A.G.-S.; writing—review and editing, A.G.-S., J.C., A.M.W. and T.K.; visualization, A.G.-S., J.C., A.M.W. and T.K.; supervision, T.K.; project administration, A.G.-S. and J.C.; funding acquisition, A.G.-S., D.N. and T.K. All authors have read and agreed to the published version of the manuscript.

Funding: This research was funded by the Medical University of Lodz, grant number 502-03/6-024-01/502-64-072. The APC was funded by grants no. 503/6-077-01/503-61-001, 564/9-905-01/564-01, and 503/6-086-01/503-61-001 from the Medical University of Lodz.

Institutional Review Board Statement: The study was conducted in accordance with the Declaration of Helsinki and approved by the Institutional Ethics Committee of the Medical University of Lodz (RNN/15/15/KE/L, 17 March 2015).

Informed Consent Statement: Informed consent was obtained from all parents or legal guardians of minor study participants involved in the study.

Data Availability Statement: The data presented in this study are available on request from the corresponding authors. The data are not publicly available to preserve privacy of minor participants.

Acknowledgments: Authors would like to thank Andrzej Olczyk from the Department of Hygiene and Health Promotion, Medical University of Lodz (MUL), students of the Faculty of Dietetics of MUL, Paulina Janiak and Przemysław Tomaszewski for their assistance in data collection, Piotr Grzelak from the Higher School of Sport in Lodz for technical assistance, Elżbieta Trafalska and Barbara Rózga-Obrębska from the Department of Nutrition and Epidemiology (MUL) for their computer diet analysis assistance, and Anna Prymont-Przymińska, from the Department of Clinical Physiology (MUL), and Agnieszka Sobczak, student of Faculty of Medical Analytics (MUL), for their laboratory support. We would also like to thank Edward Lowczowski (MUL) for language assistance.

Conflicts of Interest: The authors declare no conflicts of interest. The funders had no role in the design of the study; in the collection, analyses, or interpretation of data; in the writing of the manuscript, or in the decision to publish the results.

References

1. Lü, J.-M.; Lin, P.H.; Yao, Q.; Chen, C. Chemical and Molecular Mechanisms of Antioxidants: Experimental Approaches and Model Systems. *J. Cell. Mol. Med.* **2010**, *14*, 840–860. [CrossRef]
2. González, D.; Marquina, R.; Rondón, N.; Rodriguez-Malaver, A.J.; Reyes, R. Effects of Aerobic Exercise on Uric Acid, Total Antioxidant Activity, Oxidative Stress, and Nitric Oxide in Human Saliva. *Res. Sports Med.* **2008**, *16*, 128–137. [CrossRef] [PubMed]
3. Ostachowska-Gasior, A.; Kolarzyk, E.; Szot, W.; Lyszczarz, J. The Relation between Antioxidative Ability and the Diet of Young Swimmers. *Rocz. Akad. Med. Bialymst.* **2005**, *50* (Suppl. S1), 241–244.
4. Damirchi, A.; Saati Zareei, A.; Sariri, R. Salivary Antioxidants of Male Athletes after Aerobic Exercise and Garlic Supplementation on: A Randomized, Double Blind, Placebo-Controlled Study. *J. Oral Biol. Craniofacial Res.* **2015**, *5*, 146–152. [CrossRef]
5. Bakhtiari, S.; Azimi, S.; Mehdipour, M.; Amini, S.; Elmi, Z.; Namazi, Z. Effect of Cigarette Smoke on Salivary Total Antioxidant Capacity. *J. Dent. Res. Dent. Clin. Dent. Prospects* **2015**, *9*, 281–284. [CrossRef]
6. Neshat, F.; Shirzaiy, M.; Shademan, S. Salivary Total Antioxidant and Lipid Peroxidation Levels in Passive Smoking and Nonsmoking Adolescents. *Addict. Health* **2020**, *12*, 216–224. [CrossRef] [PubMed]
7. Rahmani, M.; Ghorchi, V.; Rezaei, F.; Vaisi-Raygani, A. Evaluation of Total Antioxidant Capacity of Saliva in High School Students. *Glob. J. Health Sci.* **2015**, *8*, 89–94. [CrossRef]

8. Matei, M.N.; Popa, P.Ș.; Covaci, A.M.; Chipirliu, O.; Earar, K.; Stoica, G.; Zaharia, A.E.; Maftei, N.M.; Gurău, G.; Lisă, E.L.; et al. The Impact of Competitive Sports on Oral Health: Exploring Their Relationship with Salivary Oxidative Stress in Children. *Healthcare* **2023**, *11*, 2927. [CrossRef] [PubMed]
9. Atsumi, T.; Tonosaki, K.; Fujisawa, S. Salivary Free Radical-Scavenging Activity Is Affected by Physical and Mental Activities. *Oral Dis.* **2008**, *14*, 490–496. [CrossRef]
10. Lin, S.-P.; Li, C.-Y.; Suzuki, K.; Chang, C.-K.; Chou, K.-M.; Fang, S.-H. Green Tea Consumption after Intense Taekwondo Training Enhances Salivary Defense Factors and Antibacterial Capacity. *PLoS ONE* **2014**, *9*, e87580. [CrossRef]
11. Gawron-Skarbek, A.; Chrzczanowicz, J.; Kostka, J.; Nowak, D.; Drygas, W.; Jegier, A.; Kostka, T. Physical Activity, Aerobic Capacity, and Total Antioxidant Capacity in Healthy Men and in Men with Coronary Heart Disease. *Oxid. Med. Cell. Longev.* **2015**, *2015*, 197307. [CrossRef]
12. Zalavras, A.; Fatouros, I.G.; Deli, C.K.; Draganidis, D.; Theodorou, A.A.; Soulas, D.; Koutsioras, Y.; Koutedakis, Y.; Jamurtas, A.Z. Age-Related Responses in Circulating Markers of Redox Status in Healthy Adolescents and Adults during the Course of a Training Macrocycle. *Oxid. Med. Cell. Longev.* **2015**, *2015*, 283921. [CrossRef]
13. Battino, M.; Ferreiro, M.S.; Gallardo, I.; Newman, H.N.; Bullon, P. The Antioxidant Capacity of Saliva. *J. Clin. Periodontol.* **2002**, *29*, 189–194. [CrossRef] [PubMed]
14. Peluso, I.; Raguzzini, A. Salivary and Urinary Total Antioxidant Capacity as Biomarkers of Oxidative Stress in Humans. *Pathol. Res. Int.* **2016**, *2016*, 5480267. [CrossRef] [PubMed]
15. Chrzczanowicz, J.; Gawron, A.; Zwolinska, A.; de Graft-Johnson, J.; Krajewski, W.; Krol, M.; Markowski, J.; Kostka, T.; Nowak, D. Simple Method for Determining Human Serum 2,2-Diphenyl-1-Picryl-Hydrazyl (DPPH) Radical Scavenging Activity-Possible Application in Clinical Studies on Dietary Antioxidants. *Clin. Chem. Lab. Med.* **2008**, *46*, 342–349. [CrossRef] [PubMed]
16. Vassalle, C.; Masini, S.; Carpeggiani, C.; L'Abbate, A.; Boni, C.; Zucchelli, G.C. In Vivo Total Antioxidant Capacity: Comparison of Two Different Analytical Methods. *Clin. Chem. Lab. Med.* **2004**, *42*, 84–89. [CrossRef]
17. Sies, H. Total Antioxidant Capacity: Appraisal of a Concept. *J. Nutr.* **2007**, *137*, 1493–1495. [CrossRef]
18. Greabu, M.; Battino, M.; Mohora, M.; Totan, A.; Spinu, T.; Totan, C.; Didilescu, A.; Duța, C. Could Constitute Saliva the First Line of Defence against Oxidative Stress? *Rom. J. Intern. Med.* **2007**, *45*, 209–213.
19. Buczko, P.; Zalewska, A.; Szarmach, I. Saliva and Oxidative Stress in Oral Cavity and in Some Systemic Disorders. *J. Physiol. Pharmacol.* **2015**, *66*, 3–9.
20. Martins, J.R.; Díaz-Fabregat, B.; Ramírez-Carmona, W.; Monteiro, D.R.; Pessan, J.P.; Antoniali, C. Salivary Biomarkers of Oxidative Stress in Children with Dental Caries: Systematic Review and Meta-Analysis. *Arch. Oral Biol.* **2022**, *139*, 105432. [CrossRef]
21. Mohideen, K.; Chandrasekaran, K.; Veeraraghavan, H.; Faizee, S.H.; Dhungel, S.; Ghosh, S. Meta-Analysis of Assessment of Total Oxidative Stress and Total Antioxidant Capacity in Patients with Periodontitis. *Dis. Markers* **2023**, *2023*, 9949047. [CrossRef]
22. Jarosz, M. *Standards of Human Nutrition*; Food and Nutrition Institute: Warsaw, Poland, 2012.
23. Stelmach, W.; Kaczmarczyk-Chałas, K.; Bielecki, W.; Drygas, W. The Impact of Income, Education and Health on Lifestyle in a Large Urban Population of Poland (Cindi Programme). *Int. J. Occup. Med. Environ. Health* **2004**, *17*, 393–401.
24. Tomaszewski, P.; Milde, K.; Stupnicki, R. Body Mass Index–Proposed Norms for Children and Youths. *Pap. Anthropol.* **2013**, *22*, 203–213. [CrossRef]
25. Kułaga, Z.; Litwin, M.; Grajda, A.; Gurzkowska, B.; Napieralska, E.; Kułaga, K. Distribution of Blood Pressure in School-Aged Children and Adolescents Reference Population. *Stand. Med.* **2010**, *7*, 853–864.
26. Fox, S.M., 3rd; Naughton, J.P.; Gorman, P.A. Physical Activity and Cardiovascular Health. 3. The Exercise Prescription: Frequency and Type of Activity. *Mod. Concepts Cardiovasc. Dis.* **1972**, *41*, 25–30. [PubMed]
27. Szponar, L.; Wolnicka, K.; Rychlik, E. *Album of Photographs of Food Products and Dishes*; National Food and Nutrition Institute: Warsaw, Poland, 2000.
28. Kunachowicz, H.; Nadolna, I.; Przygoda, B.; Iwanow, K. *Charts of Nutritive Values of Products and Foods*; PZWL: Warsaw, Poland, 2005.
29. Navazesh, M. Methods for Collecting Saliva. *Ann. N. Y. Acad. Sci.* **1993**, *694*, 72–77. [CrossRef] [PubMed]
30. Gawron-Skarbek, A.; Prymont-Przymińska, A.; Sobczak, A.; Guligowska, A.; Kostka, T.; Nowak, D.; Szatko, F. A Comparison of Native and Non-Urate Total Antioxidant Capacity of Fasting Plasma and Saliva among Middle-Aged and Older Subjects. *Redox Rep.* **2018**, *23*, 57–62. [CrossRef]
31. Atsumi, T.; Iwakura, I.; Kashiwagi, Y.; Fujisawa, S.; Ueha, T. Free Radical Scavenging Activity in the Nonenzymatic Fraction of Human Saliva: A Simple DPPH Assay Showing the Effect of Physical Exercise. *Antioxid. Redox Signal.* **1999**, *1*, 537–546. [CrossRef]
32. Evans, L.W.; Omaye, S.T. Use of Saliva Biomarkers to Monitor Efficacy of Vitamin C in Exercise-Induced Oxidative Stress. *Antioxidants* **2017**, *6*, 5. [CrossRef]
33. Gawron-Skarbek, A.; Guligowska, A.; Prymont-Przymińska, A.; Godala, M.; Kolmaga, A.; Nowak, D.; Szatko, F.; Kostka, T. Dietary Vitamin C, E and β-Carotene Intake Does Not Significantly Affect Plasma or Salivary Antioxidant Indices and Salivary C-Reactive Protein in Older Subjects. *Nutrients* **2017**, *9*, 729. [CrossRef]

34. Logan, D.; Wallace, S.M.; Woodside, J.V.; McKenna, G. The Potential of Salivary Biomarkers of Nutritional Status and Dietary Intake: A Systematic Review. *J. Dent.* **2021**, *115*, 103840. [CrossRef]
35. Zare Javid, A.; Seal, C.J.; Heasman, P.; Moynihan, P.J. Impact of a Customised Dietary Intervention on Antioxidant Status, Dietary Intakes and Periodontal Indices in Patients with Adult Periodontitis. *J. Hum. Nutr. Diet.* **2014**, *27*, 523–532. [CrossRef] [PubMed]
36. Kamodyová, N.; Tóthová, L.; Celec, P. Salivary Markers of Oxidative Stress and Antioxidant Status: Influence of External Factors. *Dis. Markers* **2013**, *34*, 313–321. [CrossRef]
37. Halliwell, B.; Gutteridge, J.M. The Definition and Measurement of Antioxidants in Biological Systems. *Free Radic. Biol. Med.* **1995**, *18*, 125–126. [CrossRef]
38. Bartosz, G. *The Second Face of Oxygen*, 2nd ed.; PWN: Warsaw, Poland, 2003.
39. Poljsak, B.; Raspor, P. The Antioxidant and Pro-Oxidant Activity of Vitamin C and Trolox in Vitro: A Comparative Study. *J. Appl. Toxicol.* **2008**, *28*, 183–188. [CrossRef]
40. Kaźmierczak-Barańska, J.; Boguszewska, K.; Adamus-Grabicka, A.; Karwowski, B.T. Two Faces of Vitamin C-Antioxidative and Pro-Oxidative Agent. *Nutrients* **2020**, *12*, 1501. [CrossRef]
41. Cahill, L.E.; El-Sohemy, A. Vitamin C Transporter Gene Polymorphisms, Dietary Vitamin C and Serum Ascorbic Acid. *J. Nutr. Nutr.* **2010**, *2*, 292–301. [CrossRef]
42. Grzesiak-Gasek, I.; Kaczmarek, U. Influence of Swimming Training Session on Selected Saliva Components in Youth Swimmers. *Front. Physiol.* **2022**, *13*, 869903. [CrossRef]
43. Mahdivand, A.; Tabar, S.F.; Dehghani, S.; Ebrahimi, F.; Moosavi, S.S.; Ghiri, E.H.; Rezaee, M. The Effect of One Session Concurrent Training on Salivary Total Antioxidant Capacity, IgA and Hormonal in Male Student-Athletes. *Int. J. Sport Stud.* **2013**, *3*, 448–455.
44. Deminice, R.; Sicchieri, T.; Payão, P.O.; Jordão, A.A. Blood and Salivary Oxidative Stress Biomarkers Following an Acute Session of Resistance Exercise in Humans. *Int. J. Sports Med.* **2010**, *31*, 599–603. [CrossRef] [PubMed]
45. Pani, S.C.; Al Khabbaz, H.J.; Bin Enayeg, S.H.; Bin Zouman, A.H. The Relationship between Examination-Related Academic Stress, Salivary Antioxidant Capacity and Exercise Patterns of Final-Year Saudi Dental Students. *Eur. J. Dent. Educ.* **2017**, *21*, e83–e88. [CrossRef]
46. Munther, S. The Effects of Cigarette Smoking and Exercise on Total Salivary Antioxidant Activity. *Saudi Dent. J.* **2019**, *31*, 31–38. [CrossRef] [PubMed]
47. Arazi, H.; Simaei, E.; Taati, B. Comparison of Responses of Salivary Antioxidant Markers to Exhaustive Aerobic Exercise in Smoker and Non-Smoker Young Girls. *J. Sports Med. Phys. Fit.* **2016**, *56*, 1132–1138.
48. Babaei, P.; Damirchi, A.; Soltani Tehrani, B.; Nazari, Y.; Sariri, R.; Hoseini, R. Effect of Exercise Training on Saliva Brain Derived Neurotrophic Factor, Catalase and Vitamin C. *Med. J. Islam. Repub. Iran* **2016**, *30*, 452.
49. Alves, R.C.C.; Ferreira, R.O.; Frazão, D.R.; de Souza Né, Y.G.; Mendes, P.F.S.; Marañón-Vásquez, G.; Royes, L.F.F.; Fagundes, N.C.F.; Maia, L.C.; Lima, R.R. The Relationship between Exercise and Salivary Oxidative Stress: A Systematic Review. *Antioxidants* **2022**, *11*, 1489. [CrossRef]
50. Safabakhsh, D.; Jazaeri, M.; Abdolsamadi, H.; Abassi, E.; Farhadian, M. Comparison of Salivary Interleukin-6, Interleukin-8, C-Reactive Protein Levels and Total Antioxidants Capacity of Obese Individuals with Normal-Weight Ones. *Rom. J. Intern. Med.* **2022**, *60*, 215–221. [CrossRef]
51. Gunjalli, G.; Kumar, K.N.; Jain, S.K.; Reddy, S.K.; Shavi, G.R.; Ajagannanavar, S.L. Total Salivary Anti-Oxidant Levels, Dental Development and Oral Health Status in Childhood Obesity. *J. Int. Oral Health* **2014**, *6*, 63–67.
52. Zalewska, A.; Kossakowska, A.; Taranta-Janusz, K.; Zięba, S.; Fejfer, K.; Salamonowicz, M.; Kostecka-Sochoń, P.; Wasilewska, A.; Maciejczyk, M. Dysfunction of Salivary Glands, Disturbances in Salivary Antioxidants and Increased Oxidative Damage in Saliva of Overweight and Obese Adolescents. *J. Clin. Med.* **2020**, *9*, 548. [CrossRef]
53. Esenlik, E.; Bolat Gümüş, E.; Eroğlu Albayrak, G.; Kumbul Doğuç, D. Does Puberty Affect Oxidative Stress Levels and Antioxidant Activity of Saliva in Patients with Fixed Orthodontic Appliances? *J. Orofac. Orthop./Fortschritte Kieferorthopädie* **2023**, *84*, 56–64. [CrossRef] [PubMed]

nutrients

MDPI

Article

Dietary and Physical Activity Correlates of Muscle Mass in 60–65-Year-Old Seniors: A Gender-Specific Analysis

Bartłomiej K. Sołtysik *, Paweł Balicki , Klaudia Kowalczyk, Aleksandra Lutostańska, Julia Dmuchowska, Małgorzata Pigłowska and Tomasz Kostka

Department of Geriatrics and Internal Medicine, Healthy Ageing Research Centre (HARC), Medical University of Lodz, Pomorska Street 251, 92-213 Lodz, Poland; pawel.balicki@umed.lodz.pl (P.B.); k.kowalczyk@csk.umed.pl (K.K.); a.lutostanska@csk.umed.pl (A.L.); j.dmuchowska@csk.umed.pl (J.D.); malgorzata.piglowska@umed.lodz.pl (M.P.); tomasz.kostka@umed.lodz.pl (T.K.)

* Correspondence: bartlomiej.soltysik@umed.lodz.pl; Tel.: +48-42-2792480

Abstract: Introduction: Sarcopenia and loss of skeletal muscle mass represent major public health concerns in aging populations. Although both diet and physical activity (PA) are recognized as modifiable determinants of muscle mass, their effects may differ by sex. This study aimed to examine dietary and behavioral correlates of muscle mass amongst community-dwelling adults aged 60–65 in Central Poland. **Methods:** The study included 134 women and 138 men. Body composition was assessed using bioelectrical impedance (Maltron Bioscan 920, Essex, UK). Dietary intake was evaluated using a 24 h recall analyzed with Dieta 5.0 software. PA was measured using the Seven-Day Physical Activity Recall Questionnaire and the Stanford Physical Activity Indices. Statistical analysis included bivariate correlations and general linear modeling performed separately for women and men. **Results:** In women, skeletal muscle mass (as a percent of body mass) showed significant positive associations with protein intake per kilogram of body weight, magnesium, phosphorus, and moderate health-related PA. Concomitantly, there was a negative correlation with lipids such as long-chain polyunsaturated fatty acids (PUFA). In multivariate models, protein intake remained the only predictor. In men, only protein intake per kilogram of body weight demonstrated a significant association with muscle mass; no other dietary or PA factors were retained in the model. **Conclusions:** The findings indicate that dietary and behavioral factors influencing muscle mass vary by sex. While muscle mass in women is linked to multiple nutritional and lifestyle factors, men appear primarily responsive to total protein intake. These sex-specific differences may underscore the importance of tailored strategies in sarcopenia prevention.

Keywords: muscle mass; nutrition; protein intake; physical activity; seniors

1. Introduction

The demographic shift towards an aging population imposes significant challenges on healthcare systems and demands refined strategies aimed at preserving health and functional independence amongst older adults. A critical component of healthy aging is the maintenance of adequate skeletal muscle mass, which serves as a key determinant of physical performance, functional capacity, and ultimately, survival. Amongst individuals transitioning into older age, particularly those in their sixth and seventh decades of life, skeletal muscle mass emerges as a vital marker of physiological reserve.

Sex-related differences in body composition—specifically in terms of lean body and muscle mass—become especially pronounced in early older age. This period is often marked by the onset of sarcopenia, a progressive and generalized loss of muscle mass and strength. Evidence suggests that a healthy dietary pattern may exert a protective role against sarcopenia in women, a finding not consistently observed in men [1]. Similarly, physical activity (PA) appears to mitigate muscle loss [2], although sex-specific differences in response remain inadequately understood.

Both nutritional intake [3–5] and PA [6–8] are established as key modifiable determinants of muscle mass. A high-protein diet, traditionally emphasizing animal-derived proteins, is associated with enhanced anabolic responses [9–11]. Nonetheless, recent studies indicate that plant-based proteins, when appropriately supplemented—particularly with leucine—may offer comparable anabolic potential [9]. Interestingly, some evidence suggests that plant-based dietary patterns may confer broader functional benefits, such as improved independence [12].

Beyond protein, other dietary components play a crucial role in muscle health. Lipid intake, specifically mono- and polyunsaturated fatty acids [13], as well as dietary fiber [14], has been implicated in modulating sarcopenia risk. However, dietary regimens that exclude high-quality protein sources—such as strict vegan diets—may lack sufficient anabolic properties to support muscle maintenance in older adults [15]. Longitudinal data indicate that a diet rich in vegetables, whole grains, and animal protein is positively associated with muscle mass over time, although such findings are derived from male-only cohorts [16].

Micronutrients also contribute to muscle integrity. According to existing reviews, selenium, calcium, magnesium, and phosphorus are inversely associated with sarcopenia prevalence [17]. Some studies amongst community-dwelling older adults reinforce these associations [18]. While magnesium supplementation shows limited impact on muscle strength in the general population, subgroup analyses indicate potential benefits in magnesium-deficient individuals, particularly seniors [19]. Emerging evidence further supports magnesium's role in attenuating age-related muscle loss, especially amongst women [20]. Another study indicated a potential effect of magnesium in the preservation of age-related muscle mass loss in a group of women [21]. The notable differences between women and men identified in this study reflect a pattern observed across multiple studies. In one research study conducted in a group of older women, low protein intake had an impact on lower muscle mass but also a higher occurrence of physical limitations [22]. A large Korean cohort study demonstrated an inverse association between healthy diet and low muscle mass in older adults; notably, this relationship was evident only in women, with no significant association observed in men [23].

PA remains the cornerstone of sarcopenia prevention and treatment. Resistance training is particularly effective in mitigating muscle atrophy associated with aging [2,7,24]. In addition, regular engagement in moderate-to-vigorous leisure-time PA appears to confer protective effects [25]. Hormonal changes, especially the decline in estrogen during menopause, significantly contribute to muscle mass loss in women [26], yet similar processes are observed in aging men [27]. Overall, PA is consistently recognized as the most robust non-pharmacological intervention to counteract sarcopenia [8].

Despite growing research in this domain, important gaps remain in understanding the interaction between dietary components, PA patterns, and sex-specific influences on muscle mass dynamics in aging populations.

To our knowledge, this study represents the first attempt to identify factors associated with skeletal muscle mass in a cohort of community-dwelling older adults residing in Central Poland. This area is characterized by particularly unfavorable aging-related health indicators, the highest advancement of the aging process and the highest values of negative health measures in the whole country [28]. Given the escalating public health implications of sarcopenia, especially in regions with limited access to preventive care, continued research in this field is of paramount importance.

2. Materials and Methods

The study reports findings from the project titled "The Occurrence of Oxidative Stress and Selected Cardiovascular Risk Factors in Relation to the Functional Status of Older Adults in the Context of Workload" (conducted by the Central Institute for Labor Protection–National Research Institute, Warsaw, Poland). The research involved community dwellers (150 men and 150 women), all age-matched during recruitment, which was conducted via local community centers and senior organizations. A total of 16 women and 12 men were not qualified for further examination because of contraindications to performing bioimpedance analysis (like implantation of a pacemaker or metal prostheses). Participants were independent, community-dwelling volunteers who met the inclusion criteria of being between 60 and 65 years old and providing informed written consent. The study received approval from the Committee on the Ethics of Research in Human Experimentation at the Medical University of Lodz (RNN/648/14/KB, dated 23 September 2014) and was conducted in accordance with the ethical principles outlined in the Helsinki Declaration.

2.1. Diet

After analyzing the participants' diets, the daily intake of individual nutrients was estimated based on a detailed analysis of their menus. Food and beverage consumption on the most representative day was assessed by a qualified dietitian using a 24 h dietary recall questionnaire, supported by a portion size folder containing graphical illustrations of typical portion sizes (e.g., several differently sized servings of the same dish). To minimize reporting errors, participants were asked in advance to prepare a list of all food products, snacks, and beverages consumed during the days of assessment. Dietary intake data were collected over three consecutive days, and the day deemed most representative of the participant's typical diet was selected for analysis. Importantly, interviewers were instructed not to influence or assess the diet themselves. The reported dietary data were analyzed using Dieta 5.0 software (National Food and Nutrition Institute, Warsaw, Poland), which was used to calculate energy and nutrient intake. This method has also been applied in previous studies [29].

2.2. Body Composition

Muscle mass, presented as a percentage of total body mass, was determined using electrical bioimpedance. (Maltron Bioscan 920, Maltron International Ltd., Rayleigh, Essex, UK). Two injector electrodes were positioned on the dorsal side of the foot and wrist, while two detector electrodes were placed between the styloid processes of the radius and ulna, as well as between the medial and lateral malleolus. Throughout the measurement, each participant lay in a supine position with their feet separated and hands resting at their sides [30]. The Maltron BioScan 920-II has demonstrated high reliability in clinical studies, particularly for assessing body composition in older adults [31,32], and in our study, the device was calibrated prior to testing the subjects to ensure measurement accuracy.

2.3. PA

The Seven-Day Physical Activity Recall Questionnaire measures weekly sleep hours and categorizes activities into light, moderate, hard, and very hard based on energy expenditure. Energy expenditure was estimated based on activity intensity, assigning specific calorie burn rates per kilogram of body mass per hour for sleep and varying physical activity levels. Each activity category was assigned a specific energy cost expressed in kilocalories (kcal) burned per kilogram of body mass per hour: 1 kcal/kg/hour for sleep,

1.5 kcal/kg/hour for low-intensity activity, 4 kcal/kg/hour for moderate-intensity activity, 6 kcal/kg/hour for vigorous-intensity activity, and 10 kcal/kg/hour for very vigorous-intensity activity. Total weekly energy expenditure was then calculated by multiplying the hours spent in each activity category by its corresponding rate and summing the results [33].

The Stanford Moderate Index assesses health-related PA behaviors through daily habits like taking stairs, walking instead of driving, or parking farther. The Stanford Hard Index evaluates vigorous activities performed regularly for at least three months, such as jogging, cycling, or swimming. These indices, scored from 0 to 6 (moderate) and 0 to 5 (hard), are summarized as PA-health-related behaviors I (PA-HRB I) and II (PA-HRB II), respectively. Standardized protocols are detailed in a previous publication [34].

2.4. Statistical Analysis

The statistical analysis of the variables was conducted using both parametric and non-parametric tests. The Shapiro–Wilk test was employed to evaluate the empirical distribution of the variables, while the Levene test was used to assess variance homogeneity. Measures of central tendency, including the arithmetic mean (m) and median (Me), were calculated, along with measures of dispersion such as standard deviation (SD) and the lower and upper quartiles. For quantitative variables, the non-parametric Mann–Whitney U test was used. Additionally, Spearman's rank correlation test (rho coefficient) was utilized to determine relationships between two quantitative variables. To compare qualitative variables, the chi-square test was used. For variables that showed statistical significance in bidirectional tests, general linear models were built, and non-significant variables were subsequently removed through stepwise elimination. Due to known sex-based differences in body composition and nutritional profiles, separate general linear models were developed for women and men to ensure appropriate interpretation of predictors. All analyses were conducted using Statistica software, version 13.3 (Statsoft, Kraków, Poland). To ensure adequate statistical power for detecting a meaningful association, a priori power analysis was conducted for the correlation test. Assuming a two-tailed significance level of $\alpha = 0.05$, a desired power of 0.80 ($1 - \beta$), and an expected small-to-moderate correlation effect size of $r = 0.20$, the estimated required sample size was calculated. The analysis indicated that a minimum of 198 participants would be necessary to reliably detect a correlation of this magnitude. The final sample size of 272 participants exceeded this requirement, ensuring sufficient statistical power for the analyses conducted.

3. Results

Table 1 presents basic nutritional data and PA parameters stratified by sex, including statistically significant differences between groups. However, the comparison between sexes was not accounted for in the subsequent analysis due to the inherently distinct dietary profiles of women and men, as well as sex-specific patterns of PA influenced by anthropometric differences. All calculated data used for the initial assessment are presented in Supplementary Materials Tables S1 and S2.

Given the number of parameters included in the table, variables that were not utilized in further analyses—due to lack of correlation or absence of effect in the multivariate model—were excluded (presented in Tables S1 and S2). The omitted variables include: animal protein [g], isoleucine [mg], leucine [mg], lysine [mg], methionine [mg], phenylalanine [mg], cystine [mg], tyrosine [mg], threonine [mg], tryptophan [mg], valine [mg], arginine [mg], alanine [mg], aspartic acid [mg], glutamic acid [mg], glycine [mg], proline [mg], serine [mg], histidine [mg], myristoleic acid [c14:1. g], pentadecanoic acid [c15:1. g], palmitoleic acid [c16:1. g], heptadecenoic acid [c17:1. g], oleic acid [c18:1. g], eicosenoic acid [c20:1. g], linoleic acid [c18:2. g], alpha-linolenic acid (ala) [c18:3. g], arachidonic acid (aa) [c20:4. g], eicosatrienoic acid [c20:3. g], butyric acid [c4:0. g], caproic acid [c6:0. g], caprylic acid [c8:0. g], capric acid [c10:0. g], lauric acid [c12:0. g], myristic acid [c14:0. g], pentadecanoic acid [c15:0. g], palmitic acid [c16:0. g], heptadecanoic acid [c17:0. g], stearic acid [c18:0. g], arachidic acid [c20:0. g], sodium [mg], potassium [mg], calcium [mg], iodine [mg], iron [mg], vitamin A [μg], retinol [μg], beta-carotene [μg], vitamin E [mg], riboflavin [mg], niacin [mg], vitamin B6 [mg], vitamin C [mg], vitamin B12 [μg], folate [μg], sucrose [g], lactose [g], cholesterol [mg], energy [kcal], water [g], ash [g] and starch [g].

Table 1. Comparison between women and men in terms of anthropometry, diet, muscle mass and physical activity.

Variable	Women N = 134		Men N = 138		p
	Mean ± SD	Median (Lower-Upper Quartile)	Mean ± SD	Median (Lower-Upper Quartile)	
Age [years]	62.39 ± 1.58	62 (61–64)	62.92 ± 1.71	63 (61–64)	0.008
BMI [kg/m^2]	28.00 ± 4.58	27.51 (24.79–30.79)	28.14 ± 4.47	27.71 (25.08–30.53)	0.81
Muscle mass [% of body mass]	26.51 ± 2.50	26.48 (24.81–28.37)	36.11 ± 2.49	35.88 (34.79–37.85)	<0.001
Total protein [g]	66.65 ± 24.83	65.88 (49.30–81.36)	83.53 ± 32.12	78.73 (61.23–97.62)	<0.001
Protein per 1 kg of body weight [g/kg]	0.96 ± 0.40	0.91 (0.67–1.22)	1.01 ± 0.46	0.93 (0.73–1.21)	0.9
Plant protein [g]	22.39 ± 8.49	21.45 (15.92–27.60)	28.18 ± 12.70	25.60 (20.09–33.36)	<0.001
Total carbohydrates [g]	213.83 ± 83.44	198.71 (151.31–268.65)	275.43 ± 110.34	253.28 (196.00–328.58)	<0.001
Dietary fiber [g]	19.71 ± 7.91	17.98 (14.54–24.65)	22.00 ± 10.05	19.20 (15.04–27.27)	0.25
Long-chain polyunsaturated fatty acids [g]	0.26 ± 0.78	0.03(0.01–0.11)	0.33 ± 0.92	0.04 (0.0–0.11)	0.49
Digestible carbohydrates [g]	194.18 ± 79.57	179.23(135.09–243.36)	253.51 ± 103.70	230.45 (177.15–306.56)	<0.001
Phosphorus [mg]	1122.80 ± 403.70	1113.69 (864.77–1382.86)	1341.27 ± 501.92	1247.15 (976.12–1635.72)	0.001
Magnesium [mg]	294.23 ± 106.12	268.42 (223.32–352.62)	335.79 ± 129.60	311.02 (240.09–383.03)	0.007
Zinc [mg]	9.11 ± 3.25	8.67 (6.96–10.83)	11.42 ± 4.55	10.44 (8.71–13.63)	<0.001
Copper [mg]	1.17 ± 0.44	1.10 (0.83–1.45)	1.29 ± 0.57	1.12 (0.90–1.54)	0.21
Manganese [mg]	5.07 ± 2.08	4.83(3.59–6.19)	5.66 ± 2.78	5.01 (3.74–7.18)	0.26
Thiamine [mg]	1.11 ± 0.54	0.98 (0.72–1.36)	1.45 ± 0.66	1.30 (0.96–1.84)	<0.001
Vitamin D [μg]	2.84 ± 5.08	1.70 (0.85–2.52)	3.52 ± 3.98	2.23 (1.24–3.66)	0.001
Vitamin B12 μg]	4.65 ± 10.80	2.53 (1.62–3.56)	5.41 ± 14.84	2.89 (1.73–4.01)	0.11
Erucic acid [C22:1. g]	0.20 ± 0.47	0.03 (0.00–0.17)	0.21 ± 0.42	0.04 (0.00–0.23)	0.86
Total monounsaturated fatty acids [g]	20.69 ± 14.87	18.24 (12.03–25.31)	29.32 ± 16.04	26.70 (17.07–37.97)	<0.001
Stearidonic acid [C18:4. g]	0.02 ± 0.06	0 (0–0)	0.02 ± 0.08	0 (0–0)	0.96
Eicosapentaenoic acid (EPA) [C20:5. g]	0.08 ± 0.24	0 (0–0.02)	0.10 ± 0.30	0 (0–0.02)	0.52
Docosapentaenoic acid (DPA) [C22:5. g]	0.03 ± 0.09	0 (0–0.01)	0.03 ± 0.07	0 (0–0.02)	0.28
Docosahexaenoic acid [DHA. C22:6. g]	0.15 ± 0.47	0.02 (0.01–0.08)	0.20 ± 0.56	0.03 (0.00–0.09)	0.56
Total polyunsaturated fatty acids [g]	8.93 ± 7.03	7.55 (4.90–10.74)	11.50 ± 8.29	9.80 (5.83–14.12)	0.001
Saturated fatty acids: total [SFA. g]	21.70 ± 17.71	19.86 (12.77–27.02)	31.59 ± 20.88	26.49 (19.02–39.90)	<0.001
Physical activity–health related behaviors moderate (PA-HRBI)	2.86 ± 1.63	3 (2–4)	2.71 ± 1.69	3 (1–4)	0.41
Physical activity–health related behaviors hard (PA-HRBII)	0.26 ± 0.71	0 (0–0)	0.25 ± 0.69	0 (0–0)	0.98
Physical activity–energy expenditure (PA-EE) [kcal/kg/day]	45.74 ± 7.09	44.55 (39.92–50.50)	44.51 ± 8.09	42.04 (37.71–50.25)	0.07

Table 2 presents the population characteristics based on occupation, residence, and marital status. Women were more frequently divorced, widowed, or single compared to men. Regarding medical history, men more often reported hypertension and myocardial infarction, while women more frequently experienced osteoporosis, gastrointestinal disorders, and depression.

Table 2. Comparison between women and men in terms of marital status, occupation, chronic diseases and medications.

Variable		Women N = 134	Men N = 138	p
Marital status	Married	71 (52.9%)	113 (81.8%)	0.001
	Divorced	25 (18.6%)	17 (12.32%)	
	Widowed	28 (20.9%)	4 (2.9%)	
	Single	10 (7.5%)	4 (2.9%)	
Place of residence	Urban	126 (94.0)	126 (91.3%)	0.38
	Rural	8 (5.9%)	12 (8.7%)	
Occupation	White collar	45 (33.6%)	45 (32.6%)	0.82
	Physical	41(30.6%)	47 (34.0%)	
	Unemployed	48 (35.8%)	36 (33.4%)	
Diseases	Arterial hypertension	61 (45.5%)	82 (59.4%)	0.02
	Hypercholesterolemia	95 (70.9%)	87 (63.0%)	0.16
	Diabetes mellitus	15 (11.1%)	18 (13.0%)	0.64
	Coronary artery disease	13 (9.7%)	21 (15.22%)	0.16
	Myocardial infarction	2 (1.5%)	11 (7.9%)	0.01
	Heart failure	20 14.9%)	13 (9.42%)	0.16
	Stroke	6 (4.48%)	5 (3.62%)	0.71
	Chronic lung disease	22 (16.4%)	14 (10.1%)	0.12
	Osteoarthritis	68 (51.1%)	61 (44.2%)	0.25
	Osteoporosis	24 (17.9%)	3 (2.2%)	<0.001
	Gastrointestinal disorders	54 (40.3%)	39 (28.3%)	0.03
	Depression	30 (22.4%)	12 (8.7%)	0.01
	Urinary incontinence	31 (23.1%)	23 (16.7%)	0.18
Medications	Anticoagulants	24 (17.9%)	20 (14.5%)	0.74
	Beta-adrenolitics	39 (29.1%)	37 (26.8%)	0.67
	Calcium channel blockers	10 (7.5%)	20 (14.5%)	0.06
	Angiotensin-converting enzyme inhibitors	30 (22.4%)	35 (25.4%)	0.56
	Angiotensin II receptors blockers	16 (11.9%)	7 (5.0%)	0.04
	Diuretics	27 (20.1%)	24 (17.4%)	0.56
	Statins	24 (17.9%	37 (26.85)	0.07

Women were also more likely to use angiotensin II receptor blockers. Among women with hypertension or diabetes mellitus, significantly lower muscle mass was observed ($z = -5.05$, $p = 0.001$; $z = -3.56$, $p = 0.001$, respectively). Additionally, women taking anticoagulants, beta-blockers, calcium channel blockers, or angiotensin-converting enzyme (ACE) inhibitors also had significantly lower muscle mass ($z = -3.17$, $p = 0.001$; $z = -3.01$, $p = 0.002$; $z = -2.75$, $p = 0.005$; $z = -3.73$, $p = 0.001$, respectively).

However, none of these variables remained significant in the general linear model.

Table 3 presents the key correlation matrices between skeletal muscle mass (expressed as a percentage of total body mass) and dietary components, as well as PA variables. In women, skeletal muscle mass was positively correlated with several nutritional and behavioral factors, including protein intake per kilogram of body weight, plant-derived protein, total carbohydrate intake, dietary fiber and digestible carbohydrates. Positive associations were also observed for selected micronutrients such as phosphorus, magnesium, zinc, copper, manganese, as well as for thiamine. Additionally, higher levels of moderate and hard health-related PA were associated with greater muscle mass. Conversely, negative correlations were identified between muscle mass and intake of vitamin D, erucic acid, stearidonic acid, eicosapentaenoic acid (EPA), docosapentaenoic acid (DPA), docosahexaenoic acid (DHA), and long-chain PUFA. In men, skeletal muscle mass showed a positive correlation with protein intake per kilogram of body weight and engagement in hard health-related PA.

Table 3. Correlation between muscle mass expressed as a percentage of body mass with diet components and physical activity.

Variable	Women N = 134		Men N = 138	
	Muscle Mass [%]	*p*	Muscle Mass [%]	*p*
Total protein [g]	0.08	ns	0.04	ns
Protein per 1 kg of body weight [g/kg]	0.41	<0.001	0.35	<0.001
Plant protein [g]	0.25	<0.01	0.08	ns
Total carbohydrates [g]	0.26	<0.01	0.10	ns
Dietary fiber [g]	0.18	<0.05	0.00	ns
Long-chain polyunsaturated fatty acids [g]	−0.24	<0.01	0.00	ns
Digestible carbohydrates [g]	0.25	<0.01	0.10	ns
Phosphorus [mg]	0.21	<0.01	0.01	ns
Magnesium [mg]	0.30	<0.001	0.00	ns
Zinc [mg]	0.22	<0.01	0.02	ns
Copper [mg]	0.20	<0.01	0.01	ns
Manganese [mg]	0.20	<0.05	0.08	ns
Thiamine [mg]	0.17	<0.05	0.02	ns
Vitamin D [μg]	−0.24	<0.01	−0.09	ns
Erucic acid [C22:1. g]	−0.20	<0.05	−0.07	ns
Total monounsaturated fatty acids [MUFA. g]	−0.01	ns	0.04	ns
Stearidonic acid [C18:4. g]	−0.23	<0.01	−0.07	ns
Eicosapentaenoic acid (EPA) [C20:5. g]	−0.21	<0.05	−0.05	ns
Docosapentaenoic acid (DPA) [C22:5. g]	−0.22	<0.05	−0.01	ns
Docosahexaenoic acid [DHA. C22:6. g]	−0.24	<0.05	−0.04	ns
Total polyunsaturated fatty acids [PUFA. g]	−0.03	ns	−0.05	ns
Saturated fatty acids: total [SFA. g]	−0.02	ns	0.07	ns
Physical activity–health related behaviors moderate (PA-HRBI)	0.23	0.01	0.14	ns
Physical activity–health related behaviors hard (PA-HRBII)	0.19	<0.05	0.20	<0.05
Physical activity–energy expenditure (PA-EE) [kcal/kg/day]	−0.01	ns	0.07	ns

ns—not significant.

In the next step, the variables significant in bivariate analyses were employed in the general linear models (calculated separately for women and men). Although numerous variables correlated with muscle mass, in the general linear model for women, the muscle mass was associated only with intake of protein per 1 kg of body mass [Equation (1)]. For men, the model indicates an association with protein intake per 1 kg of body mass

[Equation (2)]. All variables significant in univariate analysis were initially included in the multivariate model, followed by stepwise removal of non-significant ones. Protein intake remained the only consistent dietary predictor, as other nutrients lost significance after adjustment, likely due to collinearity between dietary components.

Equation (1) for muscle mass in women:

$$\text{Females muscle mass}_{[\%\ \text{of body mass}]} = 24.11 + 2.49 \times \text{Protein per 1 kg of body weight [g/kg]}, \tag{1}$$

for protein per 1 kg of body weight [g/kg] $p < 0.000001$; F = 26.048,
for whole model $p < 0.000001$; F = 2240.04,
$R^2 = 0.16$.

Equation (2) for muscle mass in men:

$$\text{Males muscle mass}_{[\%\ \text{of body mass}]} = 34.19 + 1.90 \times \text{Protein per 1 kg of body weight [g/kg]}, \tag{2}$$

for protein per 1 kg of body weight [g/kg] $p = 0.000023$; F = 19.276,
for whole model $p < 0.000001$; F = 5049.60,
$R^2 = 0.12$.

4. Discussion

To our knowledge, this is the first attempt to assess the percentage of muscle mass in a population of young older adults residing in Central Poland, with particular emphasis on the role of diet and PA patterns as contributing factors. The collected data reveal a substantial disparity between sexes, with notable differences observed in both dietary composition and PA, each of which may independently or synergistically influence muscle mass.

In women, muscle mass demonstrated significant associations with multiple dietary and lifestyle variables. According to the general linear model, muscle mass correlated positively with protein intake standardized per kilogram of body weight. However, in correlations, muscle mass was associated with numerous dietary components, such as intake of PUFAs, phosphorus, and magnesium. Additionally, moderate engagement in health-related physical activity appeared to play a contributory role.

When considering dietary components, the female participants who exhibited lower muscle mass tended to consume diets rich in shellfish, nuts and seeds, meat (e.g., liver), legumes, and dairy products. Amongst these, protein intake emerges as the most consistently validated dietary determinant of muscle mass, as confirmed by numerous studies [3,5]. However, ongoing research continues to explore the optimal type, amount, and timing of protein ingestion, particularly with an emphasis on early-day consumption, such as during breakfast, which may enhance anabolic response [35]. Despite this, some meta-analyses suggest no significant differences in outcomes when comparing plant-based versus animal-based protein sources in relation to lean mass or muscle strength [36]. In therapeutic contexts, especially concerning sarcopenia, a daily intake of 1.4 g of protein per kilogram of body weight has been linked to muscle mass preservation [37,38]. This threshold may reflect age-related declines in anabolic sensitivity and the uneven amino acid profiles found in various protein-containing foods, which complicate efficient muscle protein synthesis [39,40]. In our research, there was no differentiation for the source of protein in relation to muscle mass.

PUFAs have also been proposed as protective agents against muscle mass decline. Several studies indicate that PUFA consumption may decrease the risk of low muscle mass in the general population [41] and interventions with PUFA intake seem to improve the gait speed [42,43] or slow down the muscle loss [44]. The properties of fatty acids seem to exhibit anti-inflammatory effects, increase activation of the mTORC1 (mechanistic target of rapamycin complex 1) signaling pathway, and reduce intracellular protein degradation. Additionally, the substances promote mitochondrial formation and function, enhance amino acid transport and uptake, and modulate activity at the neuromuscular junction [45]. A meta-analysis on omega-3 supplementation in older adults supports these findings, showing improved muscle strength and functional performance [43]. Our data, however, in bidirectional analyses, indicate a negative association between some polyunsaturated fatty acids and muscle mass in the group of women. This unexpected finding may reflect reverse causality—where women with lower muscle mass might increase PUFA intake in response to health concerns—or population-specific dietary patterns. The age- and disease-related muscle loss prevention caused by PUFA has been proven [46]. A minimum intake of 2 g/day of omega-3 fatty acid is linked with muscle gain and walking speed improvement [43]. Similarly to PUFA, our study has found a negative correlation between vitamin D3 and muscle mass in women. Again, previously conducted observations indicate a positive association between vitamin D3 and muscle tissue [47] and its deficiency is one of the risk factors for developing sarcopenia [48,49]. In our research, both described relations are presented in women. There are several reasons why the results of this study might differ from the previous research. One possibility is that the people in our study are different from those in the earlier studies—for example, the earlier studies may have looked at individuals who were already at high risk for health problems, while our study involved generally healthy people who may respond differently. Another explanation could be reverse causality—people with lower muscle mass might start taking supplements in an effort to improve their health, which could make it seem like supplement use is linked to lower muscle mass, even though it is actually the result, not the cause. Nonetheless, this result demands further investigation.

In the current study, phosphorus intake was independently associated with muscle mass percentage in women. While phosphorus is primarily recognized for its role in bone health, especially in concert with calcium in the pathophysiology of osteoporosis [50], its high intake has also been linked to adverse renal outcomes [51]. Importantly, phosphorus-rich diets often overlap with high-protein dietary patterns due to their shared sources: animal and plant proteins, fish, seafood, dairy and legumes. Bidirectional analysis showed a strong positive correlation between phosphorus and muscle mass. However, in multivariate models, this relationship is not statistically significant. This may be attributed to collinearity with protein intake, which could mask or confound the independent effect of phosphorus. Alternatively, adjusted models may reflect the role of phosphorus, as some studies have found lower phosphorus concentrations amongst individuals with sarcopenia [17] or sarcopenic obesity [52]. Some hypotheses of a phosphorus- and protein-rich acidic diet contributing to bone resorption, muscle loss, and elevated risks of chronic kidney or liver disease also demand consideration [53]. Further investigation is required to elucidate these associations.

In the presented research, magnesium intake was positively associated with muscle mass, though this relationship was exclusive to the female cohort. According to a systematic review, magnesium correlates with muscle mass, strength, and physical performance and may be inversely associated with the prevalence of sarcopenia [54]. While some meta-analyses have failed to demonstrate a benefit of magnesium in the general population, its role appears more significant in older adults and high-risk subgroups [19]. In hypertensive individuals, dietary—but not supplemental—magnesium was linked to increased muscle mass [55]. Consistent results have been reported in studies from the United Kingdom, where magnesium intake was positively associated with skeletal muscle indices in middle-aged and older populations [56]. The absence of this association in the tested male subgroup remains unexplained and needs further investigation.

PA, particularly resistance training, is one of the most robust modifiers of muscle mass across all ages [2,24]. Through activation of anabolic signaling pathways and mitochondrial biogenesis, physical exercise facilitates skeletal muscle hypertrophy [57]. Nevertheless, aging is accompanied by progressive desensitization to anabolic stimuli—both nutritional and mechanical—which contributes to proteolysis and muscle fiber atrophy [58]. In the current study, a nuanced differentiation in the impact of PA was observed. Leisure-time moderate PA, categorized under health-related behaviors, had a significant association with muscle mass in women; in men, leisure-time hard PA was linked with muscle mass. In contrast, energy-expenditure-related PA, encompassing domestic and occupational activities, showed no such relationship. This relation has been previously established in studies involving middle-aged and older adults [59], and again, in our research, the relationship with PA differs by sex.

Amongst male participants, both bivariate and multivariate analyses yielded more modest associations. Only protein intake per kilogram of body mass remained significant in the general linear model. No other dietary or PA variables showed a significant relationship with muscle mass. This suggests that in males, variability in muscle mass is primarily influenced by total protein intake, with other dietary components playing a subordinate role. Furthermore, existing literature indicates that the source of amino acids may be less relevant in predicting muscle mass outcomes amongst men [4,60].

Beyond biological sex differences in muscle composition, sociocultural influences also shape PA patterns and body image expectations, contributing to distinct lifestyle choices between men and women [61,62]. The findings of the present study imply that amongst 60–65-year-old seniors, diet and PA exert differential effects on muscle mass depending on sex, underscoring the need for sex-specific interventions and recommendations.

Limitations of the Study

This study has several limitations that should be noted. First, its cross-sectional design does not allow for conclusions about cause and effect. The sample is limited to 60–65-year-old adults from central Poland, which may affect the application of the results to other populations. Two measures of PA were based on questionnaires, which can lead to errors in reporting. However, both tools used—Stanford and Seven-Day Physical Activity Recall—are well-known and have been validated. The assessment of diet may also be biased by incorrect reporting of food amounts or portion sizes. An additional limitation is the absence of biochemical markers of protein metabolism and flexibility testing, which could have provided deeper insights into physiological and functional aspects of muscle health. Lastly, the study group was relatively small, which may reduce the strength of the findings, and even though protein intake was a statistically significant predictor of muscle mass, the explained variance was modest, indicating that other unmeasured factors likely contribute to muscle mass variation.

5. Conclusions

This study highlights clear differences between women and men in factors related to muscle mass amongst 60–65-year-old adults in Central Poland. In women, muscle mass was associated with protein intake per kilogram of body weight, as well as with selected nutrients such as polyunsaturated fatty acids, phosphorus, and magnesium. Moderate PA, defined as health-related behavior, also showed a significant link in this group. In men, only protein intake showed a consistent association, with no other dietary factors reaching significance. In terms of activity-related aspects, intensive leisure time PA seems to be connotative. These findings suggest a stronger and more complex role of diet and lifestyle in women, while in men, muscle mass appears to depend more on total protein consumption alone. The collinearity between nutrients, particularly protein and micronutrients, may affect the direction and strength of observed relationships. The sex-based differences likely reflect both biological and behavioral mechanisms. Further research is needed to clarify these patterns and guide effective nutritional and activity-based interventions.

Supplementary Materials: The following supporting information can be downloaded at https://www.mdpi.com/article/10.3390/nu17111930/s1, Table S1: Comparison between women and men in terms of anthropometry, diet, muscle mass and physical activity; Table S2: Correlation between muscle mass expressed as a percent of body mass with diet components and physical activity.

Author Contributions: Conceptualization, B.K.S. and T.K.; methodology, M.P.; software, P.B. and J.D.; validation, B.K.S. and T.K.; formal analysis, B.K.S.; investigation, B.K.S. and K.K.; resources, B.K.S.; data curation, M.P. and A.L.; writing—original draft preparation, P.B. and B.K.S.; writing—review and editing, J.D. and T.K.; visualization, B.K.S. and K.K.; supervision, T.K. and M.P.; project administration, T.K.; funding acquisition, T.K. All authors have read and agreed to the published version of the manuscript.

Funding: The authors were partly supported by the Central Institute for Labour Protection—National Research Institute project (KBNSR/N/I/427/2014) and received grants funded by the Medical University of Lodz, Poland (503/6-020-01/503-61-001 and 503/6-077-01/503-61-001).

Institutional Review Board Statement: The study was conducted according to the guidelines of the Declaration of Helsinki and approved by the Committee on the Ethics of Research in Human Experimentation at the Medical University of Lodz (protocol code RNN/648/14/KB, 23 September 2014).

Informed Consent Statement: Informed consent was obtained from all subjects involved in the study.

Data Availability Statement: The original contributions presented in this study are included in the article and Supplementary Materials. Further inquiries can be directed to the corresponding author.

Conflicts of Interest: The authors declare no conflicts of interest.

References

1. Ghoreishy, S.M.; Koujan, S.E.; Hashemi, R.; Heshmat, R.; Motlagh, A.D.; Esmaillzadeh, A. Relationship between healthy eating index and sarcopenia in elderly people. *BMC Geriatr.* **2023**, *23*, 25. [CrossRef] [PubMed]
2. McKendry, J.; Coletta, G.; Nunes, E.A.; Lim, C.; Phillips, S.M. Mitigating disuse-induced skeletal muscle atrophy in ageing: Resistance exercise as a critical countermeasure. *Exp. Physiol.* **2024**, *109*, 1650–1662. [CrossRef] [PubMed]
3. Guimarães-Ferreira, L.; Cholewa, J.M.; Naimo, M.A.; Zhi, X.I.; Magagnin, D.; de Sá, R.B.; Streck, E.L.; da Silva Teixeira, T.; Zanchi, N.E. Synergistic effects of resistance training and protein intake: Practical aspects. *Nutrition* **2014**, *30*, 1097–1103. [CrossRef]
4. Morton, R.W.; Murphy, K.T.; McKellar, S.R.; Schoenfeld, B.J.; Henselmans, M.; Helms, E.; Aragon, A.A.; Devries, M.C.; Banfield, L.; Krieger, J.W.; et al. A systematic review, meta-analysis and meta-regression of the effect of protein supplementation on resistance training-induced gains in muscle mass and strength in healthy adults. *Br. J. Sports Med.* **2018**, *52*, 376–384. [CrossRef]
5. Deer, R.R.; Volpi, E. Protein intake and muscle function in older adults. *Curr. Opin. Clin. Nutr. Metab. Care* **2015**, *18*, 248–253. [CrossRef] [PubMed]
6. Distefano, G.; Goodpaster, B.H. Effects of Exercise and Aging on Skeletal Muscle. *Cold Spring Harb. Perspect. Med.* **2018**, *8*, a029785. [CrossRef]
7. Landi, F.; Marzetti, E.; Martone, A.M.; Bernabei, R.; Onder, G. Exercise as a remedy for sarcopenia. *Curr. Opin. Clin. Nutr. Metab. Care* **2014**, *17*, 25–31. [CrossRef]
8. Beaudart, C.; Dawson, A.; Shaw, S.C.; Harvey, N.C.; Kanis, J.A.; Binkley, N.; Reginster, J.Y.; Chapurlat, R.; Chan, D.C.; Bruyère, O.; et al. Nutrition and physical activity in the prevention and treatment of sarcopenia: Systematic review. *Osteoporos. Int.* **2017**, *28*, 1817–1833. [CrossRef]
9. Pandey, A.; Pearlman, M.; Bonnes, S.L.; Nour, S.I. Can We Maintain Muscle Mass on a Plant-Based Diet? *Curr. Nutr. Rep.* **2025**, *14*, 16. [CrossRef]
10. Hevia-Larraín, V.; Gualano, B.; Longobardi, I.; Gil, S.; Fernandes, A.L.; Costa, L.A.R.; Pereira, R.M.R.; Artioli, G.G.; Phillips, S.M.; Roschel, H. High-Protein Plant-Based Diet Versus a Protein-Matched Omnivorous Diet to Support Resistance Training Adaptations: A Comparison Between Habitual Vegans and Omnivores. *Sports Med.* **2021**, *51*, 1317–1330. [CrossRef]

11. López-Moreno, M.; Kraselnik, A. The Impact of Plant-Based Proteins on Muscle Mass and Strength Performance: A Comprehensive Review. *Curr. Nutr. Rep.* **2025**, *14*, 37. [CrossRef] [PubMed]
12. Ren, L.; Tang, Y.; Yang, R.; Hu, Y.; Wang, J.; Li, S.; Yu, M.; Jiang, Y.; Liu, Z.; Wu, Y.; et al. Plant-based dietary pattern and low muscle mass: A nation-wide cohort analysis of Chinese older adults. *BMC Geriatr.* **2023**, *23*, 569. [CrossRef]
13. Montiel-Rojas, D.; Santoro, A.; Nilsson, A.; Franceschi, C.; Capri, M.; Bazzocchi, A.; Battista, G.; de Groot, L.; Feskens, E.J.M.; Berendsen, A.A.M.; et al. Beneficial Role of Replacing Dietary Saturated Fatty Acids with Polyunsaturated Fatty Acids in the Prevention of Sarcopenia: Findings from the NU-AGE Cohort. *Nutrients* **2020**, *12*, 3079. [CrossRef]
14. Montiel-Rojas, D.; Nilsson, A.; Santoro, A.; Franceschi, C.; Bazzocchi, A.; Battista, G.; de Groot, L.; Feskens, E.J.M.; Berendsen, A.; Pietruszka, B.; et al. Dietary Fibre May Mitigate Sarcopenia Risk: Findings from the NU-AGE Cohort of Older European Adults. *Nutrients* **2020**, *12*, 1075. [CrossRef] [PubMed]
15. Domić, J.; Grootswagers, P.; van Loon, L.J.C.; de Groot, L. Perspective: Vegan Diets for Older Adults? A Perspective On the Potential Impact On Muscle Mass and Strength. *Adv. Nutr.* **2022**, *13*, 712–725. [CrossRef]
16. Davis, J.A.; Mohebbi, M.; Collier, F.; Loughman, A.; Staudacher, H.; Shivappa, N.; Hébert, J.R.; Pasco, J.A.; Jacka, F.N. The role of diet quality and dietary patterns in predicting muscle mass and function in men over a 15-year period. *Osteoporos. Int.* **2021**, *32*, 2193–2203. [CrossRef]
17. van Dronkelaar, C.; van Velzen, A.; Abdelrazek, M.; van der Steen, A.; Weijs, P.J.M.; Tieland, M. Minerals and Sarcopenia; The Role of Calcium, Iron, Magnesium, Phosphorus, Potassium, Selenium, Sodium, and Zinc on Muscle Mass, Muscle Strength, and Physical Performance in Older Adults: A Systematic Review. *J. Am. Med. Dir. Assoc.* **2018**, *19*, 6–11.e3. [CrossRef]
18. Scott, D.; Blizzard, L.; Fell, J.; Giles, G.; Jones, G. Associations between dietary nutrient intake and muscle mass and strength in community-dwelling older adults: The Tasmanian Older Adult Cohort Study. *J. Am. Geriatr. Soc.* **2010**, *58*, 2129–2134. [CrossRef] [PubMed]
19. Wang, R.; Chen, C.; Liu, W.; Zhou, T.; Xun, P.; He, K.; Chen, P. The effect of magnesium supplementation on muscle fitness: A meta-analysis and systematic review. *Magnes. Res.* **2017**, *30*, 120–132. [CrossRef]
20. Dominguez, L.J.; Barbagallo, M.; Lauretani, F.; Bandinelli, S.; Bos, A.; Corsi, A.M.; Simonsick, E.M.; Ferrucci, L. Magnesium and muscle performance in older persons: The InCHIANTI study. *Am. J. Clin. Nutr.* **2006**, *84*, 419–426. [CrossRef]
21. Welch, A.A.; Kelaiditi, E.; Jennings, A.; Steves, C.J.; Spector, T.D.; MacGregor, A. Dietary Magnesium Is Positively Associated With Skeletal Muscle Power and Indices of Muscle Mass and May Attenuate the Association Between Circulating C-Reactive Protein and Muscle Mass in Women. *J. Bone Miner. Res.* **2016**, *31*, 317–325. [CrossRef] [PubMed]
22. Nilsson, A.; Montiel Rojas, D.; Kadi, F. Impact of Meeting Different Guidelines for Protein Intake on Muscle Mass and Physical Function in Physically Active Older Women. *Nutrients* **2018**, *10*, 1156. [CrossRef]
23. Kim, J.; Lee, Y.; Kye, S.; Chung, Y.S.; Kim, K.M. Association between healthy diet and exercise and greater muscle mass in older adults. *J. Am. Geriatr. Soc.* **2015**, *63*, 886–892. [CrossRef]
24. Hunter, G.R.; McCarthy, J.P.; Bamman, M.M. Effects of resistance training on older adults. *Sports Med.* **2004**, *34*, 329–348. [CrossRef]
25. Pearson, A.M. Muscle growth and exercise. *Crit. Rev. Food Sci. Nutr.* **1990**, *29*, 167–196. [CrossRef]
26. Maltais, M.L.; Desroches, J.; Dionne, I.J. Changes in muscle mass and strength after menopause. *J. Musculoskelet. Neuronal Interact.* **2009**, *9*, 186–197.
27. Gharahdaghi, N.; Rudrappa, S.; Brook, M.S.; Idris, I.; Crossland, H.; Hamrock, C.; Abdul Aziz, M.H.; Kadi, F.; Tarum, J.; Greenhaff, P.L.; et al. Testosterone therapy induces molecular programming augmenting physiological adaptations to resistance exercise in older men. *J. Cachexia Sarcopenia Muscle* **2019**, *10*, 1276–1294. [CrossRef] [PubMed]
28. Kopiec, T.; Stańczyk, K.; Burzyńska, M. Assessment of Lodz Province Residents Opinions on the Needs For the Social Activation of Seniors. *Acta Univ. Lodz. Folia Oeconomica* **2022**, *6*, 4–23. [CrossRef]
29. Karolczak, K.; Guligowska, A.; Kostanek, J.; Soltysik, B.; Kostka, T.; Watala, C. The amino acid content in the daily diet of seniors negatively correlates with the degree of platelet aggregation in a sex- and agonist-specific manner. *Aging* **2022**, *14*, 7240–7262. [CrossRef]
30. Fife, E.; Kostka, J.; Kroc, Ł.; Guligowska, A.; Pigłowska, M.; Sołtysik, B.; Kaufman-Szymczyk, A.; Fabianowska-Majewska, K.; Kostka, T. Relationship of muscle function to circulating myostatin, follistatin and GDF11 in older women and men. *BMC Geriatr.* **2018**, *18*, 200. [CrossRef]
31. Sipers, W.; Dorge, J.; Schols, J.; Verdijk, L.B.; van Loon, L.J.C. Multifrequency bioelectrical impedance analysis may represent a reproducible and practical tool to assess skeletal muscle mass in euvolemic acutely ill hospitalized geriatric patients. *Eur. Geriatr. Med.* **2020**, *11*, 155–162. [CrossRef] [PubMed]
32. Gijsen, M.; Simons, E.; De Cock, P.; Malbrain, M.L.N.G.; Wauters, J.; Spriet, I. Reproducibility of fluid status measured by bioelectrical impedance analysis in healthy volunteers: A key requirement to monitor fluid status in the intensive care unit. *Anaesthesiol. Intensive Ther.* **2021**, *53*, 193–199. [CrossRef] [PubMed]

33. Bonnefoy, M.; Normand, S.; Pachiaudi, C.; Lacour, J.R.; Laville, M.; Kostka, T. Simultaneous validation of ten physical activity questionnaires in older men: A doubly labeled water study. *J. Am. Geriatr. Soc.* **2001**, *49*, 28–35. [CrossRef]
34. Sołtysik, B.K.; Karolczak, K.; Kostka, T.; Stephenson, S.S.; Watala, C.; Kostka, J. Contribution of Physical Activity to the Oxidative and Antioxidant Potential in 60–65-Year-Old Seniors. *Antioxidants* **2023**, *12*, 1200. [CrossRef]
35. Khaing, I.K.; Tahara, Y.; Chimed-Ochir, O.; Shibata, S.; Kubo, T. Effect of breakfast protein intake on muscle mass and strength in adults: A scoping review. *Nutr. Rev.* **2025**, *83*, 175–199. [CrossRef]
36. Lim, M.T.; Pan, B.J.; Toh, D.W.K.; Sutanto, C.N.; Kim, J.E. Animal Protein versus Plant Protein in Supporting Lean Mass and Muscle Strength: A Systematic Review and Meta-Analysis of Randomized Controlled Trials. *Nutrients* **2021**, *13*, 661. [CrossRef]
37. Capitão, C.; Coutinho, D.; Neves, P.M.; Capelas, M.L.; Pimenta, N.M.; Santos, T.; Mäkitie, A.; Ravasco, P. Protein intake and muscle mass maintenance in patients with cancer types with high prevalence of sarcopenia: A systematic review. *Support. Care Cancer* **2022**, *30*, 3007–3015. [CrossRef] [PubMed]
38. Wolfe, R.R.; Cifelli, A.M.; Kostas, G.; Kim, I.Y. Optimizing Protein Intake in Adults: Interpretation and Application of the Recommended Dietary Allowance Compared with the Acceptable Macronutrient Distribution Range. *Adv. Nutr.* **2017**, *8*, 266–275. [CrossRef]
39. Morais, J.A.; Chevalier, S.; Gougeon, R. Protein turnover and requirements in the healthy and frail elderly. *J. Nutr. Health Aging* **2006**, *10*, 272–283.
40. Baum, J.I.; Kim, I.Y.; Wolfe, R.R. Protein Consumption and the Elderly: What Is the Optimal Level of Intake? *Nutrients* **2016**, *8*, 359. [CrossRef]
41. Phillips, N.; Gray, S.R.; Combet, E.; Witard, O.C. Long-chain n-3 polyunsaturated fatty acids for the management of age- and disease-related declines in skeletal muscle mass, strength and physical function. *Curr. Opin. Clin. Nutr. Metab. Care* **2024**, *27*, 98–105. [CrossRef] [PubMed]
42. Isanejad, M.; Tajik, B.; McArdle, A.; Tuppurainen, M.; Sirola, J.; Kröger, H.; Rikkonen, T.; Erkkilä, A. Dietary omega-3 polyunsaturated fatty acid and alpha-linolenic acid are associated with physical capacity measure but not muscle mass in older women 65–72 years. *Eur. J. Nutr.* **2022**, *61*, 1813–1821. [CrossRef] [PubMed]
43. Huang, Y.H.; Chiu, W.C.; Hsu, Y.P.; Lo, Y.L.; Wang, Y.H. Effects of Omega-3 Fatty Acids on Muscle Mass, Muscle Strength and Muscle Performance among the Elderly: A Meta-Analysis. *Nutrients* **2020**, *12*, 3739. [CrossRef]
44. Smith, G.I.; Julliand, S.; Reeds, D.N.; Sinacore, D.R.; Klein, S.; Mittendorfer, B. Fish oil-derived n-3 PUFA therapy increases muscle mass and function in healthy older adults. *Am. J. Clin. Nutr.* **2015**, *102*, 115–122. [CrossRef]
45. Therdyothin, A.; Phiphopthatsanee, N.; Isanejad, M. The Effect of Omega-3 Fatty Acids on Sarcopenia: Mechanism of Action and Potential Efficacy. *Mar. Drugs* **2023**, *21*, 399. [CrossRef] [PubMed]
46. Troesch, B.; Eggersdorfer, M.; Laviano, A.; Rolland, Y.; Smith, A.D.; Warnke, I.; Weimann, A.; Calder, P.C. Expert Opinion on Benefits of Long-Chain Omega-3 Fatty Acids (DHA and EPA) in Aging and Clinical Nutrition. *Nutrients* **2020**, *12*, 2555. [CrossRef]
47. Bo, Y.; Liu, C.; Ji, Z.; Yang, R.; An, Q.; Zhang, X.; You, J.; Duan, D.; Sun, Y.; Zhu, Y.; et al. A high whey protein, vitamin D and E supplement preserves muscle mass, strength, and quality of life in sarcopenic older adults: A double-blind randomized controlled trial. *Clin. Nutr.* **2019**, *38*, 159–164. [CrossRef]
48. Bollen, S.E.; Bass, J.J.; Fujita, S.; Wilkinson, D.; Hewison, M.; Atherton, P.J. The Vitamin D/Vitamin D receptor (VDR) axis in muscle atrophy and sarcopenia. *Cell Signal* **2022**, *96*, 110355. [CrossRef]
49. Ma, Y.; Liu, Y.; Zheng, J.; Zheng, Z.; Li, J. Clinical significance of serum irisin, 25(OH)D3 and albumin in older adults with chronic disease and sarcopenia. *Aging Clin. Exp. Res.* **2025**, *37*, 153. [CrossRef]
50. Bellavia, D.; Costa, V.; De Luca, A.; Maglio, M.; Pagani, S.; Fini, M.; Giavaresi, G. Vitamin D Level Between Calcium-Phosphorus Homeostasis and Immune System: New Perspective in Osteoporosis. *Curr. Osteoporos. Rep.* **2024**, *22*, 599–610. [CrossRef]
51. Byrne, F.N.; Gillman, B.; Kiely, M.; Bowles, M.; Connolly, P.; Earlie, J.; Murphy, J.; Rennick, T.; Reilly, E.O.; Shiely, F.; et al. Revising Dietary Phosphorus Advice in Chronic Kidney Disease G3-5D. *J. Ren. Nutr.* **2021**, *31*, 132–143. [CrossRef] [PubMed]
52. Choi, M.K.; Bae, Y.J. Dietary calcium, phosphorus, and osteosarcopenic adiposity in Korean adults aged 50 years and older. *Arch. Osteoporos.* **2021**, *16*, 89. [CrossRef] [PubMed]
53. Carnauba, R.A.; Baptistella, A.B.; Paschoal, V.; Hübscher, G.H. Diet-Induced Low-Grade Metabolic Acidosis and Clinical Outcomes: A Review. *Nutrients* **2017**, *9*, 538. [CrossRef]
54. van Dronkelaar, C.; Fultinga, M.; Hummel, M.; Kruizenga, H.; Weijs, P.J.M.; Tieland, M. Minerals and Sarcopenia in Older Adults: An Updated Systematic Review. *J. Am. Med. Dir. Assoc.* **2023**, *24*, 1163–1172. [CrossRef] [PubMed]
55. Wang, Q.; Si, K.; Xing, X.; Ye, X.; Liu, Z.; Chen, J.; Tang, X. Association between dietary magnesium intake and muscle mass among hypertensive population: Evidence from the National Health and Nutrition Examination Survey. *Nutr. J.* **2024**, *23*, 37. [CrossRef]
56. Hayhoe, R.P.G.; Lentjes, M.A.H.; Mulligan, A.A.; Luben, R.N.; Khaw, K.T.; Welch, A.A. Cross-sectional associations of dietary and circulating magnesium with skeletal muscle mass in the EPIC-Norfolk cohort. *Clin. Nutr.* **2019**, *38*, 317–323. [CrossRef]

57. El Assar, M.; Álvarez-Bustos, A.; Sosa, P.; Angulo, J.; Rodríguez-Mañas, L. Effect of Physical Activity/Exercise on Oxidative Stress and Inflammation in Muscle and Vascular Aging. *Int. J. Mol. Sci.* **2022**, *23*, 8713. [CrossRef]
58. Wilkinson, D.J.; Piasecki, M.; Atherton, P.J. The age-related loss of skeletal muscle mass and function: Measurement and physiology of muscle fibre atrophy and muscle fibre loss in humans. *Ageing Res. Rev.* **2018**, *47*, 123–132. [CrossRef]
59. Kim, B.; Osuka, Y.; Okubo, Y.; Zhao, X.; Kim, G.M.; Oh, S. The Physical Activity Paradox in Low Muscle Mass in Middle-Aged and Older Adults. *Am. J. Prev. Med.* **2025**, *68*, 348–356. [CrossRef]
60. Tipton, K.D.; Wolfe, R.R. Exercise, protein metabolism, and muscle growth. *Int. J. Sport. Nutr. Exerc. Metab.* **2001**, *11*, 109–132. [CrossRef]
61. Nuzzo, J.L. Narrative Review of Sex Differences in Muscle Strength, Endurance, Activation, Size, Fiber Type, and Strength Training Participation Rates, Preferences, Motivations, Injuries, and Neuromuscular Adaptations. *J. Strength Cond. Res.* **2023**, *37*, 494–536. [CrossRef] [PubMed]
62. Chen, M.J.; Ko, P.S.; Lee, M.C.; Su, S.L.; Yu, S. Gender difference in appendicular muscle strength: Determinant of the quality of life in the older Taiwanese. *Aging* **2022**, *14*, 7517–7526. [CrossRef] [PubMed]

nutrients

MDPI

Article

Medium-Chain Triglyceride Dietary Supplements Reduce Glucose Metabolism of Gait-Related Skeletal Muscle in Older Adults: A Longitudinal ^{18}F-FDG PET/CT Analysis

Tatsushi Mutoh [1,2,*], Hiroki Kataoka [1], Yasuko Tatewaki [1] and Yasuyuki Taki [1]

1 Department of Aging Research and Geriatric Medicine, Institute of Development, Aging and Cancer, Tohoku University, Aoba-ku, Sendai 980-8575, Japan
2 Division of Neurocritical Care, Research Institute for Brain and Blood Vessels, Akita Cerebrospinal and Cardiovascular Center, Senshu-Kubota-machi, Akita 010-0874, Japan
* Correspondence: tmutoh@tohoku.ac.jp

Abstract: Background/Objectives: Dietary supplementation with medium-chain triglycerides (MCTs) improves walking balance and cognitive function in healthy older adults. This study aimed to determine the biological effects of MCTs on gait-related skeletal muscles in healthy older adults by analyzing muscle density and glucose metabolism. Methods: ^{18}F-FDG-PET/CT imaging data from 63 participants (18 g/day of MCTs and matching placebo in the form of a jelly stick [6 g each, ingested 3 times/day]) in a randomized clinical trial were analyzed. The three-dimensional regions of interest were set as muscles associated with walking balance (bilateral triceps, psoas, and vastus medialis). Each muscle's mean standardized uptake value (SUV_{mean}) and Hounsfield units (HU) were calculated for relative quantitative measurements. Results: MCT supplementation for 3 months decreased the SUV_{mean} ($p < 0.001$) and increased the HU of the psoas ($r = -0.61$) and vastus medialis muscles ($r = -0.59$) ($p < 0.001$); no changes were apparent in participants supplemented with long-chain triglycerides. The changes in the SUV_{mean} for each muscle were correlated negatively with those of plasma β-hydroxybutyrate in MCT-supplemented participants ($r = -0.57$ [psoas] and -0.59 [vastus medialis]; $p < 0.001$). Conclusion: A 3-month MCT supplementation suppressed glucose metabolism and increased the muscle density in gait-related skeletal muscles, consistent with previous findings that MCT supplementation stabilizes balance functions during walking in healthy older adults.

Keywords: glucose metabolism; gait; ketone; medium-chain triglyceride; elderly

1. Introduction

Establishing a good health status is an important global issue for an aging population [1]. Among healthy older adults, age-related cognitive and muscle function decline is considered frailty and is a serious societal burden [2,3]. Sarcopenia and dementia are major disorders that shorten life expectancies and increase proportionally with aging [4]. Therefore, preventing these physiological or pathological events before the onset of age-related frailty is especially important.

Ketone bodies are an alternative energy substrate for organs requiring glucose, especially in the older brain, where glucose utilization deteriorates [5]. Medium-chain triglyceride (MCT) oil comprises mixed fatty acids (predominantly the ketogenic compounds caprylic [C8] and capric acids [C10]) extracted from natural products, including milk fat, palm kernel, and coconut oils. In rodents, MCT is an immediate energy source facilitating exercise performance through activating mitochondrial biogenesis and metabolism [6]. MCT supplementation (12-18 g/day) demonstrated positive effects on cognition, both at rest and following exercise in healthy adults [7]. Combining MCTs with aerobic exercise extends its efficacy in improving muscle function and subjective physical and mental health in middle-aged and older adults with poor exercise habits or low body mass index (<24.0 kg/m^2) at high risk for frailty [8,9]. A recent double-blind, randomized clinical trial (RCT) showed that a 3-month supplementation of MCT oil (18 g/day; 3 meals/day) in healthy older adults improves gait, balance, and executive functions compared with a placebo control comprising long-chain triglyceride (LCT) oil without MCTs [10].

Physiologically, MCTs provide an energy supply to the brain via both direct and indirect (ketone bodies synthesized via β-oxidation in the liver and acylated ghrelin in the stomach) pathways of digested medium-chain fatty acids (MCFAs) [11,12]. Furthermore, MCFAs circulating in the peripheral blood can also act on skeletal muscle to enhance mitochondrial biosynthesis and mitochondrial metabolic activity [11]. However, the biological mechanisms of the MCTs' essential modulating of the muscle metabolism and function in older adults have not been elucidated.

Skeletal muscle is a primary contributor to energy expenditure because of the substantial amount of energy used to maintain gait and posture to mediate locomotion [13]. ^{18}F-2-fluoro-2-deoxy-D-glucose (FDG) positron emission tomography (PET) can quantify the metabolic activity of skeletal muscle, as well as other body organs such as the brain and liver. The PET-derived standardized uptake value (SUV) is proportional to the metabolic activity of the skeletal muscle [14], and thus the mean values (SUV_{mean}) in each region of interest (ROI) analyzed by computed tomography (CT) scan enables assessment of energy expenditure of the specific muscle area. In addition, muscle quality assessment using CT scans involves analyzing the density of skeletal muscle, measured in Hounsfield Units (HU), within specific ROIs [15]. This CT-derived skeletal muscle density provides insights into muscle health, with higher HU values indicating denser and healthier muscle tissue, and lower values suggesting infiltration of fat or other non-muscle tissues [16].

We hypothesized that dietary supplementation of MCTs would promote nutritional support of the physical elements of the elderly that regulate balance during walking. Thus, the goal of this study was to investigate the effects of MCTs on the metabolism and quality of gait-related skeletal muscles in healthy older adults.

2. Materials and Methods

2.1. Study Design and Ethics Approval

This was a randomized, double-blind, placebo-controlled, parallel-group, two-arm (1:1 ratio) trial conducted between October 2018 and December 2019, registered as the MCT SMILE (SuppleMentary for Life in the Elderly) project study (UMIN000033447). The study procedures were performed in accordance with the tenets of the Declaration of Helsinki. The study protocol was approved by the Clinical Research Ethics Committee of the Tohoku University Graduate School of Medicine (2018-2-67, date on 23 July 2018). Written informed consent was obtained from each participant.

2.2. Participants

Details of the original MCT SMILE study have been described previously [10]. Briefly, the inclusion criteria were an age of 65–80 years, right-handed, without dementia or mild cognitive impairment, and with full autonomy in activities of daily living. Participants taking nutritional supplements affecting energy metabolism or body composition were excluded from the study. Eligible participants were assigned randomly to the MCT group or a placebo control group who took a matching formula made with canola oil (LCT) as a caloric equivalent to the MCT-based vegetable oil (Figure 1). Each participant was scheduled for imaging studies, neurocognitive and physical function tests, and blood examinations before and after the 3-month intervention. A yogurt-flavored jelly stick was used (total weight, 15 g) containing 6 g of MCTs (75% C8:0 and 25% C10:0 from total fatty acids) or 6 g of LCT (64% C18:1, 19% C18:2, and 9% C18:3 from total fatty acids) [12]. In this study, participants and researchers could not distinguish between the two supplements from the appearance (created using an unlabeled silver stick), flavor, or texture. Participants were instructed to consume 3 sticks per day, one just prior to every meal, for a total of 3 consecutive months. Lifestyle, eating habits, and medications were not changed throughout the study period. Each participant maintained a daily logbook to ensure their compliance.

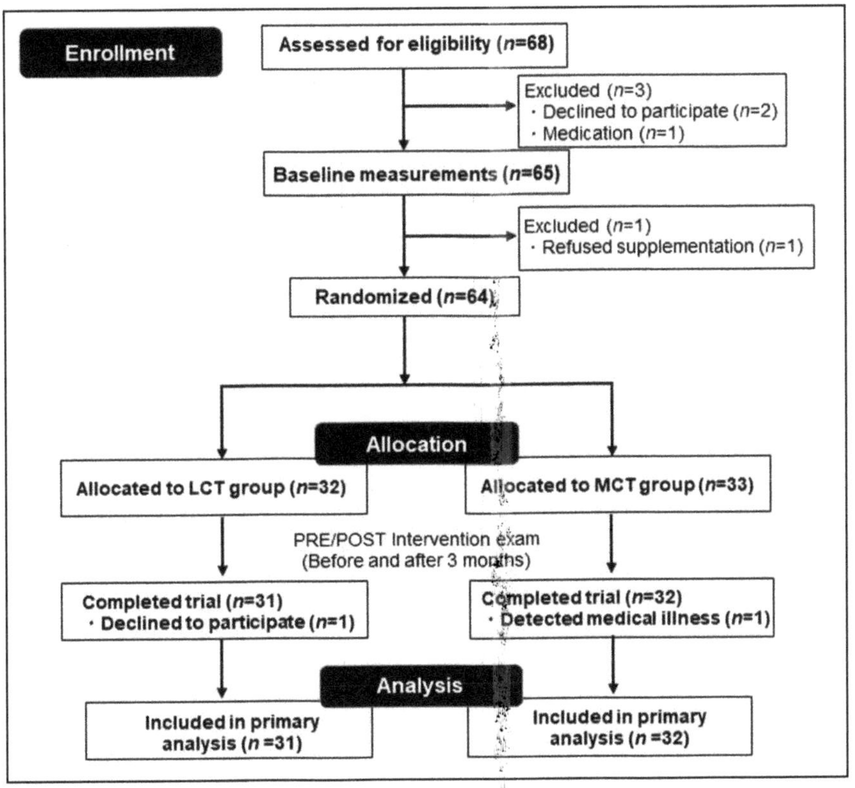

Figure 1. CONSORT diagram describing recruitment and random allocation of the participants.

2.3. *Image Acquisition*

Whole-body FDG PET/CT images were acquired on a GE Discovery PET/CT scanner (GE Healthcare, Milwaukee, WI, USA). Low-dose CT was performed at 140 kVp, 25 mAs, and a layer thickness of 2 mm. Brain PET images were acquired for 3 min in three-dimensional (3D) mode using a single bed position. The patients were required to fast for a minimum of 12 h before starting the PET scan to ensure the plasma glucose level was $\leq$6.0 mM. Image acquisition started approximately 60 min after injection of 3.7 MBq/mL/kg ^{18}F-FDG. PET images incorporating all image corrections were reconstructed using the manufacturer's software and recommended parameters (β = 200; field of view, 300 mm; matrix size, 128 $\times$ 128; layer thickness, 3.26 mm) to obtain maximum intensity projection and fused images. Imaging data were then imported into LIFEx open-source software (v7.8.0; http://www.lifexsoft.org: accessed on 17 May 2025) in the Digital Imaging and Communications in Medicine (DICOM) format to analyze the PET metabolic and CT density parameters. The SUV_{mean} of each ROI for both sides was calculated using LIFEx software. The mean SUV_{mean} for patient-based assessments was calculated by averaging the values obtained for each unilateral region.

A 3D ROI of 5.1 cm^3 was manually placed at the widest and thickest part of each relevant muscle belly identified by the PET/CT fusion image (Figure 2a,b). This study focused on the relationship between muscle density and metabolism of the major large muscles associated with walking balance (bilateral triceps, psoas, and vastus medialis) (Figure 2c–e) rather than changes in muscle quantity (mass) because we aimed to clarify the primary biological effects of MCT on skeletal muscles without muscle atrophy. As a reference and for assessing hepatic FDG phosphorylation, an ROI (3 cm in diameter) was placed in the upper right lobe of the liver (Figure 2f) [17].

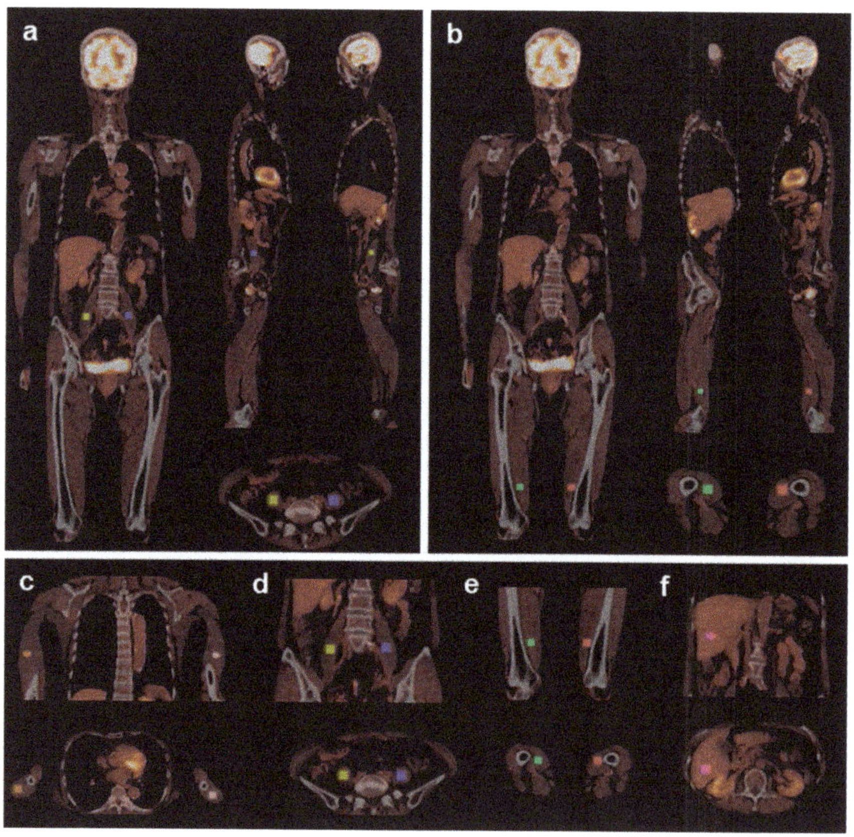

Figure 2. Representative whole-body FDG PET/CT images of ROI placement on the psoas (**a**) and vastus medialis (**b**). Three-dimensional ROIs (5.1 cm^3) are placed at the widest and thickest part of each muscle belly by confirming the coronal, sagittal, and cross-sectional images. ROI placement on the skeletal muscles and liver: The major gait-related muscles ((**c**), triceps; (**d**), psoas; (**e**), vastus medialis) are identified bilaterally on PET/CT fusion images. The liver ROI is used as the standard reference for glucose uptake (**f**). The upper and lower rows represent coronal and cross-sectional images, respectively. ROI: region of interest.

2.4. Measurements

The PET/CT-derived SUV_{mean} and HU values were measured before and 3 months after starting the intervention. Blood samples were analyzed for metabolic byproducts, including ketone bodies (β-hydroxybutyrate and acetoacetate) and glucose derived from the blood plasma samples, by a commercial clinical laboratory (SRL Inc., Tokyo, Japan) before and 3 months after intervention. The venous blood samples were taken after a 12-h overnight fast through an intravenous catheter secured for the PET study, as described [10].

2.5. Statistical Analysis

A minimum sample size of 28 was established from a previous study [18] on the cognitive effects of MCT supplementation in elderly patients, which was calculated to detect a clinically relevant effect with a 2-sided α of 0.05 and 90% power. Allowing for a 10% dropout during the intervention, the total required sample size for the present study was estimated as 31 per group. Continuous data are presented as the mean ± standard deviation. Repeated-measures two-way analysis of variance was used to determine differences within each variable. Two time points were included: the within-participant factor (effect per unit of time), and the between-participant factor (the differences between the MCT and control groups). When the group × time interaction was significant, tests of simple effects were performed to determine whether the groups differed significantly during the intervention period, using post hoc analyses adjusted for the Bonferroni correction (α level 0.025), where appropriate. Pearson's correlation coefficients were calculated to investigate the relationship between ketone body synthesis (β-hydroxybutyrate) and skeletal muscle glucose metabolism (SUV_{mean}) before and after intervention. Linear regression analyses were performed to evaluate the SUV_{mean} and muscle density (HU) association within the same ROI for each muscle. Statistical significance was set at $p < 0.05$. All analyses were performed using SPSS version 28 (IBM; Armonk, NY, USA), Bell Curve for Excel (SSRI, Tokyo, Japan), and Prism 9 (GraphPad Software; La Jolla, CA, USA).

3. Results

3.1. Characteristics of Participants

Among 68 participants, 63 (females/males: 22/10 in the MCT group and 21/10 in the placebo group) completed the study (Figure 1). The baseline demographic data of the 63 participants were not significantly different between the groups (see the demographic data of the participants for the original MCT SMILE study [10]).

3.2. Effects of MCT on Blood Ketone Bodies and Glucose Metabolism

MCT supplementation had an effect on maintaining ketone bodies after a 3-month intervention; they decreased in the placebo control group (Table 1). In the MCT group, several weak but significant correlations were found between plasma β-hydroxybutyrate and the SUV_{mean} of gait-related skeletal muscles, represented by the iliopsoas and vastus medialis; no relationships were apparent in the placebo control (Table 2).

For the MCT-treated participants, simple linear regression analysis of the longitudinal data measured before and after the intervention suggests that β-hydroxybutyrate was associated negatively with glucose metabolism in these two muscles, which are responsible for balance and posture during walking (Figure 3).

Table 1. Changes in plasma ketone bodies before (Pre) and after (Post) intervention.

	Placebo			Medium-Chain Triglycerides			Intergroup *p* Value
	Pre	Post	*p*	Pre	Post	*p*	
Total ketone bodies (μmol/L)	155 ± 96	112 ± 78	0.01	110 ± 87	90 ± 62	0.17	0.09
β-hydroxybutyrate (μmol/L)	105 ± 65	74 ± 53	0.03	74 ± 61	58 ± 46	0.46	0.05
Acetoacetate (μmol/L)	50 ± 33	38 ± 26	0.006	36 ± 28	32 ± 17	0.10	0.08
Glucose (mmol/L)	5.3 ± 0.3	5.3 ± 0.3	0.57	5.4 ± 0.5	5.5 ± 0.4	0.06	0.06

Data are expressed as the mean ± standard deviation. Statistically significant results with $p < 0.05$ are shown in bold.

Table 2. Pearson correlation coefficient between plasma β-hydroxybutyrate and gait-related skeletal muscle SUV_{mean} before and after intervention.

	Placebo			Medium-Chain Triglycerides		
	r	*95%CI*	*p*	*r*	*95%CI*	*p*
Triceps	−0.102	−0.446 0.268	0.59	−0.341	−0.617 0.008	0.056
Psoas	−0.029	−0.385 0.335	0.88	−0.571	−0.767 −0.278	0.0006
Vastus medialis	0.026	−0.337 0.383	0.89	−0.593	−0.780 −0.307	0.0004

Statistically significant results with $p < 0.05$ are shown in bold. CI: confidence interval.

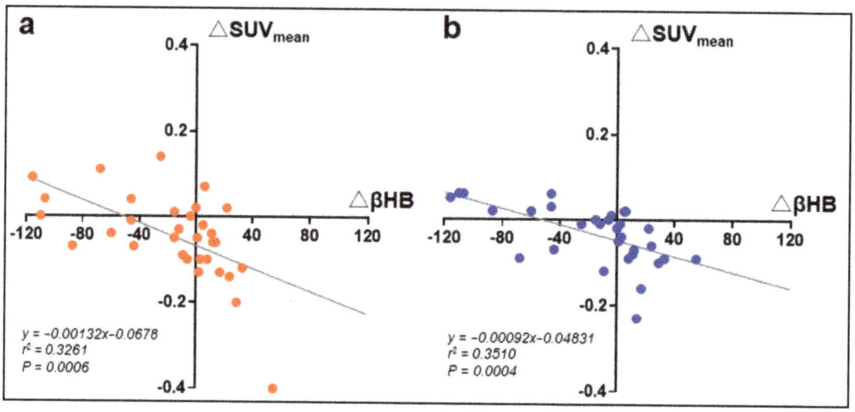

Figure 3. Scatter plots of the changes in plasma β-hydroxybutyrate and mean standardized uptake value (SUV_{mean}) of the psoas (**a**) or vastus medialis (**b**) muscles with regression lines in participants after 3-month MCT oil supplementation. βHB: plasma β-hydroxybutyrate.

3.3. Effects of MCT on Glucose Metabolism and Muscle Density

For post-intervention glucose metabolism, MCT decreased the SUV_{mean} in the lower skeletal muscles (psoas and vastus medialis), with a slight elevation in the liver (Table 3), but no significant changes in blood glucose levels (Table 1). In addition, MCT increased the post-intervention HU of these two muscles, and a significant difference was detected in the psoas muscle compared to the placebo control. For the relationship between glucose metabolism and skeletal muscle density in participants supplemented with MCT, the SUV_{mean} was negatively associated with HU values ($r = -0.613$ [95%CI: −0.793~−0.337], $p = 0.0002$ [Psoas]; $r = -0.587$ [95%CI: −0.777~−0.299, $p = 0.0004$ [Vastus medialis]) (Figure 4). No apparent changes in the metabolic or muscle parameters were detected in the placebo group.

Table 3. PET metabolic and CT density parameters before (Pre) and after (Post) intervention.

	Mean Standardized Uptake Value			Intergroup p Value	Hounsfield Units			Intergroup p Value
	Pre	Post	p		Pre	Post	p	
Triceps								
Placebo	0.64 ± 0.11	0.62 ± 0.08	0.07	0.98	60.5 ± 7.3	59.6 ± 7.9	0.36	0.06
MCT	0.63 ± 0.10	0.63 ± 0.09	0.80		63.4 ± 6.4	63.1 ± 7.8	0.73	
Psoas								
Placebo	0.60 ± 0.12	0.59 ± 0.10	0.51	0.43	54.2 ± 4.1	53.1 ± 2.9	0.30	<0.001
MCT	0.63 ± 0.08	0.59 ± 0.10	0.002		49.8 ± 3.8	53.0 ± 3.9	0.002	
Vastus medialis								
Placebo	0.60 ± 0.10	0.61 ± 0.10	0.67	0.69	46.5 ± 6.0	44.3 ± 5.1	0.15	0.11
MCT	0.63 ± 0.09	0.60 ± 0.08	0.03		42.4 ± 6.5	45.4 ± 4.8	0.04	
Liver								
Placebo	2.28 ± 0.31	2.29 ± 0.37	0.64	0.97	62.6 ± 6.4	64.3 ± 6.8	0.05	0.95
MCT	2.23 ± 0.39	2.35 ± 0.34	0.003		63.3 ± 5.9	63.4 ± 7.0	0.89	

Data are expressed as the mean ± standard deviation. Statistically significant results with $p < 0.05$ are shown in bold. PET: positron emission tomography, CT: computed tomography, MCT: medium-chain triglycerides.

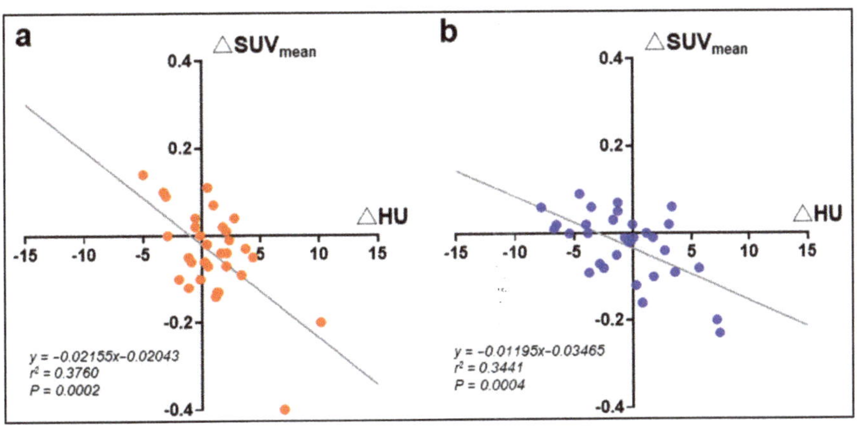

Figure 4. Scatter plots of the changes in CT mean standardized uptake value (SUV_{mean}) of the psoas (**a**) or vastus medialis (**b**) muscles with regression lines in participants after a 3-month MCT oil supplementation. βHB: plasma β-hydroxybutyrate.

4. Discussion

4.1. Mechanism by Which MCTs Modulate Energy Metabolism

Increased levels of ketone bodies attenuate glucose utilization in peripheral tissues, have anti-lipolytic effects in adipose tissue, and potentially attenuate proteolysis in skeletal muscles [19]. It is unclear why chronic MCT supplementation did not elevate but rather declined plasma ketone bodies in our participants. However, the sustained circulating β-hydroxybutyrate, the most abundant ketone body [20], observed only in the MCT supplemented participants may reflect certain beneficial metabolic changes due to MCTs. In fact, MCTs are rapidly absorbed and metabolized, converting into ketones with varied estimated plasma half-lives depending on the type (0.8 to 3.1 h for β-hydroxybutyrate and 8 to 14 h for acetoacetate) [21]. Therefore, ketone bodies sampled at least 12 h after the last MCT ingestion could have been reduced compared to their peak plasma levels.

PET image analysis showed glucose hypometabolism in the psoas and vastus medialis after a 3-month MCT intervention, indicating altered energy metabolism and glucose utilization. High-fat ketogenic diets achieved by MCTs have been shown to induce a "metabolic switch" from glycolysis to ketone body utilization in the mitochondrial citric acid cycle, preferentially in the heart, skeletal muscle, and brain tissues in healthy adults [22,23]. These observations can be explained by the inverse relationship between ketolysis and glycolysis in the lower-body skeletal muscles [19] and regional brain areas (e.g., the primary sensorimotor cortex) related to gait balance control through increased cerebellar neural connectivity [10].

4.2. Effects of MCTs on Skeletal Muscle Mass and Density

This study acquired whole-body CT fusion images simultaneously with PET scans to evaluate muscle quantity (mass) determined by the skeletal muscle area [24]. However, for healthy older adults without anatomical changes in muscle mass, the quality of the muscle seems more important than the quantity given the relatively short study period (3 months). Normal reference data regarding CT-derived muscle parameters have been reported recently, including skeletal muscle density (HU) [24,25]. As a measure of muscle quality, myosteatosis can be indirectly assessed by muscle radiodensity attenuation in the skeletal muscles of the lower extremities [26]. Notably, MCTs caused slight but significant time-course enhancement of CT densities in the psoas and vastus medialis muscles within the normal range (+30 to +150 HU) [24] and above lower thresholds (psoas, 46.1) [24]. The psoas muscle is important in dynamic function and postural support; the vastus medialis and the quadriceps provide stability during the stance phase in the gait cycle and support normal posture. Therefore, increased HU may affect muscle quality, improving gait function following MCT supplementation.

Unfortunately, segmenting multiple skeletal muscle regions in abdominal or abdominopelvic CT images is difficult for several reasons, including muscle morphology, signal intensity, and image artifacts [27]. Due to this, further image analyses incorporating magnetic resonance imaging data are expected to clarify the MCT-induced differences in regional energy metabolism, especially the reliance on oxidative phosphorylation between slow-twitch (type I) and fast-twitch (type II) fibers and their subtypes, which contribute to long-term endurance and powerful bursts of gait movement, respectively [19].

4.3. Practical Application of MCTs

Frailty and sarcopenia are major health issues among elderly people [28]. The potential of MCTs to address these age-related physical conditions is just beginning to be studied since the 2000s. We have recently reported the effect of MCTs on increasing muscle functionality without altering muscle mass in healthy older adults. Supplementation of MCTs with or without aerobic exercise improved muscle functions (e.g., knee extension strength and balance ability during walking) without changing the skeletal muscle mass compared with the placebo control using LCTs [8]. These findings have been confirmed in vivo by detecting altered glucose metabolism both in the brain (e.g., right primary sensorimotor cortex) and in some skeletal muscles responsible for gait motor functions, and increased neural connectivity between brain areas related to balance and memory functions (e.g., contralateral cerebellum to the bilateral amygdala and anterior hippocampus), using FDG-PET/CT and functional magnetic resonance imaging studies [10]. The beneficial aspects of MCTs are not limited to healthy subjects and could also be applicable to frail older adults. It is interesting to note that MCT supplementation at smaller doses (6 g/day for 3 month) has been shown to increase both muscle mass and function and to decrease fat mass with maintained or increased body weight [12], suggesting some positive "add-on" effects of MCTs on anatomical changes associated with frailty/sarcopenia.

4.4. Limitations

There are several limitations in our study. First, this study may have been underpowered for detecting the desired group differences because of a small sample size; however, its risk for bias was minimized compared to other RCTs [29]. Second, we could not target ketone body metabolism in skeletal muscles because of limited PET tracer, including ^{11}C-β-hydroxybutyrate [30]. Indeed, it is hard to determine the ketogenic shift of each muscle using only the circulating ketone bodies with shorter half-lives. Nevertheless, significant negative relationships between plasma β-hydroxybutyrate levels and imaging outcomes may, at least, support a favorable biological effect of MCTs on selected skeletal muscles responsible for walking in healthy older adults.

5. Conclusions

A 3-month MCT supplementation suppressed glucose metabolism in gait-related skeletal muscles and increased their muscle density, consistent with previous findings that it stabilizes balance functions during walking in healthy older adults [10]. Present functional/morphological imaging results extend our knowledge of MCTs' biological effect against senescent change.

Author Contributions: Conceptualization, T.M. and Y.T. (Yasuko Tatewaki); methodology, T.M. and Y.T. (Yasuko Tatewaki); formal analysis, H.K.; investigation, T.M. and Y.T. (Yasuko Tatewaki); data curation, Y.T. (Yasuyuki Taki); visualization, T.M. and H.K.; writing—original draft preparation, T.M.; writing—review and editing, T.M., H.K., Y.T. (Yasuko Tatewaki) and Y.T. (Yasuyuki Taki); supervision, Y.T. (Yasuyuki Taki); project administration, T.M. and Y.T. (Yasuko Tatewaki); funding acquisition, T.M. All authors have read and agreed to the published version of the manuscript.

Funding: This investigator-initiated trial was supported by the Industry–Academia Collaboration of The Nisshin OilliO Group, Ltd. (Kanagawa, Japan). The funder had no function in the study's design, the data collection, analysis, or interpretation, the writing of the report, or the decision to submit the article for publication.

Institutional Review Board Statement: This study was performed in accordance with the Declaration of Helsinki and national ethical standards. The Clinical Research Ethics Committee of the Tohoku University Graduate School of Medicine approved the study protocol on 29 May 2018 (approval number: 2018-2-67). This study was registered with the University Hospital Medical Information Network Clinical Trials Registry (UMIN-CTR) on 23 July 2018 (UMIN000033447).

Informed Consent Statement: Informed consent was obtained from all subjects involved in the study. Written informed consent has been obtained from the patient(s) to publish this paper.

Data Availability Statement: As this study contains only a small number of participants, some of the personal information that may assist in the deduction or reveal the identity of participants has been deleted in order to protect the privacy of these individuals.

Acknowledgments: We are grateful to Akira Arai (Kousei Sendai Clinic, Sendai, Japan) for assistance with PET data acquisition and processing. The authors thank Shinji Watanabe, Chika Sakurai, Chie Arai, and Noriyuki Yamamoto (Central Research Center, The Nisshin OilliO Group Ltd., Kanagawa, Japan) for their assistance with the foundation and continuous encouragement of this project.

Conflicts of Interest: The authors declare no conflicts of interest.

Abbreviations

The following abbreviations are used in this manuscript:

CT	Computed Tomography
FDG	^{18}F-2-fluoro-2-deoxy-D-glucose
HU	Hounsfield units
LCT	Long-chain triglyceride
MCT	Medium-chain triglyceride
PET	Positron emission tomography
RCT	Randomized clinical trial
ROI	Region of interest
SUV	Standardized uptake value
3D	Three-dimensional.

References

1. Balachandran, A.; de Beer, J.; James, K.S.; van Wissen, L.; Janssen, F. Comparison of Population Aging in Europe and Asia Using a Time-Consistent and Comparative Aging Measure. *J. Aging Health* **2020**, *32*, 340–351. [CrossRef]
2. Wang, X.; Hu, J.; Wu, D. Risk factors for frailty in older adults. *Medicine* **2022**, *101*, e30169. [CrossRef]
3. Takei, S.; Okada, Y.; Ochi, M.; Miura, S.; Shiraoka, A.; Ochi, H.; Matsumoto, S.; Igase, M.; Fujishita, S.; Ohyagi, Y. Frailty and aging are associated with cognitive decline and dermal advanced glycation end-product accumulation in older Japanese men. *Arch. Gerontol. Geriat.* **2024**, *1*, 100071. [CrossRef]
4. Arosio, B.; Calvani, R.; Ferri, E.; Coelho-Junior, H.J.; Carandina, A.; Campanelli, F.; Ghiglieri, V.; Marzetti, E.; Picca, A. Sarcopenia and Cognitive Decline in Older Adults: Targeting the Muscle-Brain Axis. *Nutrients* **2023**, *15*, 1853. [CrossRef]
5. Kapogiannis, D.; Avgerinos, K.I. Brain glucose and ketone utilization in brain aging and neurodegenerative diseases. *Int. Rev. Neurobiol.* **2020**, *154*, 79–110. [PubMed]
6. Wang, Y.; Liu, Z.; Han, Y.; Xu, J.; Huang, W.; Li, Z. Medium Chain Triglycerides enhances exercise endurance through the increased mitochondrial biogenesis and metabolism. *PLoS ONE* **2018**, *13*, e0191182. [CrossRef]
7. Ashton, J.S.; Roberts, J.W.; Wakefield, C.J.; MacLaren, D.P.M.; Marwood, S.; Malone, J.J. Medium chain triglycerides with a C8:C10 ratio of 30:70 enhances cognitive performance and mitigates the cognitive decline associated with prolonged exercise in young and healthy adults. *Physiol. Behav.* **2023**, *269*, 114284. [CrossRef] [PubMed]
8. Kojima, K.; Ishikawa, H.; Watanabe, S.; Nosaka, N.; Mutoh, T. A Randomized, Double-Blind, Controlled Trial Assessing If Medium-Chain Triglycerides in Combination with Moderate-Intensity Exercise Increase Muscle Strength in Healthy Middle-Aged and Older Adults. *Nutrients* **2023**, *15*, 3275. [CrossRef]
9. Ishikawa, H.; Kojima, K.; Watanabe, S.; Nosaka, N.; Mutoh, T. Effect of medium-chain triglycerides supplements and walking on health-related quality of life in sedentary, healthy middle-aged, and older adults with low BMIs: A randomized, double-blind, placebo-controlled, parallel-group trial. *Front. Nutr.* **2023**, *10*, 1296896. [CrossRef]
10. Mutoh, T.; Kunitoki, K.; Tatewaki, Y.; Yamamoto, S.; Thyreau, B.; Matsudaira, I.; Kawashima, R.; Taki, Y. Impact of medium-chain triglycerides on gait performance and brain metabolic network in healthy older adults: A double-blind, randomized controlled study. *Geroscience* **2022**, *44*, 1325–1338. [CrossRef]
11. Watanabe, S.; Tsujino, S. Applications of Medium-Chain Triglycerides in Foods. *Front. Nutr.* **2022**, *9*, 802805. [CrossRef] [PubMed]
12. Ezaki, O.; Abe, S. Medium-chain triglycerides (8:0 and 10:0) increase muscle mass and function in frail older adults: A combined data analysis of clinical trials. *Front. Nutr.* **2023**, *10*, 1284497. [CrossRef]
13. Zurlo, F.; Larson, K.; Bogardus, C.; Ravussin, E. Skeletal muscle metabolism is a major determinant of resting energy expenditure. *J. Clin. Investig.* **1990**, *86*, 1423–1427. [CrossRef]
14. Goncalves, M.D.; Green-McKenzie, J.; Alavi, A.; Torigian, D.A. Regional Variation in Skeletal Muscle and Adipose Tissue FDG Uptake Using PET/CT and Their Relation to BMI. *Acad. Radiol.* **2017**, *24*, 1288–1294. [CrossRef] [PubMed]
15. Looijaard, W.G.; Dekker, I.M.; Stapel, S.N.; Girbes, A.R.; Twisk, J.W.; Oudemans-van Straaten, H.M.; Weijs, P.J. Skeletal muscle quality as assessed by CT-derived skeletal muscle density is associated with 6-month mortality in mechanically ventilated critically ill patients. *Crit. Care* **2016**, *20*, 386. [CrossRef] [PubMed]
16. Engelke, K.; Museyko, O.; Wang, L.; Laredo, J.D. Quantitative analysis of skeletal muscle by computed tomography imaging-State of the art. *J. Orthop. Transl.* **2018**, *15*, 91–103. [CrossRef]
17. Zwezerijnen, G.J.C.; Eertink, J.J.; Ferrández, M.C.; Wiegers, S.E.; Burggraaff, C.N.; Lugtenburg, P.J.; Heymans, M.W.; de Vet, H.C.W.; Zijlstra, J.M.; Boellaard, R. Reproducibility of [18F]FDG PET/CT liver SUV as reference or normalisation factor. *Eur. J. Nucl. Med. Mol. Imaging* **2023**, *50*, 486–493. [CrossRef]

18. Kimoto, A.; Ohnuma, T.; Toda, A.; Takebayashi, Y.; Higashiyama, R.; Tagata, Y.; Ito, M.; Ota, T.; Shibata, N.; Arai, H. Medium-chain triglycerides given in the early stage of mild-to-moderate Alzheimer's disease enhance memory function. *Psychogeriatrics* **2017**, *17*, 520–521. [CrossRef]
19. Yakupova, E.I.; Bocharnikov, A.D.; Plotnikov, E.Y. Effects of Ketogenic Diet on Muscle Metabolism in Health and Disease. *Nutrients* **2022**, *14*, 3842. [CrossRef]
20. Moya-Garzon, M.D.; Wang, M.; Li, V.L.; Lyu, X.; Wei, W.; Tung, A.S.; Raun, S.H.; Zhao, M.; Coassolo, L.; Islam, H.; et al. A β-hydroxybutyrate shunt pathway generates anti-obesity ketone metabolites. *Cell* **2025**, *188*, 175–186.e120. [CrossRef]
21. Clarke, K.; Tchabanenko, K.; Pawlosky, R.; Carter, E.; Todd King, M.; Musa-Veloso, K.; Ho, M.; Roberts, A.; Robertson, J.; Vanitallie, T.B.; et al. Kinetics, safety and tolerability of (R)-3-hydroxybutyl (R)-3-hydroxybutyrate in healthy adult subjects. *Regul. Toxicol. Pharmacol.* **2012**, *63*, 401–408. [CrossRef] [PubMed]
22. Cunnane, S.C.; Courchesne-Loyer, A.; St-Pierre, V.; Vandenberghe, C.; Pierotti, T.; Fortier, M.; Croteau, E.; Castellano, C.A. Can ketones compensate for deteriorating brain glucose uptake during aging? Implications for the risk and treatment of Alzheimer's disease. *Ann. N. Y. Acad. Sci.* **2016**, *1367*, 12–20. [CrossRef]
23. Courchesne-Loyer, A.; Croteau, E.; Castellano, C.A.; St-Pierre, V.; Hennebelle, M.; Cunnane, S.C. Inverse relationship between brain glucose and ketone metabolism in adults during short-term moderate dietary ketosis: A dual tracer quantitative positron emission tomography study. *J. Cereb. Blood Flow Metab.* **2017**, *37*, 2485–2493. [CrossRef] [PubMed]
24. De Marco, D.; Mamane, S.; Choo, W.; Mullie, L.; Xue, X.; Afilalo, M.; Afilalo, J. Muscle Area and Density Assessed by Abdominal Computed Tomography in Healthy Adults: Effect of Normal Aging and Derivation of Reference Values. *J. Nutr. Health Aging* **2022**, *26*, 243–246. [CrossRef]
25. Amini, B.; Boyle, S.P.; Boutin, R.D.; Lenchik, L. Approaches to Assessment of Muscle Mass and Myosteatosis on Computed Tomography: A Systematic Review. *J. Gerontol. A Biol. Sci. Med. Sci.* **2019**, *74*, 1671–1678. [CrossRef]
26. Ahn, H.; Kim, D.W.; Ko, Y.; Ha, J.; Shin, Y.B.; Lee, J.; Sung, Y.S.; Kim, K.W. Updated systematic review and meta-analysis on diagnostic issues and the prognostic impact of myosteatosis: A new paradigm beyond sarcopenia. *Ageing Res. Rev.* **2021**, *70*, 101398. [CrossRef]
27. Song, G.; Zhou, J.; Wang, K.; Yao, D.; Chen, S.; Shi, Y. Segmentation of multi-regional skeletal muscle in abdominal CT image for cirrhotic sarcopenia diagnosis. *Front. Neurosci.* **2023**, *17*, 1203823. [CrossRef] [PubMed]
28. Dodds, R.; Sayer, A.A. Sarcopenia and frailty: New challenges for clinical practice. *Clin. Med.* **2016**, *16*, 455–458. [CrossRef]
29. Giannos, P.; Prokopidis, K.; Lidoriki, I.; Triantafyllidis, K.K.; Kechagias, K.S.; Celoch, K.; Candow, D.G.; Ostojic, S.M.; Forbes, S.C. Medium-chain triglycerides may improve memory in non-demented older adults: A systematic review of randomized controlled trials. *BMC Geriatr.* **2022**, *22*, 817. [CrossRef]
30. Kjaerulff, M.L.G.; Nielsen, E.N.; Gormsen, L.C.; Dias, A.H. First-in-human whole-body PET/CT imaging with the optimized ketone tracer [(11)C]β-hydroxybutyrate using a long axial field-of-view scanner. *Eur. J. Nucl. Med. Mol. Imaging* **2024**, *51*, 3802–3804. [CrossRef]

nutrients

MDPI

Article

Effects of Pomegranate Extract on Inflammatory Markers and Cardiometabolic Risk Factors in Adults Aged 55–70 Years: A Randomised Controlled Parallel Trial

Grace Farhat [1,*], Jhama Malla [2], Jay Vadher [3] and Emad A. S. Al-Dujaili [4]

[1] Faculty of Health and Education, Manchester Metropolitan University, Manchester M15 6BG, UK
[2] Faculty of Health and Medical Sciences, University of Surrey, Guildford GU2 7YH, UK
[3] Faculty of Sport and Exercise, Manchester Metropolitan University, Manchester M15 6BH, UK
[4] Centre for Cardiovascular Science, Faculty of Medicine and Veterinary Medicine, Queen's Medical Research Institute, University of Edinburgh, Edinburgh EH16 4TJ, UK
* Correspondence: g.farhat@mmu.ac.uk

Abstract: Background: Chronic inflammation increases morbidity in older adults and significantly impacts healthy ageing. Pomegranate extract (PE), rich in polyphenols, has been suggested to reduce inflammation and could prevent cardiovascular disease. However, there is limited research examining the potential of PE in disease prevention in ageing. **Methods**: A two-arm double-blind parallel trial was conducted, in which participants received either placebo capsules (maltodextrin) or pomegranate extract (740 mg) daily for 12 weeks. At baseline, week 6, and week 12, anthropometric measurements, blood pressure, and blood samples were collected. Serum inflammatory markers (IL-6, IL-1-α, IL1-β, IL-2, TNF-α, CRP and PAI-1), fasting blood glucose, and lipid levels were also measured. **Results**: A total of 86 participants met the eligibility criteria, with 76 completing the trial. A significant interaction between treatment and time was observed for the IL-6 ($p = 0.02$) and IL1-β ($p = 0.05$) levels, with both parameters significantly decreasing in the PE group. CRP and TNF-α showed a downward trend in the PE group, but it was not statistically significant ($p > 0.05$). Systolic blood pressure significantly decreased in the PE group (by 5.22 ± 1.26 mmHg (SE), $p = 0.04$), indicating potential clinical relevance, with diastolic blood pressure showing a similar downward trend (2.94 ± 1.08 mmHg (SE), $p = 0.3$). Despite being apparently healthy with no diagnosed diseases, a substantial number of participants exhibited elevated levels of inflammatory markers and systolic blood pressure. **Conclusions**: PE can lower inflammatory markers and blood pressure, which can be high in both normal-weight and overweight older adults, making it a cost-effective measure to promote healthy ageing. Further long-term studies are needed to address the limitations of this 3-month study, including the overrepresentation of normal-weight participants, and to gain a better understanding of the impact of weight on the above-mentioned outcomes.

Keywords: pomegranate extract; inflammation; ageing; inflammageing; blood pressure; overweight

1. Introduction

Ageing has been associated with increased inflammation, often referred to as "inflammageing", a chronic low-grade inflammatory state characterised by increased levels of pro-inflammatory markers such as interleukin-6 (IL-6), interleukin-1 (IL-1), C-reactive protein (CRP), and tumour necrosis factor-alpha (TNF-α) [1,2]. Inflammageing is believed to play a role in the development of various co-morbidities including cardiovascular disease,

https://doi.org/10.3390/nu17071235

diabetes, and neurodegenerative disorders [1,3]. With the global number of individuals aged over 60 years projected to reach 2.1 billion by 2050 [4], improving the health of older adults is more critical than ever. Older individuals, usually defined as those >55 years of age [5] are generally considered to be at an increased risk for cardiovascular disease [6]. Therefore, targeting this age group, rather than solely focusing on those aged 60 years and above, is crucial for preventive interventions aimed at reducing inflammation and cardiovascular risk factors and, subsequently, reducing the risk of disease in older adults.

Inflammageing is suggested to be a result of the remodelling of the immune system, leading to the production of pro-inflammatory cytokines [3]. Overweight and obesity are rising in prevalence in older adults, similarly to the rest of the population, and they can further exacerbate inflammageing and increase the risk of comorbidities [7,8]. In a previous study, overweight and obese individuals showed a decreased expression of interleukin 2 (IL-2), which was inversely correlated with CRP [9]. Therefore, this overweight population presents additional risks that warrant careful consideration.

Polyphenols have regained significant popularity in recent years, and their role in ageing has attracted attention from the scientific community, prompting efforts to find alternative and cost-effective ways to improve health. Pomegranate (*Punica granatum* L.), a fruit representing a rich source of antioxidants, such as ellagitannins (particularly punicalagin, which is unique to pomegranate), has been shown to exhibit one of the highest levels of antioxidant activity among multiple polyphenol-rich foods (e.g., green tea, wine) [10]. Pomegranate has been previously considered an exotic fruit in several Western countries [11], but its regular consumption has significantly increased over the past few years. Pomegranate is presented as a sustainable fruit as it can adapt to climate change, is drought tolerant, can be grown in a wide range of soils, and has low water and carbon footprints, resulting in low environmental impacts when adequate agricultural practices are used [12–15].

The benefits of pomegranate on inflammatory markers and cardiovascular disease risk factors have been well documented. We previously reported its benefits on blood pressure and cardiovascular risk factors in the general population [16–18]. In addition, a meta-analysis of 16 randomised clinical trials reported the effect of pomegranate in reducing inflammatory markers [19]. However, findings are limited by the short duration of several studies (<12 weeks), the heterogeneous population characteristics, and the lack of focus on prevention in older adults. Notably, with this meta-analysis indicating that the beneficial effects of pomegranate were more pronounced in overweight and obese individuals because of their elevated risk, a further exploration of this association is needed to inform future recommendations. This trial aimed to assess the effects of pomegranate extract on inflammatory markers and cardiometabolic risk factors in normal-weight and overweight adults aged 55–70 years.

2. Materials and Methods

This trial was registered with clincialtrials.gov (NCT05588479) and granted ethical approval by the Manchester Metropolitan University Faculty of Health and Education (reference number: 47627). Participants provided written informed consent prior to participation. Recruitment took place between December 2022 and June 2024.

2.1. Participants

Volunteers were identified through physical posters in GP practices, community centres, community events, gyms, university premises, and social media. Interested volunteers were then screened for eligibility, either online or in person depending on preference, and were scheduled for their first appointment at the Physiology Lab at Manchester Metropolitan University. Participants were required to be fasted for at least 8 h before each of their appointments.

The inclusion criteria included English-speaking adults of all races and socio-economic backgrounds, aged 55–70 years with the capacity to consent, and with a normal weight (BMI 18.5–24.9 kg/m^2) or overweight (BMI 25–29.9 kg/m^2) status. Obese individuals were excluded to maintain the trial focus on prevention. All genders were included. The exclusion criteria involved individuals who have been on a weight loss regimen in the past two months, those with diagnosed chronic diseases such as diabetes, hypertension, cardiovascular disease, or renal disease, and anyone taking medications that could modulate blood pressure and/or lipid levels and inflammation. Participants who were already taking antioxidant supplements were advised to discontinue use for at least 3 weeks prior to the start of the study.

2.2. Trial Design and Intervention

The trial design was described in a previous study [20]. It was a two-arm, double-blind, parallel trial in which participants were randomly assigned to receive either placebo capsules (maltodextrin) or pomegranate extract (PE) capsules (two 370 mg capsules of PE each) daily for 12 weeks. Each PE capsule contained punicalagins (36%) and ellagic acid (1.3%). The PE was microbiologically tested to ensure that it was free from pesticide residues, heavy metals, aflatoxins, and microbiological contamination, with no traces detected. PE capsules were provided by Euromed S.A, Barcelona, Spain. Random assignment was computer-generated, and groups were matched for gender and BMI. This was conducted by recruitment staff who were blinded to the intervention groups. This procedure ensured that staff were unaware of group assignments until after the baseline assessments were complete thus minimising selection bias. The pomegranate and placebo capsules looked identical and were provided to participants in two batches at baseline and week 6.

Participants attended the Physiology Lab at baseline, week 6, and week 12. During each visit, anthropometric measurements were taken; this included weight (using a digital scale: Marsden: DP2400, London, UK), height (using Seca® 711 stadiometer, Seca GmbH & Co. KG., Hamburg, Germany), waist and hip circumferences (using an elastic measuring tape), and body composition (using air displacement plethysmography (BodPod® GS-X: Cosmed, Rome, Italy). Blood pressure was measured three times following a 10 min rest, according to the WHO protocol [21], using a digital sphygmomanometer (Nissei® DS-1873, Tokyo, Japan). A 20 mL fasted venous blood sample was also collected. The blood samples were then processed and stored at −80 °C until analysis. Participants additionally answered a socio-demographic paper-based questionnaire before or during the first visit, which included information about their age, gender, occupation, ethnicity, and lifestyle habits (e.g., smoking, alcohol consumption, and physical activity habits). They were asked to note any side effects from consuming the capsules at weeks 6 and 12.

2.3. Outcome Measures and Laboratory Analysis

The primary outcome of this trial was serum IL-6 levels, while the secondary outcomes included serum CRP, TNF-α, IL-1α (Interleukin-1 alpha), IL1-β (Interleukin-1 beta), IL-2, Plasminogen Activator Inhibitor-1 (PAI-1), systolic blood pressure (SBP), diastolic blood pressure (DBP), fasting blood glucose (FBG) and lipid levels (TC (total cholesterol), HDL (high-density lipoprotein), LDL (low-density lipoprotein), and TG (triglycerides)).

The cytokines IL-6, IL-1α, IL1-β, IL-2, and TNF-α were simultaneously quantified using the Human XL Cytokine Luminex® Performance Assay Kit (Bio-tecne®, Minneapolis, MN, USA, protocol FCSTM18B-05). CRP and PAI-1 were analysed together using the Human Obesity Luminex® Performance Assay Kit (Bio-tecne®, protocol FCSTM08-2). In brief, after the serum samples were defrosted, centrifuged, and diluted according to protocol, 50 μL of the standard, control, or sample was added to each well of the 96-well plate, followed by 50 μL of a resuspended microparticle cocktail. The plate was then sealed and incubated for 2 h at room temperature on a shaker set at 800 rpm. After washing the wells 3 times with wash buffer using a magnetic device, 50 μL of a diluted biotin–antibody cocktail was added, followed by another incubation and wash. Subsequently, 50 μL of diluted streptavidin–PE was added; after another wash, the microparticles were resuspended in 100 μL of wash buffer. The final step involved reading the plate using a Luminex® analyser.

Serum FBG and lipid levels were analysed using the Cobas® 8000 c702 module (Roche Diagnostics, Basel, Switzerland) at the Manchester University NHS Foundation Trust Laboratories.

2.4. Compliance

Participants were given a paper-based diary to record the dates of capsule intake and to validate each entry with a checkmark. They were also asked during each appointment whether they had been consistent in taking the capsules daily, and notes were recorded. To monitor any changes in dietary intake during this period, participants were instructed to complete a 3-day diet diary (2 weekdays and 1 weekend) 3 times throughout the intervention (baseline, week 6, and week 12). Physical activity levels were additionally monitored throughout the intervention and translated into metabolic equivalent of task (MET) values, representing the energy expenditure of each activity relative to resting. These values were estimated using widely available guidelines for different activities [22].

2.5. Power Calculation and Statistical Analysis

A sample size of 76 participants was determined based on its ability to detect a significant difference of 12% in the IL-6 levels between the groups, achieving 90% power at $\alpha = 0.05$ (two-tailed) and allowing for stratification by weight status. Data were derived from the trial by Boldaji et al. (2009) [23]. We then aimed to recruit 38 overweight individuals and 38 controls, allowing us to reject the null hypothesis that the population means of the overweight and control groups were equal. Assuming a 10% attrition rate, a total of 84 participants were planned to be recruited.

Data were analysed using SPSS version 29 (IBM, Chicago, IL, USA) and presented as mean ± SD, unless otherwise noted as standard error (SE). Normality was assessed using the Kolmogorov–Smirnov test. For non-parametric data, variables were logarithmically transformed prior to analysis. Baseline characteristics were analysed using descriptive statistics and frequencies. The independent t-test or Mann–Whitney test was used to assess the differences in baseline characteristics between the 2 groups. For categorical variables, baseline differences were assessed using the Chi-squared exact test. The interaction between treatment (PE vs. PL) and time (baseline, week 6, and week 12) was assessed using linear mixed-effects models. For significant differences, pairwise comparisons were explored using the Bonferroni test. The impact of variables (e.g., weight status, blood pressure status) on the outcomes was assessed using a linear mixed-effects model, incorporating these variables as covariates. The correlation between outcome parameters was assessed using Pearson's or Spearman's correlation coefficient. Statistical significance was set at $p \leq 0.05$.

3. Results

A total of 355 participants responded to the advertisement, of which 38 did not reply to further communication and 60 volunteers decided not to proceed for multiple reasons (e.g., inability to commit to the dietary intervention, scheduling conflicts, and distance to the research location). Of the 257 volunteers screened, 86 were eligible for participation. Excluded participants reported taking anti-hypertensive, anti-lipemic, and/or anti-inflammatory medications (n = 128), having diabetes and/or cardiovascular disease (n = 13), taking HRT (n = 29), and having HIV (n = 1). A consort flow diagram is presented elsewhere [20] and in Figure 1.

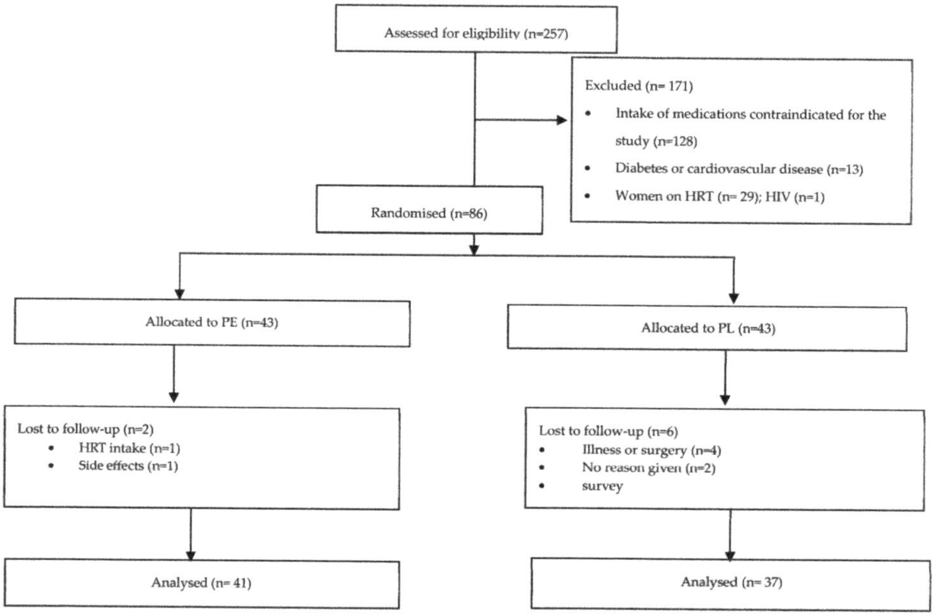

Figure 1. Consort flow diagram. Abbreviations: PE: pomegranate extract; PL: placebo; HRT: Hormone replacement therapy.

Among the 86 participants, 43 were allocated to the PE group and 43 to the PL group. Eight participants withdrew after their first appointment either due to disclosing HRT intake (n = 2), developing an illness (n = 3), having a scheduled surgery (n = 1), or noting side effects, e.g., digestive issues (n = 1). One participant did not provide a reason for withdrawal (n = 1). Two participants dropped out after completing 2 appointments for personal reasons but were still included in the analysis; 76 participants completed the full intervention. The attrition rate was estimated to be 11.63%.

Participants were predominantly females (64%) and White British (62.6%). The population had a mean BMI of 24 $\pm$ 3.21 kg/m^2, with 38.37% belonging to the overweight category. The mean SBP fell within the elevated range (128.02 $\pm$ 13.48 mmHg), despite participants being recruited with no history of hypertension or use of blood pressure medications. Characteristics of the intention-to-treat population are presented in Table 1.

An independent t-test showed no significant differences in age between the PE and PL group (p = 0.46), as well as the baseline levels of SBP (p = 0.34), DBP (p = 0.66), BMI (p = 0.78), waist circumference (p= 0.39), waist-to-hip ratio (p = 0.89), body fat percentage (p = 0.88), FBG (p = 0.92), total cholesterol (p = 0.1), HDL (p= 0.64), Triglycerides (p= 0.7), and LDL (p= 0.89) levels. No significant between-group differences in gender (p= 0.5) and ethnicity (p = 0.16) were noted.

Table 1. Baseline characteristics of the intention-to-treat population by intervention group.

Characteristics	All Participants	PE Group (n = 43)	PL Group (n = 43)
Age at baseline, y	61.26 ± 4.38	60.91 ± 4.09	61.60 ± 4.69
Sex (n)			
Female	55	27	28
Male	31	16	15
Occupation category (n)			
Professional Occupations	36	15	21
Managers, Directors, and Senior Officials	10	4	6
Health-related Professions	6	4	2
Associate Professional and Technical Occupations	5	2	3
Administrative and Secretarial Occupations	4	4	0
Unemployed	2	2	0
Sales and Customer Service Occupations	2	2	0
Skilled Trade Occupations	1	1	0
Caring, Leisure, and Other Service Occupations	1	1	0
Other	19	8	11
Ethnicity (n)			
White British	72	38	34
White Irish	3	1	2
Indian	2	0	2
Other white	2	0	2
Mixed race	2	2	3
Black	1	0	1
Other	3	2	1
Smoking status (n)			
Smoker	3	1	2
Non-smoker	83	42	41
Physical activity (MET-minutes/week)	749 (133)	746 (149)	751 (159)
BMI (kg/m^2)	24 ± 3.21	23.90 ± 3.14	24.10 ± 3.32
Waist circumference (cm)	84.59 ± 10.26	83.62 ± 9.77	85.55 ± 10.75
Waist-to-hip ratio	0.84 ± 0.69	0.83 ± 0.07	0.85 ± 0.07
Body fat percentage (%)	22.66 ± 10.02	22.75 ± 9.52	22.58 ± 10.61
SBP (mmHg)	128.02 ± 13.48	129.42 ± 14.27	126.63 ± 12.66
DBP (mmHg)	80.55 ± 8.72	80.96 ± 9.25	80.13 ± 8.24
Fasting blood glucose (mmol/L)	5.34 ± 4.66	5.35 ± 0.36	5.34 ± 0.56
Fasting lipid levels (mmol/L)			
Triglycerides	1.07 ± 0.46	1.05 ± 0.42	1.09 ± 0.50
Total cholesterol	5.79 ± 0.98	5.79 ± 1.20	5.79 ± 0.68
HDL	1.76 ± 0.43	1.79 ± 0.50	1.74 ± 0.34
LDL	3.55 ± 0.69	3.54 ± 0.72	3.56 ± 0.67

Values are reported as mean ± SD. Baseline differences between groups were analysed by independent t-test for numerical variables and Chi-squared exact test for nominal variables. No significant difference between groups was noted ($p > 0.05$). Abbreviations: PE: Pomegranate extract; PL: Placebo; SBP: Systolic blood pressure; DBP: Diastolic blood pressure; HDL: High-density lipoproteins; LDL: Low-density lipoproteins.

3.1. Effects of PE on Inflammatory Markers

No significant between-group differences in the baseline levels of IL-6 ($p = 0.49$), CRP ($p = 0.76$), TNF-α ($p = 0.17$), IL1-β ($p = 0.07$), IL1-α ($p = 0.65$), and IL-2 ($p = 0.16$) were noted.

Linear mixed model analysis revealed a significant effect of treatment and time on IL-6 levels F (1,2) = 3.97, $p = 0.02$). The PE resulted in a significant decrease in IL-6 levels compared to the placebo (by 5.47 ± 1.34 pg/mL (SE), $p < 0.001$). IL1-β levels were also shown to be significantly decreased in the PE group compared to the placebo group (F (1,2) = 2.98, $p = 0.05$). Although the CRP and TNF-α levels showed a downward trend in the PE group, this did not reach statistical significance ((F (1,2) = 0.97, $p = 0.38$) and (F (1,2) = 1.49, $p = 0.23$), respectively). No significant effects were detected for the IL1-α (F (1,2) = 1.34, $p = 0.26$), IL-2 (F (1,2) = 2.48, $p = 0.09$), and PAI-1 (F (1,2) = 0.2.19, $p = 0.12$) levels (Table 2).

Notably, there was considerable variability in the baseline IL-6 levels among the participants, ranging from 0.76 pg/mL to 34.34 pg/mL. This variability was also noted for TNF-α (0.38 to 38.86 pg/mL), IL-1α (4.56 to 34.84 pg/mL), and PAI-1 (0.1 to 19.1 pg/mL). Although clinical guidelines for normal levels of IL-6 and TNF-α have not been established, healthy levels are generally considered to be 17.4 pg/mL and 8.1 pg/mL, respectively [24,25]. Based on these thresholds, 65.5% of participants exhibited elevated IL-6 levels, and 45.5% exhibited high TNF- α levels; 96.1% of participants fell within the normal range of CRP, defined as below 1mg/dL [26].

Table 2. Effect of pomegranate extract on inflammatory markers compared to control.

		Baseline		Week 6		Week 12	
		Mean ± SD	**N**	**Mean ± SD**	**N**	**Mean ± SD**	**N**
IL-6 (pg/mL)	PL	21.27 ± 5.97	37	23.43 ± 12.16	37	23.69 ± 10.01	36
	PE	20.17 ± 7.69	40	17.42 ± 10.12	40	14.32 ± 9.78 *	39
CRP (mg/dL)	PL	0.21 ± 0.21	37	0.23 ± 0.24	37	0.22 ± 0.11	36
	PE	0.26 ± 0.41	40	0.20 ± 0.49	40	0.13 ± 0.1	39
TNF-α (pg/mL) [1]	PL	8.44 ± 9.77	36	10.5 ± 12.61	37	10.9 ± 7.86	36
	PE	10.87 ± 8.29	40	10.78 ± 8.01	40	8.93 ± 4.55	39
IL1-α (pg/mL) [1]	PL	10.88 ± 5.48	36	10.72 ± 4.54	37	13.55 ± 8.66	36
	PE	12.78 ± 6.88	40	12.02 ± 4.76	40	12.23 ± 5.41	39
IL1-β (pg/mL)	PL	5.67 ± 2.01	36	4.82 ± 1.51	37	5.58 ± 1.82	36
	PE	6.59 ± 2.35	40	5.99 ± 1.97	40	5.38 ± 1.82 *	38
IL-2 (pg/mL) [1]	PL	5.07 ± 1.22	36	5.12 ± 1.36	37	4.75 ± 1.58	36
	PE	4.84 ± 1.19	40	5.39 ± 1.61	40	5.66 ± 2.36	39
PAI-1 (ng/mL) [1]	PL	4.96 ± 4.42	36	4.88 ± 3.83	37	6.01 ± 9.26	36
	PE	5.3 ± 4.26	40	4.42 ± 4.54	39	5.17 ± 6.91	39

Data were analysed using linear mixed-effects model. [1] Data were analysed via linear mixed-effects model after logarithmic transformation of data (non-parametric data). Mean ± SD is added to facilitate comparison with other studies. * $p < 0.05$. Significant decrease from baseline. Abbreviations: IL-6: Interleukin 6; CRP: C-Reactive Protein; TNF-α: Tumour Necrosis Factor-alpha; IL1-α: Interleukin 1 alpha; IL1-β: Interleukin 1 beta; IL-2: Interleukin 2; PAI-1: Plasminogen Activator Inhibitor-1.

3.2. *Effects of PE on Blood Pressure*

The analysis showed a significant interaction between treatment and time and SBP (F (1,2) = 3.35, $p = 0.04$). SBP significantly decreased by 5.22 ± 1.26 (SE) mmHg at week 12 compared to baseline, while no significant differences were noted in the PL group. As for DBP, the results showed a trend towards a decrease in DBP in the PE group by 2.94 ± 1.08 (SE) mmHg, yet it did not reach statistical significance (F (1,2) = 1.2, $p = 0.3$) (Figure 2).

The assessment of blood pressure status in this population revealed that 79.5% of the population had elevated blood pressure (SBP between 120 and 129 mmHg). Stratifying the population based on blood pressure status showed that the significant decrease in SBP was only significant in those with elevated SBP ($p = 0.03$).

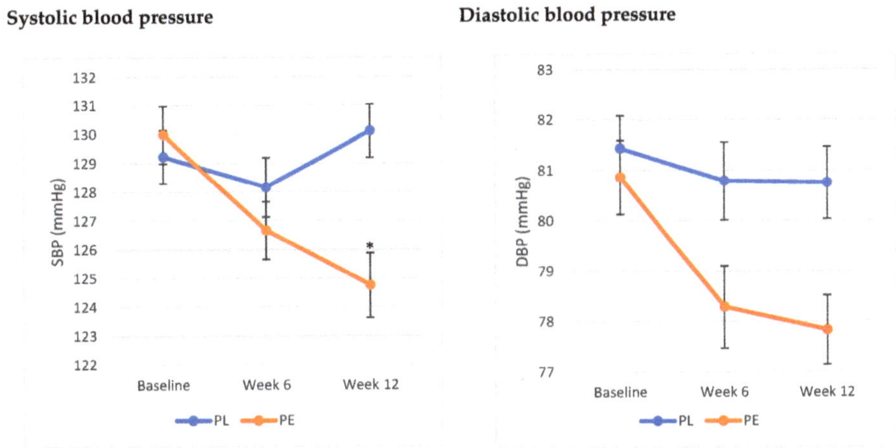

Figure 2. Effects of pomegranate extract on systolic and diastolic blood pressure compared to placebo. * Significant difference from baseline ($p < 0.05$). Values are expressed as mean ± SE. Results were analysed using linear mixed-effects model. The PE group exhibited a significant decrease in systolic blood pressure from baseline ($p < 0.05$), while it showed a trend toward a decrease in diastolic blood pressure ($p = 0.3$). Abbreviations: SBP: systolic blood Pressure; DBP: diastolic blood Pressure; PE: pomegranate extract; PL: placebo.

3.3. Effect of the Intervention on Anthropometric Measurements and Other Metabolic Health Outcomes

Analysis via the linear mixed-effects models showed no significant interactions between treatment and time and the anthropometric measurements, fasting blood glucose, and lipid levels ($p > 0.05$) (Table 3). Based on the clinical guidelines [27], 89.3% of participants had high TC levels (above 5 mmol/L) and 80.26% had high LDL levels (above 3 mmol/L). Additionally, 10.7% had elevated TG levels (above 1.7 mmol/L). However, the majority of participants had normal HDL levels, with only 4% of participants falling below the threshold of 1 mmol/L for men and 1.2 mmol/L for women; FBG levels were above the 5.4 mmol/L threshold [28] in 47.4% of participants.

Table 3. Effect of pomegranate extract on multiple outcome parameters.

		Baseline		**Week 6**		**Week 12**	
		Mean ± SD	**N**	**Mean ± SD**	**N**	**Mean ± SD**	**N**
BMI (Kg/m^2)	PL	24.13 ± 3.28	37.00	24.15 ± 3.23	37.00	23.69 ± 3.70	36.00
	PE	23.88 ± 3.22	41.00	23.75 ± 3.09	41.00	23.73 ± 3.13	40.00
WC (cm)	PL	86.02 ± 10.43	37.00	85.88 ± 10.43	37.00	86.12 ± 10.46	36.00
	PE	83.86 ± 9.94	41.00	83.79 ± 9.95	41.00	84.18 ± 10.10	40.00
WHR	PL	0.85 ± 0.06	37.00	0.85 ± 0.06	37.00	0.86 ± 0.06	36.00
	PE	0.84 ± 0.07	41.00	0.84 ± 0.07	41.00	2.01 ± 7.38	40.00
BF%	PL	22.14 ± 10.99	37.00	22.02 ± 10.31	37.00	24.35 ± 17.02	36.00
	PE	22.49 ± 9.49	41.00	22.66 ± 9.66	40.00	22.98 ± 8.15	38.00

Table 3. *Cont.*

		Baseline		Week 6		Week 12	
		Mean ± SD	N	Mean ± SD	N	Mean ± SD	N
FBG (mmol/L)	PL	5.34 ± 0.58	37.00	5.48 ± 0.51	35.00	5.49 ± 0.38	36.00
	PE	5.35 ± 0.37	40.00	5.37 ± 0.47	36.00	5.35 ± 0.39	36.00
HDL (mmol/L)	PL	1.75 ± 0.36	37.00	1.78 ± 0.43	35.00	1.72 ± 0.39	35.00
	PE	1.77 ± 0.51	39.00	1.71 ± 0.58	37.00	1.68 ± 0.45	36.00
LDL (mmol/L)	PL	3.54 ± 0.65	37.00	3.43 ± 0.72	35.00	3.29 ± 0.65	35.00
	PE	3.57 ± 0.72	39.00	3.39 ± 0.66	36.00	3.55 ± 0.67	36.00
TC (mmol/L)	PL	5.81 ± 0.65	36.00	5.72 ± 0.76	35.00	5.55 ± 0.83	36.00
	PE	5.80 ± 1.22	40.00	5.38 ± 1.43	37.00	5.76 ± 0.99	36.00
TG (mmol/L)	PL	1.11 ± 0.51	37.00	1.07 ± 0.45	35.00	1.12 ± 0.61	34.00
	PE	1.07 ± 0.42	40.00	1.25 ± 0.73	37.00	1.25 ± 0.46	36.00

Data were analysed using linear mixed-effects model. None of the parameters reported a significant difference ($p > 0.05$). Abbreviations: PE: pomegranate extract; PL: placebo; WC: waist circumference; WHR: waist-to-hip ratio; BF%: body fat percentage; FBG: fasting blood glucose; HDL: high-density lipoprotein; LDL: low-density lipoprotein; TC: total cholesterol; TG: triglycerides.

3.4. Impact of Weight Status on the Outcomes

3.4.1. Inflammatory Markers

The results showed no significant correlation between BMI and the different inflammatory markers ($p > 0.05$), showing that the high levels of certain markers did not increase positively with increased body weight.

The linear mixed-effects model analysis using BMI as a covariate showed that it did not have an impact on the outcomes for IL-6 ($F(1,2) = 0.63$, $p = 0.53$), TNF-α (($F(1,2) = 0.7$, $p = 0.5$), CRP ($F(1,2) = 0.25$, $p = 0.09$), IL-α ($F(1,2) = 1.46$, $p = 0.23$), IL-2 ($F(1,2) = 0.006$, $p = 0.99$), PAI ($F(1,2) = 2.57$, $p = 0.08$), and IL1-β ($F(1,2) = 1.35$, $p = 0.09$); the decrease in IL-6 and IL1-β levels were therefore irrespective of weight status.

3.4.2. Blood Pressure, Fasting Lipid and Glucose Levels

Pearson's correlation analysis showed no significant correlation between BMI and SBP ($p = 0.56$) or DBP ($p = 0.24$). Additionally, weight status did not seem to affect the outcomes of PE on both SBP (F (1,2), 0.4, $p = 0.67$) and DBP ($F(1,2) = 0.84$, $p = 0.43$). Similar results were noted for FBG and the fasting lipid levels (TC, TG, HDL, and LDL).

3.5. Compliance

The participants demonstrated a high level of compliance, estimated at approximately 87%. Only two individuals, both from the PL group, experienced an upset stomach during the intervention. A random review of the diet diaries from 30 participants indicated no significant variations in energy intake over the course of the intervention ($p = 0.31$ for the PL group and $p = 0.24$ for the PE group). Furthermore, there were no notable differences in macronutrient consumption, including protein, fat, and carbohydrates ($p > 0.05$). Similarly, physical activity levels remained stable throughout the intervention ($p = 0.67$ for the PL group and $p = 0.28$ for the PE group).

4. Discussion

This trial aimed to assess the effects of daily PE supplementation (740 mg) on inflammatory markers and cardiometabolic risk factors in adults aged 55–70 years, as well as its potential in preventing age-related diseases. We reported significant lowering effects of the extract on IL-6, IL1-β, and SBP, with a trend towards a decrease in CRP, TNF-α, and

DBP levels. While the trial population consisted of apparently healthy older adults with no diagnosed diseases, they exhibited higher levels of inflammatory markers compared to the estimated normal values; this is consistent with studies reporting increased levels of IL-6 and TNF-α in healthy older individuals without acute infection [29,30]. This, together with the elevated SBP reported in most participants, make our findings particularly relevant for supporting healthier ageing, irrespective of weight status.

The results of this trial align with a body of evidence that supports the beneficial effects of PE on inflammatory markers. A meta-analysis of 16 randomised clinical trials including 572 individuals reported a significant decrease in IL-6 levels [19], yet it was limited by the different dosages and formulations (use of either juice or extract), as well as trial design and the population's health state. Although we identified trends in the decrease in TNF-α and CRP that did not reach statistical significance, and several inflammatory factors showed no reduction, these effects may be typical of plant-based interventions, which generally lead to smaller and more gradual benefits than pharmacological agents. While the effects are moderate, they provide promising results for including PE in a broader health strategy focused on preventing age-related inflammation.

The blood pressure-lowering effects of pomegranate have been widely documented. In our previous short-term studies, we observed significant reductions in blood pressure among healthy individuals [15–18]. Additionally, a recent meta-analysis of 22 randomised controlled trials found that pomegranate was associated with significant reductions in both SBP and DBP, with greater reduction in those who have higher SBP at baseline [31], an outcome that is consistent with our findings. The significant decrease in SBP after 12 weeks of PE supplementation (by 5.22 ± 1.26 (SE) mmHg) may have important clinical relevance as it has been reported that a 5 mmHg reduction in SBP can reduce the risk of major cardiovascular events by 10% [32]. This finding may have significant implications for clinical practice as it may help to support hypertension prevention in older adults. This highlights the need for replicated studies to establish these results, together with exploring underlying mechanisms. Improved endothelial function and increasing nitric oxide availability have been suggested as potential pathways. Notably, ellagitannins in PE have been reported to enhance endothelial function by reducing oxidative stress and promoting endothelial nitric oxide synthase (eNOS) activity, leading to better vasodilation and lower blood pressure [33,34].

Our results add to the substantial evidence indicating no significant effects of PE on lipid levels or fasting blood glucose [35,36], despite a considerable number of our participants showing elevated levels of these parameters. This supports the notion that PE may not directly benefit fasting blood glucose and lipid levels. While PE has demonstrated anti-inflammatory and blood pressure-lowering effects, its impact on lipid and glucose metabolism appears limited. Understanding the mechanisms of action of the bioactive components involved may help enhance the potential of PE in future interventions.

We reported that both normal weight and overweight individuals exhibited elevated inflammatory markers typically associated with ageing. The lack of correlation between body weight and inflammatory markers suggests that other factors, such as lifestyle factors, may influence this association [37]. However, the lower representation of overweight participants compared to normal-weight individuals, as well as the small sample size in the stratified analysis, could partly explain this observation. Additionally, as we excluded individuals with obesity due to the focus on prevention, this may have influenced our findings, as elevated inflammatory markers may be more commonly associated with obesity than with being overweight. Future studies can explore this association.

This trial has several strengths. This is the first trial to investigate the preventive effects of PE on age-related diseases in the specific age group of 55–70 years. It has a robust sample size and involves a comprehensive analysis of inflammatory markers and several cardiometabolic risk factors. However, we note several limitations including the overrepresentation of females and normal-weight participants, which reflects the profile of individuals typically interested in participating in such research. This may have restricted the ability to evaluate the influence of gender and BMI on the outcomes. Additionally, the reliance on self-reported data regarding diet and physical activity presents another potential limitation. The large variability in parameter levels between the participants may have affected the outcomes. Lastly, while the trial was 3 months long, it still does not reflect the long-term effects of PE on inflammatory markers and cardiometabolic risk factors.

5. Conclusions

This trial demonstrates that PE may be beneficial in reducing inflammatory markers and blood pressure among older adults, where these factors are often elevated. The consumption of pomegranate extract may offer a valuable, non-pharmacological strategy to promote healthy ageing. However, confirmation in larger, long-term trials with more diverse populations is needed. Future research should additionally investigate its practical application in clinical settings while assessing its long-term benefits.

Author Contributions: G.F. and E.A.S.A.-D. designed the trial; J.M. conducted the research, including data collection and entry, with valuable assistance from J.V.; G.F. performed laboratory analysis, statistical analysis, and wrote the paper. G.F. had the primary responsibility of assessing the final content. G.F. and E.A.S.A.-D. had overall trial oversight, with J.M. contributing to the oversight under their guidance. All authors have read and agreed to the published version of the manuscript.

Funding: The trial was funded by Euromed S.A., which had no role in trial design, data collection, interpretation of data, or writing of the report.

Institutional Review Board Statement: The study was conducted in accordance with the Declaration of Helsinki and approved by the Institutional Review Board at Manchester Metropolitan University Faculty of Health and Education (reference number: 47627, 28 November 2022).

Informed Consent Statement: Informed consent was obtained from all participants involved in the study.

Data Availability Statement: Data described in the manuscript will not be made available due to being required for ongoing research and analysis.

Acknowledgments: We would like to thank all participants who took part in the study and extend our gratitude to all staff who provided technical support for the study.

Conflicts of Interest: The authors declare that this study received funding from Euromed S.A. The funder was not involved in the study design, collection, analysis, interpretation of data, the writing of this article or the decision to submit it for publication.

Abbreviations

The following abbreviations are used in this manuscript:

PE	Pomegranate extract
IL-6	Interleukin-6
IL-1α	Interleukin-1 alpha
IL-1β	Interleukin-1 beta
IL-2	Interleukin-2
TNF-α	Tumour Necrosis Factor-alpha
CRP	C-Reactive Protein
PAI-1	Plasminogen Activator Inhibitor-1

SBP	Systolic Blood pressure
DBP	Diastolic blood pressure
TC	Total Cholesterol
TG	Triglycerides
LDL	Low-Density Lipoprotein
HDL	High-Density Lipoprotein
SBP	Systolic Blood pressure
DBP	Diastolic blood pressure

References

1. Minciullo, P.L.; Catalano, A.; Mandraffino, G.; Casciaro, M.; Crucitti, A.; Maltese, G.; Basile, G. Inflammaging and anti-inflammaging: The role of cytokines in extreme longevity. *Arch. Immunol. Ther. Exp.* **2016**, *64*, 111–126. [CrossRef] [PubMed]
2. Franceschi, C.; Campisi, J. Chronic inflammation (inflammaging) and its potential contribution to age-associated diseases. *J. Gerontol. A Biol. Sci. Med. Sci.* **2014**, *69* (Suppl. S1), S4–S9. [CrossRef] [PubMed]
3. Franceschi, C.; Capri, M.; Monti, D.; Giunta, S.; Olivieri, F.; Sevini, F.; Salvioli, S. Inflammaging and anti-inflammaging: A systemic perspective on aging and longevity emerged from studies in humans. *Mech. Ageing Dev.* **2007**, *128*, 92–105. [CrossRef]
4. Ageing and Health. Available online: https://www.who.int/news-room/fact-sheets/detail/ageing-and-health (accessed on 17 October 2024).
5. Li, L.; Scott, C.A.; Rothwell, P.M. Association of younger vs older ages with changes in incidence of stroke and other vascular events, 2002–2018. *JAMA* **2022**, *328*, 563–574. [CrossRef] [PubMed]
6. Nadia, H.Z.; Mahdavi, M.M.; Hashemi, N.S.S.; Haji, G.E.; Nozari, B.; Mahdavi, A. Pattern of coronary artery disease risk factors in population younger than 55 years and above 55 years: A population fchi of 31,999 healthy individuals. *Acta Medica Iran.* **2011**, *49*, 368–374.
7. Thomas, A.L.; Alarcon, P.C.; Divanovic, S.; Chougnet, C.A.; Hildeman, D.A.; Moreno-Fernandez, M.E. Implications of inflammatory states on dysfunctional immune responses in aging and obesity. *Front. Aging* **2021**, *2*, 732414. [CrossRef]
8. Frasca, D.; Blomberg, B.B.; Paganelli, R. Aging, obesity, and inflammatory age-related diseases. *Front. Immunol.* **2017**, *8*, 1745. [CrossRef]
9. Vargas, R.; Ryder, E.; Diez-Ewald, M.; Mosquera, J.; Durán, A.; Valero, N.; Fernández, E. Increased C-reactive protein and decreased Interleukin-2 content in serum from obese individuals with or without insulin resistance: Associations with leukocyte count and insulin and adiponectin content. *Diabetes Metab. Syndr. Clin. Res. Rev.* **2016**, *10*, S34–S41. [CrossRef]
10. Gil, M.I.; Tomás-Barberán, F.A.; Hess-Pierce, B.; Holcroft, D.M.; Kader, A.A. Antioxidant activity of pomegranate juice and its relationship with phenolic composition and processing. *J. Agric. Food Chem.* **2000**, *48*, 4581–4589. [CrossRef]
11. Muñoz, J.A. Harvest, manipulation and commercialisation systems of pomegranate (*Punica granatum* L.). *Options Méditerr. Sér. A Sémin. Méditerr.* **2000**, *42*, 37–39.
12. Tatari, M.; Jadidi, E.; Shahmansouri, E. Study of some physiological responses of different pomegranate (*Punica granatum* L.) cultivars under drought stress to screen for drought tolerance. *Int. J. Fruit Sci.* **2020**, *20* (Suppl. S2), 1798–1813. [CrossRef]
13. Tinebra, I.; Scuderi, D.; Sortino, G.; Mazzaglia, A.; Farina, V. Pomegranate cultivation in Mediterranean climate: Plant adaptation and fruit quality of 'Mollar de Elche' and 'Wonderful' cultivars. *Agronomy* **2021**, *11*, 156. [CrossRef]
14. Vázquez-Rowe, I.; Kahhat, R.; Santillán-Saldívar, J.; Quispe, I.; Bentín, M. Carbon footprint of pomegranate (*Punica granatum*) cultivation in a hyper-arid region in coastal Peru. *Int. J. Life Cycle Assess.* **2017**, *22*, 601–617. [CrossRef]
15. Chawla, R.; Sheokand, A.; Rai, M.R.; Sadawart, R. Impact of climate change on fruit production and various approaches to mitigate these impacts. *Pharma Innov. J.* **2021**, *10*, 564–571.
16. Stockton, A.; Al-Dujaili, E.A.S.; McDougall, G.J.; Davidson, I.; Drummond, S.; Wyness, L. Effect of pomegranate extract consumption on cardiovascular disease risk factors, stress hormones, and quality of life in human volunteers: An exploratory randomized, double-blind, placebo-controlled trial. *EC Nutr.* **2015**, *2*, 396–411.
17. Stockton, A.; Farhat, G.; McDougall, G.J.; Al-Dujaili, E.A.S. Effect of pomegranate extract on blood pressure and anthropometry in adults: A double-blind, placebo-controlled, randomized clinical trial. *J. Nutr. Sci.* **2017**, *6*, e39. [CrossRef]
18. Al-Dujaili, E.A.S.; Casey, C.; Stockton, A. Antioxidant properties and beneficial cardiovascular effects of a natural extract of pomegranate in healthy volunteers: A randomized preliminary single-blind controlled study. *Antioxidants* **2022**, *11*, 2124. [CrossRef] [PubMed]
19. Wang, P.; Zhang, Q.; Hou, H.; Liu, Z.; Wang, L.; Rasekhmagham, R.; Yao, G. The effects of pomegranate supplementation on biomarkers of inflammation and endothelial dysfunction: A meta-analysis and systematic review. *Complement. Ther. Med.* **2020**, *49*, 102358. [CrossRef]

20. Farhat, G.; Malla, J.; Vadher, J.; Al-Dujaili, E.A.S. Impact of Pomegranate Extract Supplementation on Physical and Cognitive Function in Community-Dwelling Older Adults Aged 55–70 Years: A Randomised Double-Blind Clinical Trial. *Geriatrics* 2025, *in press*.
21. WHO. Available online: https://www.who.int/publications/i/item/9789240002654 (accessed on 27 October 2024).
22. Ainsworth, B.E.; Haskell, W.L.; Herrmann, S.D.; Meckes, N.; Bassett, D.R., Jr.; Tudor-Locke, C.; Greer, J.L.; Vezina, J.; Whitt-Glover, M.C.; Leon, A.S. 2011 Compendium of Physical Activities: A second update of codes and MET values. *Med. Sci. Sports Exerc.* **2011**, *43*, 1575–1581. [CrossRef]
23. Barati Boldaji, R.; Akhlaghi, M.; Sagheb, M.M.; Esmaeilinezhad, Z. Pomegranate juice improves cardiometabolic risk factors, biomarkers of oxidative stress and inflammation in hemodialysis patients: A randomized crossover trial. *J. Sci. Food Agric.* **2020**, *100*, 846–854. [CrossRef] [PubMed]
24. Vitkauskaite, A.; Urboniene, D.; Celiesiute, J.; Jariene, K.; Paskauskas, S.; Vaitkiene, D.; Vitkauskiene, A. Expression of inflammation depending on the stage of cervical cancer. *Medicina* **2024**, *60*, 349. [CrossRef] [PubMed]
25. Wu, H.; Wen, Y.; Yue, C.; Li, X.; Gao, R. Serum TNF-α level is associated with disease severity in adult patients with immunoglobulin A vasculitis nephritis. *Dis. Markers* **2020**, *2020*, 5514145. [CrossRef] [PubMed]
26. Nehring, S.M.; Goyal, A.; Patel, B.C. C reactive protein. In *StatPearls*; StatPearls Publishing: Treasure Island, FL, USA, 2023. [PubMed]
27. Heart UK. Available online: https://www.heartuk.org.uk/cholesterol/understanding-your-cholesterol-test-results- (accessed on 27 October 2024).
28. Diabetes.co.uk. Available online: https://www.diabetes.co.uk/diabetes_care/fasting-blood-sugar-levels.html (accessed on 3 November 2024).
29. Wei, J.; Xu, H.; Davies, J.L.; Hemmings, G.P. Increase of plasma IL-6 concentration with age in healthy subjects. *Life Sci.* **1992**, *51*, 1953–1956. [CrossRef]
30. Fagiolo, U.; Cossarizza, A.; Scala, E.; Fanales-Belasio, E.; Ortolani, C.; Cozzi, E.; Paganelli, R. Increased cytokine production in mononuclear cells of healthy elderly people. *Eur. J. Immunol.* **1993**, *23*, 2375–2378. [CrossRef] [PubMed]
31. Bahari, H.; Omidian, K.; Goudarzi, K.; Rafiei, H.; Asbaghi, O.; Hosseini Kolbadi, K.S.; Hosseini, A. The effects of pomegranate consumption on blood pressure in adults: A systematic review and meta-analysis. *Phytother. Res.* **2024**, *38*, 2234–2248. [CrossRef] [PubMed]
32. Rahimi, K.; Bidel, Z.; Nazarzadeh, M.; Copland, E.; Canoy, D.; Ramakrishnan, R.; Davis, B.R. Pharmacological blood pressure lowering for primary and secondary prevention of cardiovascular disease across different levels of blood pressure: An individual participant-level data meta-analysis. *Lancet* **2021**, *397*, 1625–1636. [CrossRef]
33. Delgado, N.T.; Rouver, W.N.; Dos Santos, R.L. Protective effects of pomegranate in endothelial dysfunction. *Curr. Pharm. Des.* **2020**, *26*, 3684–3699. [CrossRef]
34. Ignarro, L.J.; Byrns, R.E.; Sumi, D.; de Nigris, F.; Napoli, C. Pomegranate juice protects nitric oxide against oxidative destruction and enhances the biological actions of nitric oxide. *Nitric Oxide* **2006**, *15*, 93–102. [CrossRef]
35. Aziz, Z.; Huin, W.K.; Hisham, M.D.B.; Ng, J.X. Effects of pomegranate on lipid profiles: A systematic review of randomized controlled trials. *Complement. Ther. Med.* **2020**, *48*, 102236. [CrossRef]
36. Huang, H.; Liao, D.; Chen, G.; Chen, H.; Zhu, Y. Lack of efficacy of pomegranate supplementation for glucose management, insulin levels, and sensitivity: Evidence from a systematic review and meta-analysis. *Nutr. J.* **2017**, *16*, 67. [CrossRef] [PubMed]
37. Kjerulff, B.; Dowsett, J.; Jacobsen, R.L.; Gladov, J.; Larsen, M.H.; Lundgaard, A.T.; Erikstrup, C. Lifestyle and demographic associations with 47 inflammatory and vascular stress biomarkers in 9876 blood donors. *Commun. Med.* **2024**, *4*, 50. [CrossRef] [PubMed]

nutrients

MDPI

Article

Assessing Lifestyle in a Large Cohort of Undergraduate Students: Significance of Stress, Exercise and Nutrition

Daniela Lucini [1,2,*], Ester Luconi [3], Luca Giovanelli [1], Giuseppe Marano [4,5], Giuseppina Bernardelli [2,6], Riccardo Guidetti [7], Eugenio Morello [8], Stefano Cribellati [9], Marina Marzia Brambilla [10] and Elia Mario Biganzoli [4,5]

1 BIOMETRA Department, University of Milan, 20129 Milan, Italy; luca.giovanelli@unimi.it
2 Exercise Medicine Unit, Istituto Auxologico Italiano IRCCS, 20135 Milan, Italy; g.bernardelli@unimi.it
3 Department of Biomedical Sciences for Health, University of Milan, 20157 Milan, Italy; ester.luconi@unimi.it
4 Medical Statistics Unit, Department of Biomedical and Clinical Sciences L. Sacco, "Luigi Sacco" University Hospital, University of Milan, 20157 Milan, Italy; giuseppe.marano@unimi.it (G.M.); elia.biganzoli@unimi.it (E.M.B.)
5 Data Science Research Center, University of Milan, 20157 Milan, Italy
6 DISCCO Department, University of Milan, 20122 Milan, Italy
7 Dipartimento di Scienze Agrarie e Ambientali—Produzione, Territorio, Agroenergia—University of Milan, 20133 Milan, Italy; riccardo.guidetti@unimi.it
8 Laboratorio di Simulazione Urbana Fausto Curti, Dipartimento di Architettura e Studi Urbani, Polytechnic of Milan, 20133 Milan, Italy; eugenio.morello@polimi.it
9 SEGE Srl, 20146 Milan, Italy; stefano.cribellati@se-ge.com
10 Department of Language Mediation Sciences and Intercultural Studies, University of Milan, 20122 Milan, Italy; marina.brambilla@unimi.it
* Correspondence: daniela.lucini@unimi.it

Abstract: Background/Objectives: Lifestyle (in particular, nutrition and exercise) determines present and future youths' health. The goal of the present study was to identify specific student groups who deserve precise lifestyle improvement interventions, tailored to their characteristics. Methods: An anonymous web-based questionnaire to assess lifestyle was posted on the websites of two main Italian Academic Institutions, and 9423 students voluntarily participated. A personalised immediate report was provided to improve compliance/motivation. We assessed age, sex, affiliation, anthropometrics, lifestyle components (nutrition, exercise, sedentariness, stress perception, smoking, alcohol, sleep), and the desire to be helped with lifestyle improvement. Cluster analysis was performed to identify healthy lifestyle groups among the students. Results: In total, 6976 subjects [age: 21 (20, 23) yrs; 3665 female, 3300 male] completed the questionnaire and were included. Of these students, 73.9% expressed the need for lifestyle improvement help, particularly for becoming physically active (66.7%), managing stress (58.7%), and improving nutrition (52.7%). We unveil three clusters of subjects, each corresponding to a distinct lifestyle pattern. The clusters are differentiated by exercise level and perceptions of stress/fatigue/somatic symptoms (cluster 1: 74.8% meet international exercise guidelines (IEGs), 67.4% have high stress perception, 49.1% drink 1–3 glasses of wine/beer per week, and 63.3% drink 0–1 glass of spirits per week; cluster 2: 75.6% meet IEGs, 75.7% have low/medium levels of stress perception, and 65.8% have low alcohol consumption; cluster 3: 72.5% do not meet IEGs, 77.6% have high stress perception, and 67.5% have low alcohol consumption). More active students present lower stress/somatic symptoms perception. Interestingly, the AHA diet score (nutrition quality) was not in the ideal range in any cluster (nevertheless, obesity was not of concern), being worst in cluster 3, characterized by higher stress perception (59.7% had poor nutrition quality). Those who were physically active but showed a high stress/fatigue perception were used to drinking alcohol. Conclusions: Students desire help to improve their lifestyle, and this approach might help identify specific student groups to whom LIs in Academic Institutions can be tailored to foster well-being and promote health.

Keywords: well-being; physical activity; tailored intervention; stress management; public health; lifestyle assessment; physical activity; nutrition quality

1. Introduction

Undergraduate students (approximately 18–26 years) are typically in the phase of young adulthood, a pivotal time of life. They are different from older adults and adolescents in ways that affect their decision-making, behaviour, and health choices [1]. During these years, they complete their education and pursue endeavours which will shape their adult personal and working life. They also shape their attitude towards behaviours which may dramatically impact their well-being and health in the present and future, and the scientific literature [2] depicts this age as one of the best periods in the lifespan for health promotion and the primary prevention of chronic non-communicable diseases. Nevertheless, motivating young people to adopt a healthy lifestyle (defined as individual behaviours having a significant impact on health and well-being, such as nutrition, physical activity, stress management, sleep hygiene, and consuming risky substances, for example smoke and alcohol) is demanding since they frequently exhibit health behaviours below public health recommendations [3,4]. A recent study on a large Spanish student population [5] conducted during the COVID-19 pandemic revealed that a lack of time and laziness were indicated as the main reasons for giving up or not taking up physical activity. Other recent studies addressing nutrition in students have shown that a "healthy diet" pattern is present only in subjects who exercise on a regular basis [6], that there is evidence of a correlation between poor diet quality in students with elevated BMI and smoking, stress level, alcohol consumption, and poorer sleep quality [7], and that there is an association between healthy diet and physical activity [8].

Generally, young people consider themselves healthy individuals and are more prone to focusing "on the present" instead of "on the future", at least regarding health issues. To promote healthy behaviours among young populations, it might be particularly interesting to draw their attention to the "immediate" benefits of a healthy lifestyle; among these benefits, the perception of well-being and improved quality of life may play a pivotal role [9]. It might be particularly appropriate to change young adults' "point of view" [10–12] via preventive strategies, focusing more on well-being and the promotion of healthy behaviours (in particular, a physically active life, healthy nutrition, non-smoking, stress management, and sleep hygiene) than solely on reducing traditional cardio-metabolic risk factors (such as high cholesterol level, high blood pressure, overweight/obesity, etc), which often are within the normal range. Recently, we have shown [9] that young employees present a worse lifestyle than older ones, even without alterations in anthropometric, metabolic, lipid, and haemodynamic parameters. Unveiling unhealthy behaviours (for instance, poor quality of nutrition, smoking, or sedentariness) before the appearance of abnormal clinical parameters (such as those related to metabolic syndrome and low-grade chronic inflammation, such as hyperglycaemia, obesity, and high cholesterol level) may help young people to reconsider their habits and modify them as soon as possible.

It is important to underline that the worsening of psychological well-being linked to anxiety and stress is particularly interesting in youth. Stress and depression represent an emerging health issue [13,14], especially in young populations. They live in a rapidly changing and demanding world, where individual and global sources of stress contribute to the feeling that continually increasing performance is a necessity, which may not be counterbalanced by enough individual and community coping resources. The link between stress and lifestyle is complex, and many pieces of evidence suggest that stress may worsen lifestyle [11,14,15], with those affected favouring poor nutrition, sedentariness, smoking, alcohol, drug abuse, etc., as coping strategies, with a negative consequence on cardiometabolic–oncological health. On the other hand, lifestyle improvement has been shown to be a pivotal strategy to prevent chronic diseases, improve well-being, and manage stress [11,14–17]. Becoming/remaining physically active plays a central role in this context [11,16]. Many Academic Institutions [18,19] offer their students services to promote and improve well-being, including psychological support and lifestyle improvements, and some scientific papers have been devoted to the study of students' lifestyles. For instance, one study [20] showed, in a large cohort of Brazilian students, that the odds of depression and anxiety symptoms were higher in students characterized by sedentary behaviour; another study [21] revealed in German students that lower sedentary time and higher physical activity were associated with reduced levels of perceived stress. Another one [22], using cluster analysis, showed that students that smoked were more likely to report higher stress.

Considering the great importance of fostering health and well-being in young people, our hypothesis was that tailored approaches would be more effective in improving lifestyles than "generic" intervention. The present study aimed to define groups of students characterized by specific lifestyles to better tailor preventive strategies and educational procedures to favour well-being and health during academic years. To this end, we used data collected by means of a web-based anonymous questionnaire [11,23,24], filled in by a large cohort of undergraduate students from the two largest universities in the northern area of Italy (Lombardy), to investigate lifestyle components, with particular regard to nutrition habits, physical activity, perception of stress, fatigue, somatic-stress-related symptoms, the consumption of alcoholic beverages, smoking habits, and sleep.

2. Materials and Methods

2.1. Participants

This study is part of a project of the University of Milano and the Polytechnic of Milano; the goal is to put in place some best practices to improve quality of life, well-being, and sustainable lifestyle in the city area where the two big Academic Institutions are located. The promotion of healthy lifestyle behaviours has a role of paramount importance and may be considered a real sustainable tool. To take action today (to improve individual behaviour) is to preserve a great good (health) that, otherwise, might disappear [25,26]. This specific topic was ideated through a multidisciplinary collaboration between the Head and members of the residency program of Sports Medicine and Physical Exercise, several professors and experts in various areas of personal health and well-being from the University of Milan, and the Governance and University Administration. A web-based questionnaire, completely anonymous, was posted on the website of the two Academic Institutions in 2019. All the students of the Polytechnic, students of select courses at the University of Milan (Medicine and Surgery, Medical Biotechnologies, Medical Biotechnology and Molecular Medicine, Nursing, Audiometric Techniques, Viticulture and Enology, Foodservice Science and Technology, Exercise Sport and Health Sciences, Philosophy, Philosophic Sciences, International Studies and European Institutions, and Political Sciences), and all students enrolled in their first year of any course were invited to fill it out. An email explaining the purposes and goals of the questionnaire and the possibility of disseminating the results derived from the anonymous analysis was sent to the students. A personalized immediate report was provided to improve compliance/motivation. We have already described [23] the methodology employed to create the questionnaire. During the pandemic period, we offered students online healthy lifestyle promotion programs [26].

2.2. Instruments and Procedure

We collected anthropometric data (weight, height, waist circumference), age, sex, and university affiliation.

Lifestyle Assessment:

Physical activity (total activity volume) was assessed by a modified version of the commonly employed short version of the International Physical Activity Questionnaire (IPAQ) [27], which focuses on the intensity (nominally estimated in Metabolic Equivalents—METs—according to the type of activity) and duration (in minutes) of physical activity. We considered the following levels: activities of moderate intensity (≈4.0 METs/minute) and activities of vigorous intensity (≈8.0 METs/minute). These levels were used to calculate the weekly exercise volume of structured exercise (METsMV; MV—moderate and vigorous) using the following equations:

$$\text{METsMV} = 4 \times \text{M} \times \text{dM} + 8 \times \text{V} \times \text{dV}, \qquad (1)$$

where METsMV stands for weekly moderate and vigorous physical activity volume expressed in METs minutes/week; M is the number of minutes/day of moderate-intensity activity; dM is the number of days/week of moderate-intensity activity; V is the number of minutes/day of vigorous-intensity activity; and dV is the number of days/week of vigorous-intensity activities. The quantity in (1) may then be considered the total weekly volume of structured exercise.

We also assessed the frequency of regular strength and flexibility exercises, considering the following scale: never; sometimes; 1 session/week; 2–3 sessions/week; more than 3 sessions/week.

Sedentary behaviour was assessed by asking the number of hours spent in sedentary behaviour (for instance, studying, sitting, driving, TV viewing, computer or smart device usage) during weekly working days and weekend days.

Nutrition was assessed using the American Heart Association (AHA) Diet Score [28], taking into consideration fruit/vegetable, fish, sweetened beverage, whole grain, and sodium consumption (the assessment of the latter was adapted to Italian eating habits and considered as a score of "nutrition quality") [23].

Perceptions of stress, fatigue, and subjective somatic-stress-related symptoms (short 4SQ) were assessed using a self-administered questionnaire [23] with nominal self-rated Likert scales from 0 ("no perception") to 10 ("highest perception") for each measure. We considered a short version of the 4SQ, taking into account 3 somatic symptoms (perception of heart beating, perception of muscle tension, perception of knot in stomach); thus, the total score ranged from 0 to 30.

Smoking behaviour: We considered all subjects who reported to have never smoked or to have stopped smoking for more than one year as non-smokers.

We enquired about the usage of alcohol, considering Italian habits, asking the number of glasses of wine or beer consumed per week and the number of glasses of spirits consumed per week.

Perceptions of quality of sleep, quality of health, and quality of life were assessed with nominal self-rated Likert scales from 0 ("bad") to 10 ("very good") for each measure.

Desire to be helped with lifestyle change was inquired considering two options: yes or no.

2.3. Data Analysis

A quality check of the collected data was performed to remove non-realistic answers from the dataset and to identify conditions with a high percentage of non-response. All participants voluntarily provided anonymous data. The study protocol was approved by the Institutional Ethics Committee of the University of Milan (Allegato 4 Comitato Etico 25.05.18; Repertorio pareri Comitato Etico: parere numero 21/18) and by the Institutional Ethics Committee of the Polytechnic of Milan (Parere 11/2018 dated 26 July 2018).

Statistics: The data consisted of records of 9423 students who filled out the questionnaire; 2447 students who had more than five missing values were excluded. Categorical variables were summarized by counts and percentages, and numerical variables were summarized using the median and the first and third quartiles due to the asymmetry of the distributions. Comparisons between genders were carried out using quantile regression methods for numerical variables and logistic regression for categorical variables with binary or multiple response options. p-values were corrected for the multiplicity of comparisons using the Bonferroni rule. The primary aim was to identify healthy lifestyle groups among the students; to this aim, cluster analysis was performed. The following variables were used: waist circumference, AHA diet score, METs for moderate and vigorous activities, BMI, sedentary time during week days, sedentary time during weekends, hours of sleep, smoking habits, perceptions of stress, fatigue, and subjective somatic-stress-related symptoms (s4SQ), consumption of wine and beer, and consumption of spirits. All the numerical variables for the above were converted into categorical variables using the following classifications for the cluster analysis:

1. Waist circumference (WC) was coded as green (<80 cm and <94 cm, respectively, for female and male students), yellow (80–87.9 cm and 94–100.9 cm for female and male students, respectively), or red (>87.9 cm and >101.9 cm, respectively) [29]. Students who declared WC < 60 cm or >130 (female) and WC < 70.5 cm or >130 (male) were excluded from the analysis.
2. BMI (body mass index) was coded as underweight/normal weight (<25 Kg/m^2), overweight (25–29.9 Kg/m^2), or obese (30 Kg/m^2) [28].
3. METs for moderate and vigorous activity were codified as "insufficient levels of exercise" if <600 (MET·min/week), or otherwise as "adequate" [27].
4. Weekly hours spent in sedentary activity (during working days and weekends) were coded as "active habits" (<9 h/week) or "sedentary habits" (otherwise) [30].
5. Hours of sleep were considered "adequate" if ≥7 per day or "insufficient" otherwise [31].
6. Consumption of wine and beer was coded as 0 glasses/week, 0.1–1 glasses/week, 1.1–2.9 glasses/week, or >2.9 glasses/week.
7. Consumption of spirits: 0 glasses/week, 0.1–1 glasses/week, or >1 glasses/week.
8. Perception of subjective stress-related somatic symptoms (s4SQ) was coded into five classes in the following quintiles: 0–3, 4–6, 7–10, 11–15, and 16–30.
9. Perceptions of stress and fatigue were coded, separately, into the following five classes: 0–2, 3–4, 5–6, 7–8, and 9–10.
10. Smoking habits were coded as "smoker, ex-smoker, electronic cigarettes, or non-smoker".

Eleven subjects who declared "other gender" were excluded due to the impossibility of obtaining the classes for waist circumference, which considered only values for male and female categories. Cluster analysis was performed on 5861 subjects with complete records of the variables above. In a preliminary step, the association among the variables above was evaluated by multiple correspondence analysis [32]. The clustering algorithm used was K-modes [33] because it is suited for categorical variables. In addition, it is optimal for survey research applications because it can handle large datasets with a high number of categories of variables. The algorithm was run many times (6000 runs for k = 3 to 10 clusters), and the optimal number of clusters was chosen according to the maximum of the average silhouette width index [34]. Clusters were described using graphical representation (heatmap) and textual description. To investigate the degree of separateness of the clusters, we applied Principal Coordinates Analysis (PCoA) methods, as described by Bakker [35]. The analysis was performed using R software version 4.0.4 [36] with the packages FactoMineR [37], KlaR [38], and vegan [39] added.

3. Results

The questionnaire was filled out by 9423 subjects. Of these, 7036 were Polytechnic students (74.6%), 2205 were students of the University of Milan (23.4%), and 182 (2.0%) did not specify affiliation. Based on the pre-defined criteria (see statistical analysis), 6976 (74.03%) subjects were included in the analysis. The features of these students are summarized in Table 1.

Table 1 shows that the majority of students are normoweight, though the percentages of male students in the overweight and obesity classes are slightly greater than those of female students. Male students are slightly more active than female students who, instead, present a higher perception of stress, fatigue, and somatic symptoms. The majority of students are non-smokers and are occasional alcohol consumers, with the percentage of subjects who do not drink any alcohol being slightly greater in female students.

Table 1. Anthropometric and lifestyle data collected from all subjects (total) and divided by gender.

	Total (n = 6976)	Female (n = 3665)	Male (n = 3300)	p-Value
Affiliation:				
University of Milan	1782 (25.5%)	1221 (33.3%)	556 (16.8%)	
Polytechnic of Milan	5128 (73.5%)	2396 (65.4%)	2727 (82.5%)	
Other (not specified)	66 (0.9%)	48 (1.3%)	17 (0.5%)	
Age [y]	21 (20, 23)	21 (20, 23)	21 (20, 23)	ns
Weight [Kg]	63 (55, 72)	57 (52, 62)	71 (65, 78)	$p < 0.0001$
Height [cm]	172 (165, 179)	166 (161, 170)	179 (174, 183)	$p < 0.0001$
BMI [Kg/m^2]	21.3 (19.6, 23.2)	20.5 (19.1, 22.3)	22.2 (20.6, 24.1)	$p < 0.0001$
Underweight/normal weight (<25 Kg/m^2)	6125 (87.8%)	3353 (91.5%)	2762 (83.7%)	
Overweight (25–29.9 Kg/m^2)	713 (10.2%)	258 (7.0%)	454 (13.8%)	
Obese (≥30 Kg/m^2)	138 (2.0%)	54 (1.5%)	84 (2.5%)	
Waist circumference [cm] *	79 (70, 87)	71 (66, 80)	84 (80, 93)	$p < 0.0001$
Green	4342 (74.1%)	2378 (72.6%)	1964 (75.8%)	
Yellow	856 (14.6%)	467 (14.3%)	389 (15.0%)	
Red	664 (11.3%)	427 (13.1%)	237 (9.2%)	
METsMV [MET·min/week]	800 (200, 1800)	640 (120, 1440)	1200 (320, 2200)	$p < 0.0001$
Insufficient (<600 METs)	2845 (40.8%)	1736 (47.4%)	1104 (33.5%)	
Adequate (≥600 METs)	4131 (59.2%)	1929 (52.6%)	2196 (66.5%)	
Frequency of strength exercise:				$p < 0.0001$
Never	3719 (53.3%)	2137 (58.3%)	1577 (47.8%)	
Sometimes	889 (12.7%)	454 (12.4%)	434 (13.2%)	
1 session/week	580 (8.3%)	328 (8.9%)	249 (7.5%)	
2–3 sessions/week	1346 (19.3%)	619 (16.9%)	725 (22.0%)	
More than 3 sessions/week	442 (6.3%)	127 (3.5%)	315 (9.5%)	
Frequency of flexibility exercise:				$p < 0.0001$
Never	3271 (46.9%)	1574 (42.9%)	1695 (51.4%)	
Sometimes	1546 (22.2%)	900 (24.6%)	643 (19.5%)	
1 session/week	806 (11.6%)	495 (13.5%)	309 (9.4%)	
2–3 sessions/week	1003 (14.4%)	527 (14.4%)	474 (14.4%)	
More than 3 sessions/week	350 (5.0%)	169 (4.6%)	179 (5.4%)	
Sedentary Behaviour:				
Week days [hours/week]	45 (35, 55)	45 (35, 55)	45 (35, 55)	ns
Weekend days [hours/week]	12 (10, 18)	12 (10, 16)	14 (10, 18)	$p < 0.0001$
AHA Diet Score [a.u.]	2 (1, 3)	2 (1, 3)	2 (1, 2)	ns
Smoking habits:				ns
Non-smoker	5268 (75.5%)	2737 (74.7%)	2525 (76.5%)	
Ex-smoker	421 (6.0%)	227 (6.2%)	193 (5.8%)	
Electronic cigarette smoker	43 (0.6%)	21 (0.6%)	22 (0.7%)	
Smoker	1244 (17.8%)	680 (18.6%)	560 (17.0%)	
Coffee [cups/day]:				ns
0	2181 (31.3%)	1093 (29.8%)	1084 (32.8%)	
1–2	3495 (50.1%)	1881 (51.3%)	1611 (48.8%)	
3+	1300 (18.6%)	691 (18.8%)	605 (18.3%)	
Wine and beer [glass/week]:				$p < 0.0001$
0	2027 (29.1%)	1253 (34.2%)	772 (23.4%)	
>0–3	3675 (52.7%)	1943 (53%)	1727 (52.3%)	
4-	845 (12.1%)	336 (9.2%)	508 (15.4%)	
7+	428 (6.1%)	132 (3.6%)	293 (8.9%)	

Table 1. *Cont.*

	Total ($n = 6976$)	Female ($n = 3665$)	Male ($n = 3300$)	p-Value
Spirits [glass/week]:				
0	3842 (55.1%)	2133 (58.2%)	1704 (51.6%)	
>0–3	2992 (42.9%)	1489 (40.6%)	1500 (45.5%)	$p < 0.0001$
4–6	115 (1.6%)	32 (0.9%)	82 (2.5%)	
7+	27 (0.4%)	11 (0.3%)	14 (0.4%)	
Short 4SQ score [au]	8 (3, 13)	9 (5, 15)	6 (2, 11)	$p < 0.0001$
Stress perception [au]	6 (3, 8)	7 (4, 9)	5 (3, 8)	$p < 0.0001$
Fatigue perception [au]	7 (4, 9)	8 (5, 9)	6 (4, 8)	$p < 0.0001$
Sleep [hours/night]	7 (6, 8)	7 (6, 8)	7 (7, 8)	ns
Perception of sleep quality [au]	7 (6, 8)	7 (6, 8)	7 (6, 8)	ns
Perception of health quality [au]	7 (6, 8)	7 (5, 8)	7 (6, 8)	ns
Perception of quality of life [au]	7 (5, 8)	7 (5, 8)	7 (6, 8)	ns
Presence of chronic disease	630 (9.0%)	387 (10.6%)	241 (7.3%)	$p < 0.0001$
Desire to be helped with lifestyle change	5155 (73.9%)	2861 (78.1%)	2288 (69.3%)	$p < 0.0001$
Desire to improve nutrition	3677 (52.7%)	1864 (50.9%)	1807 (54.8%)	$p = 0.0297$
Desire to improve exercise	4652 (66.7%)	2617 (71.4%)	2030 (61.5%)	$p < 0.0001$
Desire to improve stress management	4098 (58.7%)	2380 (64.9%)	1715 (52.0%)	$p < 0.0001$

Data are presented as counts and proportions for categorical variables and medians and quartiles (Q1, Q3) for continuous ones. Eleven subjects declared to belong to the "other" gender; thus, they were accounted for only in the total group (column 2). * For waist circumference, results were calculated from data of 5862 students (3272 female, 2590 male) whose responses were considered reliable (see methods). Abbreviations: BMI = body mass index; AHA = American Heart Association; MET = Metabolic Equivalent; 4SQ = subjective somatic-stress-related symptoms questionnaire; au = arbitrary units; ns = not significant.

Notably, the majority of students were characterized by a normal BMI and normal waist circumference classes ("green"). Nevertheless, the median of the AHA diet score corresponded to "intermediate health" [28], suggesting a quality of nutrition deemed in need of improvement. Moreover, while most students reported meeting international physical activity guidelines [40] regarding endurance exercise, only a tiny percentage (more evident in male subjects) performed strength/flexibility exercises regularly (2/3 sessions/week), as per the guidelines. Notably, 78.1% of female and 69.3% of male students desired help with making a lifestyle change, particularly for improving exercise (66.7%), managing stress (58.7%), and improving nutrition (52.7%).

Investigation of Lifestyle Patterns

The association between the 13 variables used for assessing students' lifestyles (see Methods section for their definition) was evaluated via MCA (Figure S1). The first dimension (Dim. 1) and the second dimension (Dim. 2) together explained 78.3% of the variance. Dim.1 (*X*-axis) explained 61.4% of the total variability, and three variables showed high coordinates in this dimension (s4SQ, fatigue, and stress level), suggesting that these three variables are associated. Dim. 2 (*Y*-axis) explained 16.9%. Wine and beer, spirits, and (to a lesser extent) smoking showed a high coordinate on this axis, suggesting another association.

More details about the associations can be derived from Figure 1 (MCA map). There is an association between low fatigue scores, low stress scores, and low perceptions of somatic symptoms (s4SQ score), all represented on the right side of the plot. In contrast, higher levels of the same variables are all represented on the left side, indicating that they are associated with each other. Dim.1 (*X*-axis) separated subjects with a low perception of stress, fatigue, and somatic symptoms from subjects with a high level of these perceptions. At the same time, Dim.2 (*Y*-axis) separated subjects with a high consumption of wine/beer and spirits (and smokers) (observed in the top part) from subjects with low levels of the same variables (observed in the bottom part), suggesting that the consumption of alcohol and smoke are slightly associated with one another.

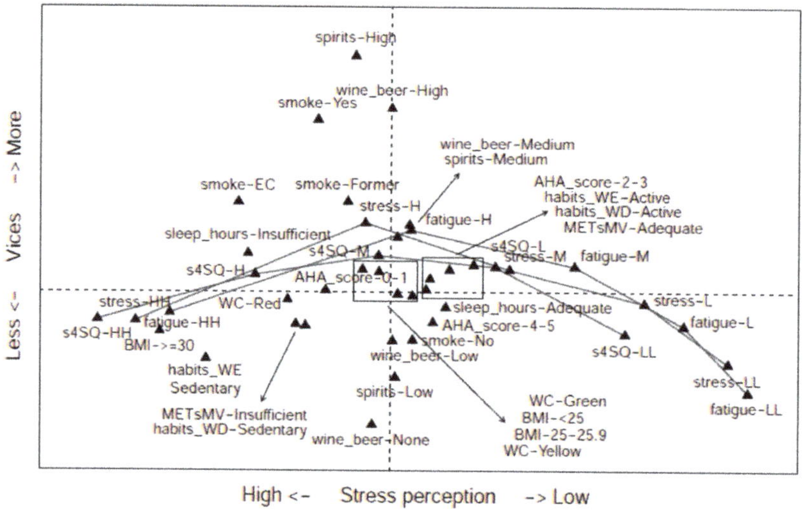

Figure 1. Multiple Correspondence Analysis map. The plot shows the modalities of the investigated variables (see the legend below) in the space spanned by the axes determined by MCA. The grey segments connect the modalities of the variables related to stress perception, namely s4SQ, stress, and fatigue. WC = waist circumference; AHA_Score = AHA nutrition score.; BMI = body mass index; METsMV = moderate and vigorous physical activity volume (adequate if $\geq$600 MET·min/week, otherwise insufficient); _WD = sedentary behaviour during working days (active if <9 h/week, otherwise sedentary); _WE = sedentary behaviour during weekends (active if <9 h/week, otherwise sedentary); sleep_hours = hours of sleep (adequate if $\geq$7 h/day, insufficient otherwise); stress: LL (low: 0–2), L (moderate/low: 3–4 points), M (moderate: 5–6 points), H (moderate/high = 7–8 points), HH (high: 9–10 points); fatigue: LL (low: 0–2), L (moderate/low: 3–4 points), M (moderate: 5–6 points), H (moderate/high = 7–8 points), HH (high: 9–10 points); s4SQ = short questionnaire on subjective somatic-stress-related symptoms: LL (low: 0–3 points), L (moderate/low: 4–6 points), M (moderate: 7–10 points), H (moderate/high: 11–15 points), HH (high: 16–30 points); smoke = smoking habits: SM (smoker), FSM (former smoker), EC (electronic cigarettes), and NS (non-smoker); Wine_beer = wine and beer consumption: none (0 glass/week), low, medium, high (0, 0.1–1, 1.1–2.9, and >2.9 glasses/week); spirits = spirit consumption: none (0 glasses/week), low (0.1–1 glasses/week), high (>1 glasses/week). The modalities of the variables of interest (e.g., smoker, non-smoker) are represented by points, and the presence of points close to one another reveals that the corresponding modalities are tendentially observed together. On the right side of the plot (*X*-axis), the following variables are found: fatigue = LL (very low), L (moderate/low), and M (moderate); stress = LL (very low), L (moderate/low), and M (moderate); and s4SQ = LL (very low) and L (moderate/low). Higher levels of the same variables are observed in the left part. Note that the different classes for perceptions of stress, fatigue, and somatic symptoms are in progressive order, as evidenced, respectively, by the lines. In the top part of the figure (*Y*-axis) and near each other, the following variables are found: smokers (also smokers of electronic cigarettes, represented by the label EC), former smokers, and the highest levels of wine and beer (represented by the label Wine_Beer-High) and spirit (Spirits-High) consumption. The lowest levels of the same variables are observed in the bottom part.

Subsequently, cluster analysis was performed. According to the average silhouette width, 5861 students were grouped into three clusters (Figure S2). Each cluster corresponds to a distinct lifestyle pattern. Figure 2 shows the characterization of clusters in terms of student's features, and the corresponding textual description is reported in Figure 3. It may be seen that the major degree of association among the variables of interest (which emerged from the MCA) is reflected in the clusters' composition. Subjects in clusters 1 and 3 present high stress and fatigue perception, along with medium–high perceptions of somatic stress-related symptoms; subjects in cluster 2 report low perceptions of somatic-stress-related symptoms and low perceptions of stress. Similarly, wine/beer and spirit consumption are connected in each of the three clusters. In the clusters, we do not find an association between smoking habits and alcohol consumption; however, this is likely due to the low degree of association.

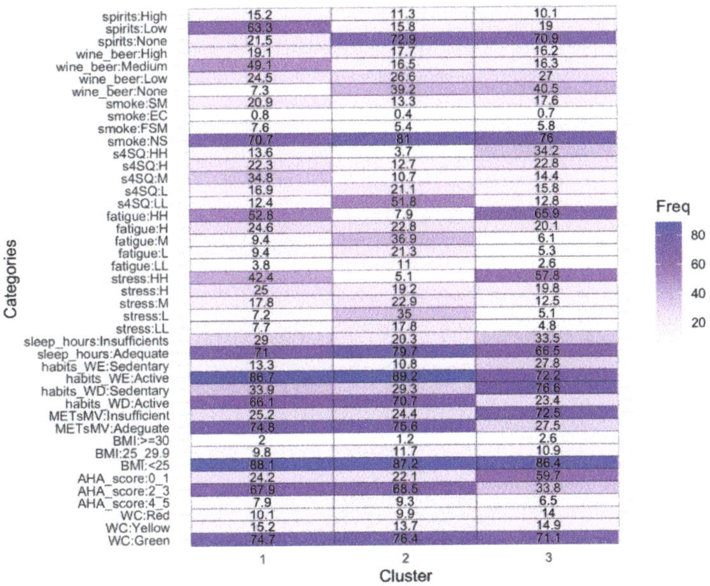

Figure 2. Heatmap showing distributions of the student's features for each cluster. The *X*-axis represents the three clusters. The *Y*-axis represents all the possible modalities of the 13 variables used for cluster analysis. The numbers in the cells express the percentages of students, showing the modalities of the variables for each cluster. See the legend of Figure 1 for abbreviations.

From Figure 2, it may be seen that all the variables contribute to defining distinct lifestyle patterns, except five variables, which are smoking habit (in fact, in all three clusters, the highest frequency is "non-smoker"), waist circumference ("green" category common to all the clusters), body mass index (<25 Kg/m^2 common to all the clusters), hours of sleep ("adequate" category common to all clusters), and sedentariness during weekends.

Figure 3 shows the three unveiled clusters of students. Students in cluster 1 are physically active, present a high perception of stress, and drink alcohol; 67.9 of them are characterized by an AHA diet score of 2–3, corresponding to "intermediate health" [28]. Cluster 2 is composed of students characterized by the best lifestyle pattern: being physically active, presenting a low stress perception, and not drinking alcohol. Nevertheless, 68.5% of them are characterized by an AHA diet score of 2–3, corresponding to "intermediate health" [28], suggesting a quality of nutrition deemed in need of improvement. Students in cluster 3 are sedentary, exercise less than recommended by international guidelines [40], and present a high perception of stress. Notably, 59.7% of them are characterized by an AHA diet score of 0–1, corresponding to "poor health" [28], suggesting a quality of nutrition deemed in need of great improvement.

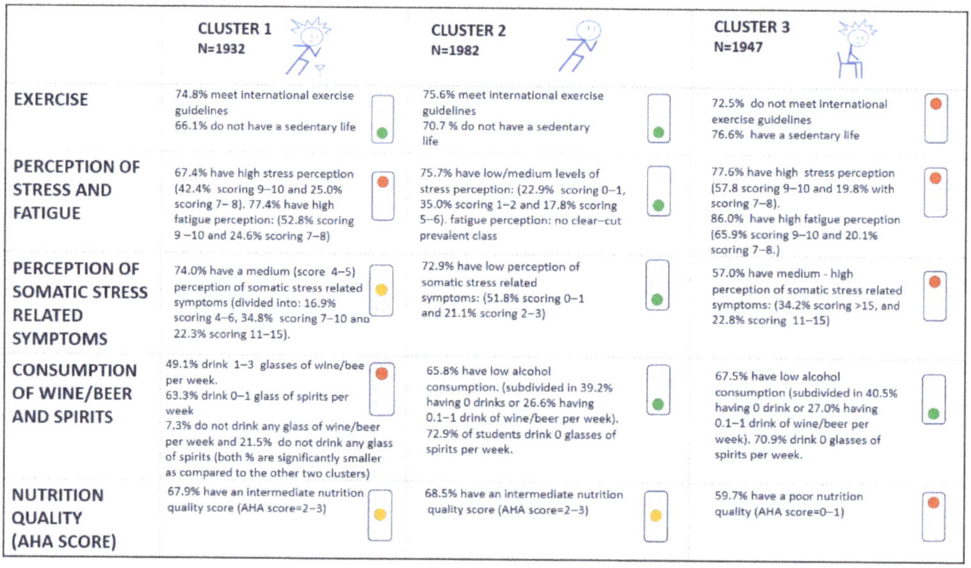

Figure 3. Characterization of students' lifestyles according to the three clusters. AHA = American Heart Association.

Remarkably, more active students present lower stress perception; moreover, students in cluster 1, who are physically active but show a high perception of stress/fatigue, are used to drinking alcohol.

PCoA was performed to investigate the degree of separateness of the three clusters. Figure 4 depicts that the clusters show some degree of separateness, even though some overlapping occurs in the central part of the figure.

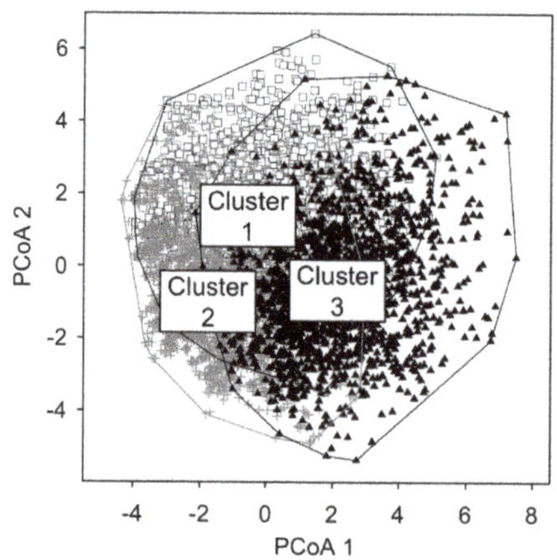

Figure 4. PCoA plot. The figure shows students represented in two-dimensional spaces that preserve the highest possible number of differences (goodness—of—fit index equal to 18.8%). Distinct labels represent students belonging to distinct clusters: empty squares for cluster 1, grey crosses for cluster 2, and black triangles for cluster 3.

Concerning the relationships between lifestyle and "external" features, we note the following: In cluster 1, 56% (C.I. 53–58%) are female and 44% are male. In cluster 2, 47% are female and 53% (C.I. 51–56%) are male. In cluster 3, 65% are female and 35% are male. Moreover, the median of the judgement on quality of health is higher in cluster 2 (eight points) as compared to clusters 1 and 3 (seven points for each one), but the difference among the three groups was not statistically significant (Wald test: $p = 0.38$)

4. Discussion

We hypothesized that the possibility of defining specific student groups, characterized by different lifestyle patterns, might help to better outline tailored intervention programs to be offered to the undergraduate students of two main Academic Institutions in northern Italy. Therefore, cluster analysis was employed to identify groups of students with similar lifestyles to better plan interventions aimed at lifestyle change.

In this paper, by employing an anonymous web-based questionnaire and a large cohort of undergraduate students, we unveil three major clusters of subjects, each corresponding to a distinct lifestyle pattern. Clusters are differentiated particularly in relation to exercise behaviour and perceptions of stress, fatigue and somatic-stress-related symptoms; more active students present lower perceptions of stress and somatic symptoms. Interestingly, we observed that the AHA diet score (considered a marker of nutrition quality) was not in the ideal range in any cluster (nevertheless, obesity was not of concern in this sample), being worst in the cluster characterized by higher perceptions of stress; students in cluster 1, who were physically active but showed a high perception of stress and fatigue, were more used to drinking alcohol. Notably, a great percentage of students desired to be helped with lifestyle improvement, particularly in terms of becoming more physically active, managing stress, and improving nutrition.

Lifestyle represents an important tool to promote health, prevent/manage chronic non-communicable diseases [12,28,40,41], and improve prognosis even in communicable diseases such as COVID-19 [42]. In addition, it is of paramount importance to foster well-being and manage stress [43,44]. Thus, improving lifestyle choices is valuable and essential for everyone, but particularly young people. Unfortunately, young people are often characterized by poor lifestyles, reduced well-being, and increased stress perception [13,14,44]—conditions which drive them to ask for help. In this paper, we observed that at least 60% of the students who filled in the lifestyle questionnaire desired to be helped in managing stress, and at least three-quarters of them in improving their lifestyle, particularly in terms of becoming physically active and having healthier nutrition. This observation suggests that institutions, particularly academic ones, should have a critical role in this regard. Many of them guarantee their students services to foster well-being [18,45–47] and promote healthy lifestyles. The possibility to tailor interventions to specific groups may represent a critical approach toward an efficacious result. Simple generic counselling may not always drive a real behavioural change [48]; on the contrary, tailored, specifically designed interventions considering group or individual characteristics and needs may be beneficial [49]. In this study, we unveiled specific student clusters characterized by specific lifestyles, considering lifestyle data collected by means of a simple web-based questionnaire. Notably, students with high stress perceptions are the least active and have the worst nutrition quality (cluster 3), while students who present similarly high stress perceptions but are physically active (cluster 1) drink more alcohol. On the other hand, students of cluster 2, who have a healthier lifestyle, may deserve attention in improving the quality of their nutrition, which, while being better than in cluster 3, was not ideal (as recommended by guidelines) [28] (poor = score 0–1; intermediate = score 2–3; ideal = score 4–5). The observation that the quality of nutrition may be suboptimal in normal-weight subjects may merit a specific note, in light of the importance of addressing this specific issue in preventive campaigns or in well-being-promoting campaigns; as such, placing attention only on overweight and obesity could be misleading.

It may be particularly useful for young subjects to design stress management and/or stress prevention campaigns that also include interventions based on lifestyle improvement; in this context, exercise may play a pivotal role [50]. On the other hand, it is important to educate students about the different benefits/risks of exercise and sport. For instance, excessively encouraging the pursuit of only high-level sports performance might lead to abandoning sports (if reached performances are not considered of note), increased risk of injuries, and promoting risky behaviours such as alcohol use, especially in subjects who present high stress perception. Vice versa, fighting sedentariness might be important to prevent the adoption of this unhealthy behaviour, which is frequently associated with stress and might accompany the student for life. Also, campaigns aimed at promoting healthy nutrition may have a significant role in stress management interventions. The link between stress and overweight and obesity is well known; interestingly, in this paper, we observed that poor nutrition quality, stress perception, insufficient exercise, and sedentariness clustered together (cluster 3), even though obesity was not of concern in these subjects. Educating young people before the appearance of clear signs of disease, such as elevated body weight, could represent a meaningful intervention, particularly in students characterized by elevated stress perception, a condition which might favour malnutrition.

The possibility of unveiling different student clusters identified by diverse lifestyle characteristics might be useful to tailor interventions and avoid general campaigns that might be suboptimal in fostering lifestyle changes.

Assessing lifestyle in undergraduate students represents an important research topic due to the possible translational implications for intervention designs in the academic setting. Several researchers have addressed this topic in different countries [5–8,20,21,51–54], using many different approaches. These studies consider that students' lifestyles are shaped by various factors, including financial opportunities [22], access to health resources, and social norms that influence their approach to health, physical activity, nutrition, stimulants, and mental health. To the best of our knowledge, most of these studies were descriptive surveys, showing the following: most of the students analysed were characterized by normal weight (with male students being slightly overweight [51–53]); male students are slightly more physically active [4] than female students; stress is of concern, particularly for female students [9,55,56]; and the majority of students are non-smokers and are occasional alcohol consumers [4,51–53]. Of particular interest is that, a more sophisticated approach, utilized in some of these papers, permitted the unveiling of important practical aspects, such as the relationship between depression and anxiety symptoms and sedentary behaviour [20]; the relationship between smoking habits and reported stress [22]; and the relationship between a healthy diet and regular exercise [6].

Notably, two major aspects were assessed in the literature: the association between physical activity and stress and the association between nutrition/diet patterns and physical activity. This issue assumes particular importance considering the strong roles of stress and unhealthy nutrition in worsening health/well-being and in many chronic diseases. On the other hand, regular aerobic exercise represents a pillar of the strategies to improve health and treat/prevent chronic disease, but also to help manage stress and nutrition patterns.

In the present study, we confirm some of the observations of other studies and add a new interesting aspect: the differences in lifestyle patterns among different clusters of students, corroborating the importance of tailoring interventions based on specific characteristics. We applied a multidimensional approach to the lifestyle assessment and cluster analysis, which allowed us to unveil that the main factors capable of distinguishing the different clusters of students were exercise, stress perception, nutrition quality, and alcohol. This approach allowed us to identify groups of students with distinct healthy behaviours and characterize them in terms of exercise, stress perception, nutrition quality, and alcohol consumption.

The numerosity of the study sample may also be of note. The majority of previous studies considered small student cohorts, except for few of them [8,20], while our study analysed data from thousands of subjects, and this numerosity allowed us to obtain reliable results.

Academic health promotion and health management may grant benefits which result in improvements in undergraduate students' lifestyles; in fact, education efforts to promote healthy lifestyles may be disseminated to academic employees and the general population. Moreover, undergraduate students may serve as models in their present and future lives [57], when (presumably) they will fill an important professional role. Lastly, specific training on lifestyle approaches for students of courses directly involved in the management of diseases and health promotion (such as medical students, nurses, physiotherapists, exercise physiologists, etc.) could become mandatory [58].

The employed questionnaire had already been used in other campaigns outside academia [11,23,24] to define the lifestyles of employees [11,23] or patients. It has been found to be capable of revealing an association between active habits and low stress perception both in healthy subjects [23] and breast cancer survivors; of revealing the betterment of different lifestyle components after a period of physical training in metabolic syndrome patients [25] and in stress management interventions [59]; of showing that young employees are characterized by poor lifestyle compared to older employees [9]; and of demonstrating an association between stress perception and markers of sympathetic overactivity [25,59]. The possibility to easily quantify stress perception using just three questions inquiring about stress from both a cognitive (directly asking about stress perception: "Do you feel stressed?") and somatic (asking questions regarding perceptions of fatigue and other somatic symptoms, such as palpitations or muscular tension) point of view may offer a simple metric for assessing and monitoring interventions [25,59].

Limitations: This study presents some limitations. In general, the data obtained through self-reported questionnaires might be of suboptimal quality. On the other hand, the high number of respondents and the quality of data analysis may help control this aspect [23]. Moreover, the questionnaire was completely anonymous, and we provided participants with a personalized, immediate report based on the filled information, hence increasing their likelihood of compliance [23] to insert trustful data on their present condition. The questionnaire was filled out voluntarily, although a sampling selection bias is expected, meaning that caution should be taken when extending the results to the overall student population of the two universities. Nevertheless, the number of respondents was relatively high for such an investigation, and we observed an extensive range of scores for all questions. Another limitation of our study should be acknowledged: we focus our attention only on the possibility of unveiling specific student clusters (using cluster analysis), possibly losing the opportunity to report on other results relevant to the community that would require different statistical approaches. Our large dataset could have permitted in-depth analysis. Nevertheless, we decided to focus our attention only on a specific goal: to define groups of students characterized by specific lifestyles to better tailor interventions aimed at improving health and well-being, answering a precise question of our Academic Institutions. Future lines of data analysis will definitely consider different statistical approaches, such as other types of parametric tests, the use of inferential statistics, etc., granting results that will be more generalizable to other contexts.

5. Conclusions

In conclusion, we report that students of the two main public universities in North Italy desire help with lifestyle improvement, mainly to be more physically active, to be capable of managing stress, and to have better nutrition. By using an ad hoc web-based lifestyle questionnaire, we revealed the presence of three main clusters of subjects characterised by different lifestyle patterns. Students who reported high perceptions of stress, fatigue, and somatic-stress-related symptoms were also less physically active and had the worst nutrition quality (cluster 3). Moreover, students with higher perceptions of stress but that were physically active (cluster 1) were those who consumed alcohol. However, students who were physically active and reported low perceptions of stress, fatigue, and somatic-stress-related symptoms (cluster 2) showed a need to improve nutrition quality. This approach might help identify specific student groups to tailor interventions fostering well-being and promoting health in academic settings.

Supplementary Materials: The following supporting information can be downloaded at: https://www.mdpi.com/article/10.3390/nu16244339/s1, Figure S1: Association between the variables used to perform clustering according to MCA; Figure S2: average silhouette width to choose the number of clusters for the Kmodes algorithm.

Author Contributions: Conceptualization, D.L., R.G., E.M., M.M.B. and E.M.B.; methodology, D.L., S.C. and E.M.B.; software, S.C., E.L., G.M. and E.M.B.; formal analysis, D.L., E.L., G.M., S.C. and E.M.B.; investigation, D.L., L.G., G.B., R.G. and E.M.; resources, D.L., R.G., E.M., S.C. and M.M.B.; data curation, D.L., S.C. and E.M.B.; writing—original draft preparation, D.L. and E.M.B.; writing—review and editing, D.L., E.L., G.M., L.G., G.B., R.G., E.M., S.C., M.M.B. and E.M.B.; supervision, D.L. and E.M.B.; project administration, D.L. and E.M.B.; funding acquisition, D.L., E.M. and M.M.B. All authors have read and agreed to the published version of the manuscript.

Funding: This research was partially funded by the Italian Ministry of Health.

Institutional Review Board Statement: The study protocol was approved by the Institutional Ethics Committee of the University of Milan (Allegato 4 Comitato Etico 25.05.18; Repertorio pareri Comitato Etico: parere numero 21/18) and by the Institutional Ethics Committee of the Polytechnic of Milan (Parere 11/2018 dated 26 July 2018).

Informed Consent Statement: All participants voluntarily provided anonymous data.

Data Availability Statement: Data will be available on justified request. We have not yet uploaded the data because they are part of an ongoing study on students' lifestyles and we are preparing other papers using them.

Conflicts of Interest: The authors declare no conflicts of interest.

References

1. Bonnie, R.J.; Stroud, C.; Breiner, H. *Investing in the Health and Well-Being of Young Adults*; National Academies Press: Washington, DC, USA, 2015.
2. Turco, J.V.; Inal-Veith, A.; Fuster, V. Cardiovascular Health Promotion: An Issue That Can No Longer Wait. *J. Am. Coll. Cardiol.* **2018**, *72*, 908–913. [CrossRef] [PubMed]
3. Wald, A.; Muennig, P.A.; O'Connell, K.A.; Garber, C.E. Associations between Healthy Lifestyle Behaviors and Academic Performance in U.S. Undergraduates: A Secondary Analysis of the American College Health Association's National College Health Assessment Ii. *Am. J. Health Promot.* **2014**, *28*, 298–305. [CrossRef] [PubMed]
4. Llorent-Bedmar, V.; Torres-Zaragoza, L.; Navarro-Granados, M.; Ballesteros-Moscosio, M.Á. Healthy Lifestyle Habits Among Students at the University of Seville, Spain. *J. Educ. Community Health* **2022**, *9*, 208–214. [CrossRef]
5. Carballo-Fazanes, A.; Rico-Díaz, J.; Barcala-Furelos, R.; Rey, E.; Rodríguez-Fernández, J.E.; Varela-Casal, C.; Abelairas-Gómez, C. Physical Activity Habits and Determinants, Sedentary Behaviour and Lifestyle in University Students. *Int. J. Environ. Res. Public Health* **2020**, *17*, 3272. [CrossRef] [PubMed]
6. Cheema, S.; Maisonneuve, P.; Abraham, A.; Chaabna, K.; Yousuf, W.; Mushannen, T.; Ibrahim, H.; Tom, A.; Lowenfels, A.B.; Mamtani, R. Dietary Patterns and Associated Lifestyle Factors among University Students in Qatar. *J Am. Coll. Health* **2023**, *71*, 2795–2803. [CrossRef] [PubMed]
7. Doak, S.; Kearney, J.M.; McCormack, J.M.; Keaver, L. The Relationship between Diet and Lifestyle Behaviours in a Sample of Higher Education Students; a Cross-Sectional Study. *Clin. Nutr. ESPEN* **2023**, *54*, 293–299. [CrossRef]
8. Lonati, E.; Cazzaniga, E.; Adorni, R.; Zanatta, F.; Belingheri, M.; Colleoni, M.; Riva, M.A.; Steca, P.; Palestini, P. Health-Related Lifestyles among University Students: Focusing on Eating Habits and Physical Activity. *Int. J. Environ. Res. Public Health* **2024**, *21*, 626. [CrossRef]
9. Lucini, D.; Pagani, E.; Capria, F.; Galiano, M.; Marchese, M.; Cribellati, S.; Parati, G. Age Influences on Lifestyle and Stress Perception in the Working Population. *Nutrients* **2023**, *15*, 399. [CrossRef]
10. Kraus, W.E.; Bittner, V.; Appel, L.; Blair, S.N.; Church, T.; Després, J.P.; Franklin, B.A.; Miller, T.D.; Pate, R.R.; Taylor-Piliae, R.E.; et al. The National Physical Activity Plan: A Call to Action from the American Heart Association A Science Advisory from the American Heart Association. *Circulation* **2015**, *131*, 1932–1940. [CrossRef] [PubMed]
11. Lucini, D.; Pagani, M. Exercise Prescription to Foster Health and Well-Being: A Behavioral Approach to Transform Barriers into Opportunities. *Int. J. Environ. Res. Public Health* **2021**, *18*, 968. [CrossRef]

12. Virani, S.S.; Newby, L.K.; Arnold, S.V.; Bittner, V.; Brewer, L.P.C.; Demeter, S.H.; Dixon, D.L.; Fearon, W.F.; Hess, B.; Johnson, H.M.; et al. 2023 AHA/ACC/ACCP/ASPC/NLA/PCNA Guideline for the Management of Patients with Chronic Coronary Disease: A Report of the American Heart Association/American College of Cardiology Joint Committee on Clinical Practice Guidelines. *J. Am. Coll. Cardiol.* **2023**, *82*, 833–955. [CrossRef]
13. Evans, T.M.; Bira, L.; Gastelum, J.B.; Weiss, L.T.; Vanderford, N.L. Evidence for a Mental Health Crisis in Graduate Education. *Nat. Biotechnol.* **2018**, *36*, 282–284. [CrossRef] [PubMed]
14. Pascoe, M.C.; Hetrick, S.E.; Parker, A.G. The Impact of Stress on Students in Secondary School and Higher Education. *Int. J. Adolesc. Youth* **2020**, *25*, 104–112. [CrossRef]
15. Yorks, D.M.; Frothingham, C.A.; Schuenke, M.D. Effects of Group Fitness Classes on Stress and Quality of Life of Medical Students. *J. Am. Osteopath. Assoc.* **2017**, *117*, e17–e25. [CrossRef]
16. Herbert, C. Enhancing Mental Health, Well-Being and Active Lifestyles of University Students by Means of Physical Activity and Exercise Research Programs. *Front. Public Health* **2022**, *10*, 849093. [CrossRef] [PubMed]
17. Curran, F.; Blake, C.; Cunningham, C.; Perrotta, C.; Van der Ploeg, H.; Matthews, J.; O'Donoghue, G. Efficacy, Characteristics, Behavioural Models and Behaviour Change Strategies, of Nonworkplace Interventions Specifically Targeting Sedentary Behaviour; a Systematic Review and Meta-Analysis of Randomised Control Trials in Healthy Ambulatory Adults. *PLoS ONE* **2021**, *16*, e0256828. [CrossRef] [PubMed]
18. Okanagan Charter: An International Charter for Health Promoting Universities and Colleges (2015). Available online: https://www.healthpromotingcampuses.org/okanagan-charter (accessed on 9 December 2024).
19. Washington, A.E.; Coye, M.J.; Boulware, L.E. Academic Health Systems' Third Curve: Population Health Improvement. *JAMA J. Am. Med. Assoc.* **2016**, *315*, 459–460. [CrossRef] [PubMed]
20. Barbosa, B.C.R.; de Menezes-Júnior, L.A.A.; de Paula, W.; Chagas, C.M. dos S.; Machado, E.L.; de Freitas, E.D.; Cardoso, C.S.; de Carvalho Vidigal, F.; Nobre, L.N.; da Silva, L.S.; et al. Sedentary Behavior Is Associated with the Mental Health of University Students during the Covid-19 Pandemic, and Not Practicing Physical Activity Accentuates Its Adverse Effects: Cross-Sectional Study. *BMC Public Health* **2024**, *24*, 1860. [CrossRef]
21. Nowak, P.F.; Bożek, A.; Blukacz, M. Physical Activity, Sedentary Behavior, and Quality of Life among University Students. *BioMed Res. Int.* **2019**, *2019*, 9791281. [CrossRef]
22. El Ansari, W.; Sebena, R.; El-Ansari, K.; Suominen, S. Clusters of Lifestyle Behavioral Risk Factors and Their Associations with Depressive Symptoms and Stress: Evidence from Students at a University in Finland. *BMC Public Health* **2024**, *24*, 1103. [CrossRef] [PubMed]
23. Lucini, D.; Solaro, N.; Lesma, A.; Gillet, V.B.; Pagani, M. Health Promotion in the Workplace: Assessing Stress and Lifestyle with an Intranet Tool. *J. Med. Internet Res.* **2011**, *13*, e88. [CrossRef] [PubMed]
24. Lucini, D.; Zanuso, S.; Blair, S.; Pagani, M. A Simple Healthy Lifestyle Index as a Proxy of Wellness: A Proof of Concept. *Acta Diabetol.* **2015**, *52*, 81–89. [CrossRef]
25. Lucini, D.; Malacarne, M.; Gatzemeier, W.; Pagani, M. A Simple Home-Based Lifestyle Intervention Program to Improve Cardiac Autonomic Regulation in Patients with Increased Cardiometabolic Risk. *Sustainability* **2020**, *12*, 7671. [CrossRef]
26. Lucini, D.; Gandolfi, C.E.; Antonucci, C.; Cavagna, A.; Valzano, E.; Botta, E.; Chiari, M.; Mameli, L.; Nahum, M.; Brambilla, M.M.; et al. #StayHomeStayFit: UNIMI's Approach to Online Healthy Lifestyle Promotion during the COVID-19 Pandemic. *Acta Biomed.* **2020**, *91*, e2020037. [CrossRef]
27. Craig, C.L.; Marshall, A.L.; Sjöström, M.; Bauman, A.E.; Booth, M.L.; Ainsworth, B.E.; Pratt, M.; Ekelund, U.; Yngve, A.; Sallis, J.F.; et al. International Physical Activity Questionnaire: 12-Country Reliability and Validity. *Med. Sci. Sports Exerc.* **2003**, *35*, 1381–1395. [CrossRef] [PubMed]
28. Lloyd-Jones, D.M.; Hong, Y.; Labarthe, D.; Mozaffarian, D.; Appel, L.J.; Van Horn, L.; Greenlund, K.; Daniels, S.; Nichol, G.; Tomaselli, G.F.; et al. Defining and Setting National Goals for Cardiovascular Health Promotion and Disease Reduction: The American Heart Association's Strategic Impact Goal through 2020 and Beyond. *Circulation* **2010**, *121*, 586–613. [CrossRef] [PubMed]
29. Alberti, K.G.M.M.; Eckel, R.H.; Grundy, S.M.; Zimmet, P.Z.; Cleeman, J.I.; Donato, K.A.; Fruchart, J.C.; James, W.P.T.; Loria, C.M.; Smith, S.C. Harmonizing the Metabolic Syndrome: A Joint Interim Statement of the International Diabetes Federation Task Force on Epidemiology and Prevention; National Heart, Lung, and Blood Institute; American Heart Association; World Heart Federation; International. *Circulation* **2009**, *120*, 1640–1645. [CrossRef] [PubMed]
30. Ekelund, U.; Tarp, J.; Steene-Johannessen, J.; Hansen, B.H.; Jefferis, B.; Fagerland, M.W.; Whincup, P.; Diaz, K.M.; Hooker, S.P.; Chernofsky, A.; et al. Dose-Response Associations between Accelerometry Measured Physical Activity and Sedentary Time and All Cause Mortality: Systematic Review and Harmonised Meta-Analysis. *BMJ* **2019**, *366*, l4570. [CrossRef] [PubMed]
31. Watson, N.F.; Badr, M.S.; Belenky, G.; Bliwise, D.L.; Buxton, O.M.; Buysse, D.; Dinges, D.F.; Gangwisch, J.; Grandner, M.A.; Kushida, C.; et al. Recommended Amount of Sleep for a Healthy Adult: A Joint Consensus Statement of the American Academy of Sleep Medicine and Sleep Research Society. *Sleep* **2015**, *38*, 843–844. [CrossRef] [PubMed]

32. Husson, F.; Lê, S.; Pagès, J. *Exploratory Multivariate Analysis by Example Using R*; CRC Press: Boca Raton, FL, USA, 2011; Volume 15.
33. Chaturvedi, A.; Foods, K.; Green, P.E.; Carroll, J.D. K-Modes Clustering. *J. Classif.* **2001**, *18*, 35–55. [CrossRef]
34. Rousseeuw, P.J. Silhouettes: A Graphical Aid to the Interpretation and Validation of Cluster Analysis. *J. Comput. Appl. Math.* **1987**, *20*, 53–65. [CrossRef]
35. Bakker, J.D. PERMDISP. In *Applied Multivariate Statistics in R*; University of Washington Libraries: Washington, DC, USA, 2024.
36. R Core Team. R: A Language and Environment for Statistical Computing. R Foundation for Statistical Computing, Vienna, Austria. 2021. Available online: https://www.r-project.org/ (accessed on 9 December 2024).
37. Lê, S.; Josse, J.; Husson, F. FactoMineR: An R Package for Multivariate Analysis. *J. Stat. Softw.* **2008**, *25*, 1–18. [CrossRef]
38. Weihs, C.; Ligges, U.; Luebke, K.; Raabe, N. KlaR Analyzing German Business Cycles. In *Data Analysis and Decision Support*; Springer: Berlin/Heidelberg, Germany, 2005; pp. 335–343. [CrossRef]
39. Oksanen, J.; Simpson, G.; Blanchet, F.; Kindt, R.; Legendre, P.; Minchin, P.; O'Hara, R.; Solymos, P.; Stevens, M.; Szoecs, E.; et al. Vegan: Community Ecology Package (R Package Version 2.6-2). 2022. Available online: https://cran.r-project.org/web/packages/vegan/index.html (accessed on 9 December 2024).
40. Bull, F.C.; Al-Ansari, S.S.; Biddle, S.; Borodulin, K.; Buman, M.P.; Cardon, G.; Carty, C.; Chaput, J.P.; Chastin, S.; Chou, R.; et al. World Health Organization 2020 Guidelines on Physical Activity and Sedentary Behaviour. *Br. J. Sports Med.* **2020**, *54*, 1451–1462. [CrossRef]
41. Visseren, F.; Mach, F.; Smulders, Y.M.; Carballo, D.; Koskinas, K.C.; Bäck, M.; Benetos, A.; Biffi, A.; Boavida, J.M.; Capodanno, D.; et al. 2021 ESC Guidelines on Cardiovascular Disease Prevention in Clinical Practice. *Eur. Heart J.* **2021**, *42*, 3227–3337. [CrossRef] [PubMed]
42. Wang, S.; Li, Y.; Yue, Y.; Yuan, C.; Kang, J.H.; Chavarro, J.E.; Bhupathiraju, S.N.; Roberts, A.L. Adherence to Healthy Lifestyle Prior to Infection and Risk of Post-COVID-19 Condition. *JAMA Intern. Med.* **2023**, *183*, 232–241. [CrossRef] [PubMed]
43. Schnermann, M.E.; Schulz, C.A.; Ludwig, C.; Alexy, U.; Nöthlings, U. A Lifestyle Score in Childhood and Adolescence Was Positively Associated with Subsequently Measured Fluid Intelligence in the DONALD Cohort Study. *Eur. J. Nutr.* **2022**, *61*, 3719–3729. [CrossRef]
44. Douwes, R.; Metselaar, J.; Pijnenborg, G.H.M.; Boonstra, N. Well-Being of Students in Higher Education: The Importance of a Student Perspective. *Cogent Educ.* **2023**, *10*, 2190697. [CrossRef]
45. University of British Columbia Wellbeing Strategic Framework. Available online: https://wellbeing.ubc.ca/framework (accessed on 28 June 2024).
46. Together for Students' Well-Being in Europe: The WISE Project EUF. Available online: https://uni-foundation.eu/2022/06/21/together-students-project/ (accessed on 28 June 2024).
47. DfE How We're Supporting University Students with Their Mental Health—The Education Hub. Available online: https://educationhub.blog.gov.uk/2023/06/09/how-supporting-university-students-mental-health/ (accessed on 28 June 2024).
48. Song, Z.; Baicker, K. Effect of a Workplace Wellness Program on Employee Health and Economic Outcomes: A Randomized Clinical Trial. *JAMA-J. Am. Med. Assoc.* **2019**, *321*, 1491–1501. [CrossRef] [PubMed]
49. Milani, R.V.; Lavie, C.J. Health Care 2020: Reengineering Health Care Delivery to Combat Chronic Disease. *Am. J. Med.* **2015**, *128*, 337–343. [CrossRef] [PubMed]
50. Mitchell, J.J.; Bu, F.; Fancourt, D.; Steptoe, A.; Bone, J.K. Longitudinal Associations between Physical Activity and Other Health Behaviours during the COVID-19 Pandemic: A Fixed Effects Analysis. *Sci. Rep.* **2022**, *12*, 15956. [CrossRef] [PubMed]
51. Gallè, F.; Sabella, E.A.; Da Molin, G.; Liguori, G.; Montagna, M.T.; Orsi, G.B.; Valerio, G.; Napoli, C. A Cross-Sectional Study Investigating Lifestyle and Weight Perception of Undergraduate Students in Southern Italy. *BMC Public Health* **2019**, *19*, 1316. [CrossRef] [PubMed]
52. Wei, C.N.; Harada, K.; Ueda, K.; Fukumoto, K.; Minamoto, K.; Ueda, A. Assessment of Health-Promoting Lifestyle Profile in Japanese University Students. *Environ. Health Prev. Med.* **2012**, *17*, 222–227. [CrossRef] [PubMed]
53. Carter, A.O.; Elzubeir, M.; Abdulrazzaq, Y.M.; Revel, A.D.; Townsend, A. Health and Lifestyle Needs Assessment of Medical Students in the United Arab Emirates. *Med. Teach.* **2003**, *25*, 492–496. [CrossRef] [PubMed]
54. Suwalska, J.; Kolasińska, K.; Łojko, D.; Bogdański, P. Eating Behaviors, Depressive Symptoms and Lifestyle in University Students in Poland. *Nutrients* **2022**, *14*, 1106. [CrossRef]
55. Stefaniak, A.R.; Blaxton, J.M.; Bergeman, C.S. Age Differences in Types and Perceptions of Daily Stress. *Int. J. Aging Hum. Dev.* **2022**, *94*, 215–233. [CrossRef]
56. Jiang, D. Perceived Stress and Daily Well-Being During the COVID-19 Outbreak: The Moderating Role of Age. *Front. Psychol.* **2020**, *11*, 571873. [CrossRef]
57. Frank, E. Physician Health and Patient Care. *JAMA* **2004**, *291*, 637. [CrossRef]

58. Hivert, M.F.; Arena, R.; Forman, D.E.; Kris-Etherton, P.M.; McBride, P.E.; Pate, R.R.; Spring, B.; Trilk, J.; Van Horn, L.V.; Kraus, W.E. Medical Training to Achieve Competency in Lifestyle Counseling: An Essential Foundation for Prevention and Treatment of Cardiovascular Diseases and Other Chronic Medical Conditions: A Scientific Statement from the American Heart Association. *Circulation* **2016**, *134*, e308–e327. [CrossRef] [PubMed]
59. Pagani, E.; Gavazzoni, N.; Bernardelli, G.; Malacarne, M.; Solaro, N.; Giusti, E.; Castelnuovo, G.; Volpi, P.; Carimati, G.; Lucini, D. Psychological Intervention Based on Mental Relaxation to Manage Stress in Female Junior Elite Soccer Team: Improvement in Cardiac Autonomic Control, Perception of Stress and Overall Health. *Int. J. Environ. Res. Public Health* **2023**, *20*, 942. [CrossRef]

nutrients

MDPI

Review

The Use of Nutritional Interventions to Enhance Genomic Stability in Mice and Delay Aging

Ivar van Galen [1,2,3], Jan H. J. Hoeijmakers [1,2,4,5] and Wilbert P. Vermeij [1,2,*]

1 Princess Máxima Center for Pediatric Oncology, 3584 CS Utrecht, The Netherlands; ivar.vangalen@maastrichtuniversity.nl (I.v.G.); j.hoeijmakers@erasmusmc.nl (J.H.J.H.)
2 Oncode Institute, 3521 AL Utrecht, The Netherlands
3 Laboratory for Experimental Orthopedics, Department of Orthopedic Surgery, Maastricht University, 6229 ER Maastricht, The Netherlands
4 Department of Molecular Genetics, Erasmus MC Cancer Institute, Erasmus University Medical Center Rotterdam, 3015 GD Rotterdam, The Netherlands
5 Institute for Genome Stability in Ageing and Disease, Cologne Excellence Cluster for Cellular Stress Responses in Aging-Associated Diseases (CECAD), University of Cologne, 50931 Cologne, Germany
* Correspondence: w.p.vermeij@prinsesmaximacentrum.nl

Abstract

Background/Objectives: Metabolism is fundamental to all living organisms. It comprises a highly complex network of fine-tuned chemical reactions that sustain life but also generate by-products that damage cellular biomolecules, including DNA, thereby contributing to aging and disease. As metabolism can be largely modified by dietary alterations, it has the potential to positively or negatively affect health and disease. Interestingly, many aging-associated illnesses known to be influenced by diet also show a causal relation with DNA damage. As DNA keeps all instructions for life, and DNA lesions, if unrepaired, interfere with vital processes such as DNA replication and transcription, DNA damage may be an important mediator of the impact of nutrition on health and aging. **Methods:** Here, we discuss the genome-protective effects of various oral interventions in mice, aiming to elucidate which nutritional alterations lower DNA damage and promote overall health. **Results:** Our analysis covers a wide range of interventions with reported positive impacts on genomic stability, including modified diets (e.g., dietary restriction, probiotics, micronutrients, fatty acids, and hormones), NAD+ precursors (e.g., nicotinamide riboside), plant derivatives, and synthetic drugs. Among these, caloric and dietary restriction emerge as the most potent, generic modulators of DNA damage and repair processes, enhancing aspects of repair efficiency through metabolic recalibration and improved cellular resilience. Other interventions, like NAD+ precursors, activate partly similar pathways without necessitating reduced food intake. **Conclusions:** While many interventions show promise, their effects are often less pronounced or are process-specific compared to caloric or dietary restriction. Additionally, many substances lack comprehensive exploration of their genome-protective effects in mice, with often only a small number of studies examining their impact on genome stability. Moreover, the heterogeneity between studies limits direct comparison. However, the observed overlap in mechanistic effects between treatments lends credibility to their potential efficacy. Ultimately, a deeper understanding of these mechanisms could pave the way for translating these findings into, e.g., combination treatments to promote healthy aging in humans.

Keywords: dietary interventions; DNA damage and repair; aging

 https://doi.org/10.3390/nu18020246

1. Introduction

Metabolism consists of an intricate network of chemical reactions that sustain life and serve as the foundation of biological functionality across all living organisms [1]. The fundamental role of metabolism extends beyond mere survival, growth, and development, as it also influences health status and disease trajectories by modulating the body's internal environment and maintaining homeostasis in the face of exogenous stressors [2]. Dietary patterns significantly affect metabolic pathways, thereby impacting energy balance, metabolic fitness, the amount and type of reactive by-products of metabolism, and overall health [3–5]. Furthermore, these metabolic processes are both consequences and drivers of the aging process, and may elicit anti-aging effects, implicating both longevity and quality of life [6,7].

Many age-related chronic diseases, such as cardiovascular disorders, neurodegeneration, and cancer, share a causal process; DNA damage (DD) [8–10]. DD generally occurs in a stochastic manner and is highly heterogeneous, ranging from small oxidation products (e.g., 8-oxo-dG) and abasic sites (induced by spontaneous hydrolysis, occurring ~10^4 times per cell per day), to helix-distorting bulky adducts, intrastrand and interstrand crosslinks, and protein–DNA crosslinks, and various forms of single- and double-strand breaks [11]. Each of these types of lesions is counteracted by one or more specialized DNA repair mechanisms [11]. Base excision repair (BER) corrects small, non-helix-distorting base lesions, while nucleotide excision repair (NER) and transcription-coupled repair (TCR) remove bulky adducts that distort the DNA helix and/or physically impede elongating RNA polymerases, resp. More disruptive lesions, like double-strand breaks, are repaired either by homologous recombination (HR), when the (proliferating) cell is in S-phase or G2, which restores the original sequence using the replicated intact copy as a template, or by non-homologous end joining (NHEJ), which directly ligates the broken DNA ends but is less error-free.

Not all DD is repaired perfectly, and the accumulation of DD over time, caused by both endogenous (e.g., reactive metabolic by-products) and exogenous factors, is now recognized as a major hallmark of aging (Table 1). This accumulation influences both the genetic and epigenetic landscape, disrupting cellular homeostasis and driving processes such as senescence and apoptosis, ultimately manifesting as age-related physiological decline [12,13]. Notably, progeroid DNA repair-deficient mouse models such as $Xpg^{-/-}$ and $Ercc1^{\Delta/-}$ mice, in which DD persists, resulting in an accelerated and shortened lifespan, exhibit epigenetic alterations, transcriptional changes, systemic biomarker shifts, and multi-organ functional decline that closely mirror those observed during natural aging, supporting their use as mechanistic models of physiological aging [12,13]. However, accurately measuring physiological (i.e., low) levels of DD and reliably assessing DNA repair activity remains technically challenging (Table 1). Methods such as the comet assay require delicate handling, and many genome maintenance interventions lack robust evidence due to methodological limitations. Additionally, antibody-based γH2AX detection is widely used to quantify DNA double-strand breaks; however, these lesions are rare, and γH2AX can also mark dying cells, complicating data interpretation. Still, growing evidence suggests that environmental and lifestyle factors, particularly diet, influence the accumulation of DD.

https://doi.org/10.3390/nu18020246

Table 1. Major types of DNA damage and their predominant characteristics [12–25].

	Base Modifications	SSBs	DSBs	Helix-Distorting Lesions	Interstrand Crosslinks
Causes	Deamination, ROS, alkylation, and UV radiation	ROS, ionizing radiation, and topoisomerase I inhibitors	Ionizing radiation, replication fork collapse, and topoisomerase II inhibitors	UV radiation, polycyclic aromatic hydrocarbons, ROS, and chemotherapeutics	Endogenous aldehydes and chemotherapy
Consequences	Mutations and altered epigenetic regulation	Replication-induced DSBs	Chromosomal aberrations, cell cycle arrest, apoptosis, and senescence	Transcription and replication stalling, mutagenesis, and cell death	Transcription and replication stalling, cell cycle arrest, cell death, and senescence
Repair Mechanisms	BER and direct reversal	SSBR (specialized BER)	NHEJ, HR, alt-EJ, and single-strand annealing	NER and TCR	FA pathway, NER, and HR
Biomarker Examples $	8-OHdG, N7-methylguanine (alkylation), and abasic (AP) sites	XRCC1 foci and PAR-polymers $	γH2AX foci $, 53BP1 foci $, RAD51 foci $, and ATM/ATR activation $	CPDs, (6-4) photoproducts, R-loops $, and GLTD $	FANCD2 foci and DNA interstrand crosslinks
Detection Methods [1–3]	ELISA [2], mass spectrometry [1], IF [2], IHC [2], and comet assay (FpG, Endo III) [3]	IF [2], alkaline comet assay [3], and FADU assay [3]	IF [2], IHC [2], Western blot [2/3], neutral comet assay [3], pulsed-field gel electrophoresis [2], and FADU assay [3]	IF [2], IHC [2], sequencing [1], UDS assay [1], Recovery RNA/DNA synthesis [1], and GLTD [1/2]	IF [2] and crosslinking comet assay [3]
Effect on Aging *	+	++	+++	+++	++

SSBs = single-strand breaks, DSBs = double-strand breaks, ROS = reactive oxygen species, 8-OHdG = 8-hydroxyguanosine, ELISA = enzyme-linked immunosorbent assay, FpG = formamidopyrimidine DNA glycosylase, IHC = immunohistochemistry, IF = immunofluorescence, FADU = fluorometric analysis of DNA unwinding, Endo = endonuclease, BER = base excision repair, SSBR = SSB repair (specialized BER), NHEJ = non-homologous end joining, HR = homologous recombination, alt-EJ = alternative end joining, NER = nucleotide excision repair, TCR = transcription-coupled repair, FA = Fanconi anemia, CPDs = cyclobutane pyrimidine dimers, GLTD = gene length-dependent transcriptional decline, UDS = unscheduled DNA synthesis. $ DNA damage biomarkers that have broad specificity or can be secondary to other lesions. [1–3] degree of accuracy/reliability of the detection method (1 high; 2 intermediate or depending on antibody specificity; 3 lower/variable). * pluses indicate an estimated relative contribution of each lesion type to aging (weak (+), moderate (++), and strong (+++) effects), inferred from available experimental and clinical evidence.

Depending on diet, health and lifespan can be positively or negatively influenced [26]. Notably, altering metabolism through dietary interventions offers a promising approach to enhancing genomic stability. Nutritional components can either provoke or protect against DD through multiple, partially overlapping mechanisms such as (i) direct effects on DD formation or repair capacity, (ii) changes in metabolic rate and energy flux that alter the production of endogenous genotoxic stress, and (iii) enhanced cellular and organismal resilience, which could indicate, for example, improved tolerance to damage without necessarily reducing lesion burden or enhanced DD response signaling. For instance, certain nutrients act as cofactors in enzymatic reactions that repair DNA, while others may modulate gene expression and mitigate cellular stress [27]. Conversely, dietary excesses of protein, simple carbohydrates, and fat can induce metabolic stress and inflammation, thereby facilitating genomic instability [28–30].

The interplay between diet, metabolism, and DD is particularly critical as it represents a modifiable factor in the aging process. With the global population aging at an unprecedented rate [31], there is a pressing need to understand and harness these relationships to devise dietary strategies capable of decelerating the aging process and prolonging a healthy lifespan [32,33].

2. Materials and Methods

This review focuses on various nutritional interventions aimed at reducing DD induction and/or improving repair mechanisms in the contexts of health and longevity in mice. Relevant literature published on PubMed was collected using two automated search queries using a semi-systematic approach without formal quality assessment. The first search consisted of all applicable PubMed papers (excluding pre-prints) up to 1 March 2023, which was supplemented with a second search for all papers published between 1 March 2023

https://doi.org/10.3390/nu18020246

and 1 November 2025 (see Supplementary Files S1–S3 for the search queries and results). Search queries included at least one primary keyword related to DNA damage and repair, one secondary keyword related to aging and health, and one tertiary keyword specific for the type of nutritional intervention, all restricted to Mus musculus (Supplementary File S1). Entries were examined in a semi-systematic review format and supplemented with articles, e.g., based on references not identified by the original search parameters. Articles were screened for relevance by assessing their inclusion of data related to DD or DD repair, and studies lacking well-defined oral treatments or involving non-edible interventions were excluded. This approach was chosen to maximize the global overview and identification of potentially relevant literature, as many studies likely contain or assessed only one type of nutritional intervention or DNA damage detection method, or looked at specific mouse models or tissue types. Although no formal quality assessment was performed, yielding a potential bias, all included studies were peer-reviewed, and articles for which authors declared a potential conflict of interest are highlighted with ‡. Ambiguities regarding these selection criteria were resolved through evaluation by a second assessor. The final dataset comprises 69 studies on dietary interventions including restrictive diets, 111 on supplements, 14 on oral medications, and 17 on other miscellaneous interventions, all with a focus on beneficial effects related to DD and its repair (Figure 1). Ultimately, this review aims to identify consumable interventions that improve genomic stability in mice and may reduce chronic diseases in humans.

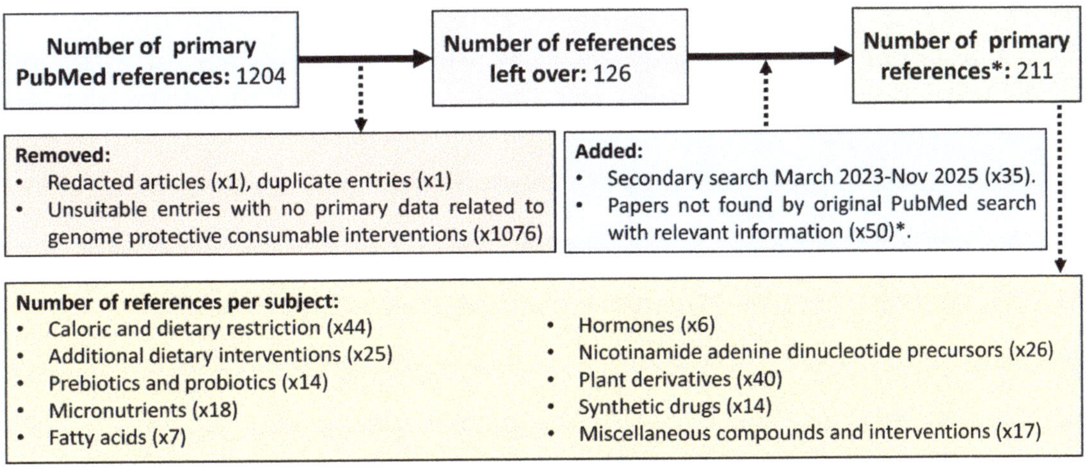

Figure 1. Schematic representation of the reference selection used in this review. PubMed references obtained from the query-based search were filtered based on relevance to genome-protective consumable interventions, with unsuitable and duplicate entries removed. Relevant articles identified after our primary search were subsequently added. The total number of references is highlighted per subject, while allowing for potential overlap. * excluding references exclusively used in Sections 1 and 4.

3. Results

3.1. Caloric and Dietary Restriction

The oldest known and most extensively studied nutritional intervention is dietary restriction (DR), where total food intake is typically reduced by 10–40% without causing malnutrition [34–36]. Caloric restriction (CR) is often used synonymously, but technically refers to a reduction in caloric intake without altering total micronutrient intake, like vitamins and minerals, which is in contrast to DR, where both macro- and micronutrient composition may vary [37]. Here, we will use the term "dietary restriction" to refer to

https://doi.org/10.3390/nu18020246

studies where total food consumption was reduced, and "caloric restriction" when this was compensated with additional micronutrients.

Both CR and DR trigger reduced energy expenditure by, e.g., lowering growth hormone, insulin-like growth factor (IGF1), thyroid hormone (receptor), mTOR, glucose, insulin levels, and body temperature [38,39]. The resulting recalibration of energy metabolism under a negative energy balance is associated with reversed age-related decline in mitochondrial activity by restoring oxidative capacity, leading to improved efficiency and redox homeostasis without increasing mitochondrial mass [38]. Consequently, oxidative damage, as measured by FpG- and Endo III-sensitive breaks in a comet assay [40], and 8-oxo-2′-deoxyguanosine (8-OHdG) oxidative biomarker levels, is lowered in various tissues, including muscle, brain, kidney, and liver [38,41]; however, in hippocampal subfields of aged wild-type C57BL/6J mice, 8-OHdG levels have been reported to increase [42]. This amelioration appeared more pronounced in post-mitotic tissues and after extended duration of the dietary intervention. Interestingly, 10 months of CR, the only period tested, demonstrated protective effects against clofibrate, an indirect liver carcinogen and oxidative stress-inducing agent specific for rodents [43], likely due to improved stress resilience and/or enhanced DNA repair.

By affecting cellular processes, 30% DR and CR are able to extend median and maximum lifespan by approximately 15–30% in wild-type mice, although considerable variation has been noted between different laboratory mouse strains [34,44]. Interestingly, these lifespan-extending effects are even more pronounced in prematurely aging DNA repair mutants [45]. In *Ercc1*$^{\Delta/-}$ and *Xpg*$^{-/-}$ mice, which carry deficiencies in multiple DNA repair pathways, including nucleotide excision and transcription-coupled repair, and mimic features of human progeroid syndromes, DR increases median remaining lifespan by ~200% and ~80%, respectively. These increases are associated with improved tissue function and histological parameters in various organs, including muscle, liver, kidney, bone, vasculature, and most prominently, the nervous system [45–50]. As these mutant mice are genetically defective in their DNA repair capacity, their heightened response to the protective effects of DR is most logically explained by a reduced DD load. One strong piece of evidence for this comes from studies showing that DR leads to lower genome-wide DD, as reflected by reduced γH2AX foci and diminished gene length-dependent transcription stress [14,45]. Since these genetic mutants are, in part, functionally defective in DNA repair pathways and no significant back-up repair systems are known, this reduction in DD is unlikely to result from enhanced repair activity. Instead, it is more plausibly attributed to a decreased metabolic production of DD or an improved ability of cells to tolerate and manage cellular stress [46].

In addition to limiting the production of endogenous DNA-damaging agents, DR has been reported to alter DNA repair activity and the expression of related proteins. Specifically, short-term intervention (4 weeks) in 3–5-month-old wild-type C57BL/6J mice increased DNA-PK and SIRT6 levels and the efficiency of NHEJ in skin, lung, kidney, and brain [51]. Similarly, DR protected against chemical mutagenesis and improved base excision repair (BER) in the brain, liver, kidney, spleen, and testes, possibly by preventing the age-related decline in the levels and activity of key proteins, such as the BER rate-limiting enzyme DNA polymerase beta [52,53]. Conversely, BER activity in the mitochondria of kidney and brain was significantly downregulated, suggesting organelle-specific changes [53]. DR reduced the level of *Igf1*, which was inversely correlated with *Dclre1a* [54], a gene whose protein product plays an important role in degrading chemically modified DNA during ICL and DSB repair [55]. DR has also been reported to downregulate the expression of various genes related to DNA repair in skeletal muscle, including, *Ddb2*, *Rad50*, and *Polb* [39]. In contrast, DR upregulated several DNA repair pathways and related proteins

https://doi.org/10.3390/nu18020246

in heart, liver, and brain tissue [56–58], suggesting tissue-specific expression differences. Furthermore, DR does not seem to influence the quantity of single-strand breaks in the brain, kidney, and liver of old wild-type animals, as measured by fluorometric analysis of DNA unwinding [59]. Together, these findings highlight the diverse effects of DR and CR on genomic stability and repair, several of which demonstrate their potential to optimize repair processes and mitigate damage in a tissue-specific manner.

The idea of improved genomic stability by DR is further supported by old preliminary studies using unscheduled DNA synthesis (UDS), which reflects a cell's ability to perform global genome nucleotide excision repair (GG-NER) [60]. For example, UVC irradiation of freshly isolated skin cells from mice on 40% DR increased UDS by 48–65% compared to AL controls [61]. Similarly, while UVC generates transcription-blocking bulky lesions, DR reduced the age-associated decline in enzyme activity and fidelity of DNA polymerase α and β in hepatocytes [62,63]. Additionally, in wild-type C57BL/6J mice, 30% DR reduced UVB-induced skin damage, histological changes, and inflammatory responses, but refeeding 24 h after irradiation partially reversed these benefits [64]. However, it also delayed γH2AX repair, suggesting that while DR limits initial damage, it also partially appears to slow recovery, possibly by reducing proliferation and the activity of replication-dependent DNA repair mechanisms like HR and XLR [64,65]. How DR affects transcription-associated DNA repair mechanisms is yet unknown. However, we have previously reported that age-related, DD-induced, gene length-dependent transcriptional decline (GLTD) was alleviated in DNA repair-deficient mutant animals when on DR, compared to ad libitum animals. This indicates that DR reduced transcription-blocking lesions genome-wide, consistent with the idea that DR lowers the overall DD load as at least one way by which it delays systemic aging [45,49,66].

Besides UV protection, DR confers protection against multiple types of genomic insults. In wild-type C57BL/6J mice, 30% DR reduced tumor incidence at necropsy [67], likely because DR reduces genomic mutation rates [68,69]. Additionally, 30% DR has been shown to protect against toxicity induced by fine ambient particulate matter, as evidenced by reduced DD, oxidative stress markers, inflammation, and improved lung tissue morphology [70].

Concurrent with the attenuation of genomic damage and the enhancement of DNA repair pathways, DR reduces natural age-related apoptotic markers and damage-inducible transcripts in the heart, such as *Bax*, *Bad*, *Casp9*, *Casp11*, and *Gadd45a* [57]. Furthermore, long-term DR reduces senescence, inflammation, and γH2AX foci in multiple tissues and cell types, including brain, adipose, corneal epithelium, and hematopoietic stem cells (HSCs) [71–75], although these effects are less pronounced in short-term DR [75]. Interestingly, many of these markers remain lowered for at least three months following a return to AL feeding after nine months of 40% DR in wild-type C57BL/6J mice [76], suggesting a prolonged protective effect.

In conclusion, CR and DR exhibit a profound and multifaceted impact on genomic stability by mitigating age-related DD and enhancing the efficiency of repair pathways, thereby contributing to improved tissue function and an extended lifespan (Figure 2). The tissue- and stressor-specific protective effects further underscore the potential of these interventions as powerful modulators of aging and genomic integrity.

https://doi.org/10.3390/nu18020246

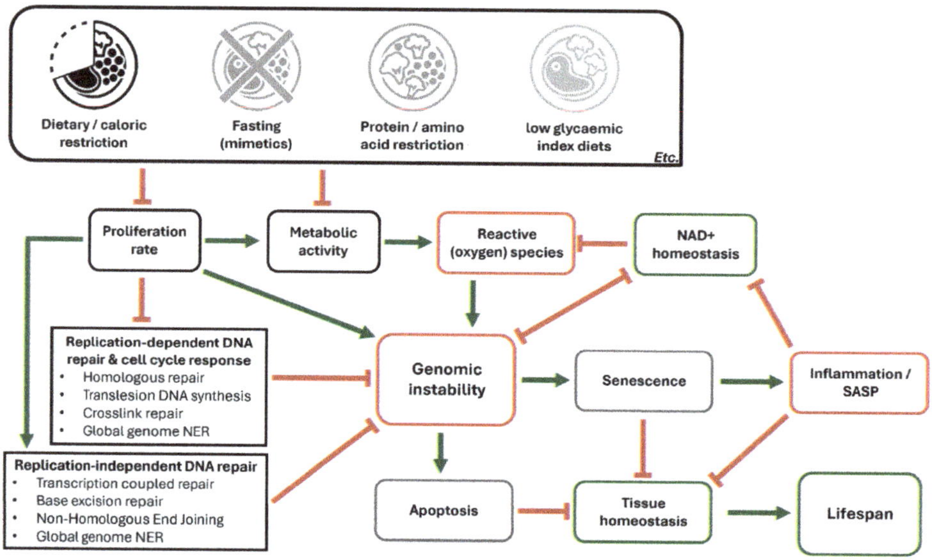

Figure 2. Dietary interventions influence genome integrity and aging-associated processes. Schematic overview of how dietary interventions modulate cellular metabolism and genomic maintenance. As caloric/dietary restriction yields the most robust effects, other diets are depicted in lighter tones. Interventions reduce proliferation and metabolic activity, lowering reactive oxygen species while improving replication-independent DNA repair, which together limit genomic instability. Enhanced DNA repair and reduced oxidative stress reduces apoptosis, senescence, and inflammation, contributing to improved tissue homeostasis and lifespan extension. Green arrows indicate promoting effects; red blunt lines indicate inhibition. Green and red outlines indicate positive and negative processes, respectively.

3.2. Additional Dietary Interventions

Other dietary modifications that affect genome stability in mice have been identified, though the evidence remains limited. Both short-term fasting and fasting-mimicking diets reduce caloric intake and are suggested to trigger protective mechanisms similar to those found in DR. Both diet types have been associated with a range of beneficial health outcomes, including enhanced stem cell regeneration and reduced inflammation across various organisms [77–80]. Likewise, alternate-day fasting reduced spindle structure abnormalities and chromosome segregation errors while restoring antioxidant defense capacity and eliminating excess reactive oxygen species (ROSs) [81]. Furthermore, fasting for a single day has been observed to improve survival rates, accompanied by increased expression of various DNA repair genes and a reduction in γH2AX foci in small intestinal epithelial stem cells, following a dose of the DNA-damaging chemotherapeutic etoposide that is lethal to fed littermates [82,83]. Together, these findings suggest that fasting, like CR/DR, may have genome-protective effects, consistent with previous reports regarding improved health in mice and other organisms [84].

Similarly, low glycemic index (GI) diets, which prioritizes the consumption of foods that induce a slower and more gradual release of glucose into the bloodstream, have been associated with improved health, likely by improving lipid metabolism and lowering postprandial hyperglycemia-associated ROS [85–87]. For instance, a study with wild-type Balb/c mice demonstrated that implementing a low GI diet late in life (20 months of age) still extended median lifespan by 12% while reducing plasma glucose levels, abasic site frequency, and levels of the DD proxy 8-OHdG [88]. Importantly, the average food

https://doi.org/10.3390/nu18020246

intake remained constant while digestible energy was only 3.5% lower in the GI diets, thus minimizing confounding effects due to CR/DR-like effects.

Macronutrients (carbohydrates, proteins, and fats) play an important role in shaping the dietary impact on health and disease. While high-fat diets (without ketone induction) are often utilized to investigate the harmful effects of obesity, modifications in dietary protein, such as the restriction of specific amino acids, enhanced both health and lifespan in wild-type mice [89–91]. For instance, methionine restriction in progeroid Hutchinson–Gilford progeria syndrome (HGPS) mutant mice extended median and maximal lifespan, and reversed transcriptomic alterations linked to inflammation and DNA repair pathways [92]. These beneficial effects are likely mediated by metabolic changes, as several associated pathways, including fatty acid metabolism, were also normalized [92]. This is further supported by studies in *Ercc1*$^{\Delta/-}$ mutant and wild-type mice indicating that adjusting macronutrient ratios, particularly the balance between carbohydrates and proteins, can enhance metabolic health and aging outcomes [30,93,94].

Curiously, despite the beneficial effects associated with protein restriction, an increase in protein intake through twice-daily supplementation of whey peptides (200–400 mg/kg) in wild-type mice also yielded positive outcomes. This supplementation protected against UVB irradiation-induced photoaging, as indicated by reduced cutaneous thickening, wrinkle formation, and melanin granules, while also preserving cutaneous elasticity, likely by reducing levels of collagen-degrading metalloproteinase-2 [95]. Furthermore, whey peptide supplementation significantly decreased the presence of Ki-67 and 8-OHdG-positive cells in the stratum basale of these chronically UVB-irradiated mice, indicating a potential role in mitigating cellular proliferation and oxidative DD, potentially mediated by VEGF [95]. While protein intake is generally associated with reduced food intake [96], the study above did not report on food intake or whey peptide-induced skin changes without chronic UVB irradiation, warranting caution and further investigation into the effects of whey peptides on genomic stability.

Integrating findings from the broader literature, we propose a (simplified) scenario for the effects of various forms of dietary interventions, particularly CR/DR, on lifespan and health, at least in part by influencing DD and DNA repair mechanisms, as presented in Figure 2, while recognizing interactive mechanisms, such as hormesis-induced resilience, likely modulate these processes both directly and indirectly. Several of the above-indicated diets overall reduce the proliferation rate of healthy body cells, which distinctively affects replication-dependent DNA repair processes like HR and XLR, as well as replication-independent DNA repair processes such as TCR and NHEJ. Combined with the suppression of metabolic activity and ROS levels, this results in a global reduction in genomic instability, lowering the incidence of cells undergoing apoptosis or entering a state of cellular senescence, preventing systemic inflammaging and functional decline in tissues [25–27,35,41,45,46,49,51,52,56,61,64,69,71–76] (Figure 2). Furthermore, factors like sex, genotype, and the specific type of dietary intervention likely influence efficacy as well, with variations in duration, meal timing, and intensity further modulating these outcomes [44,48,97,98]. Future research should examine the influence of these factors and move beyond mere correlation by directly assessing DD markers under diverse conditions to determine the causal role of these interventions on genomic stability and longevity.

3.3. Prebiotics and Probiotics

The impact of diet on the microbiota is well-documented, with numerous studies highlighting how dietary choices shape microbial communities [99–101]. Notably, aging-associated physiological changes (e.g., immune system decline and intestinal permeability) can shift the microbiota towards a less diverse and more pro-inflammatory composi-

https://doi.org/10.3390/nu18020246

tion, which has been associated with both inflammaging and frailty, further accelerating this shift [102,103]. Furthermore, this shift causally contributes to increased levels of γH2AX in the liver and heart through inhibition of DD repair and decreased antioxidant capacity [104,105], suggesting that reversal of microbiota composition through probiotic interventions might improve genomic stability.

Recent work supports this notion, where supplementation with the prebiotic neoagarotetraose in aged mice extended lifespan, reduced neuronal DD, and shifted the gut microbiota toward a more youthful, health-associated composition, resulting in increased short-chain fatty acid production and reduced neuroinflammation [106]. Similarly, specific probiotic strains such as Bifidobacterium bifidum BGN4 and Bifidobacterium longum BORI were found to reduce the number of γH2AX positive neurons in the hippocampus of aged wild-type mice [107] ‡. In another study, supplementation with Lactobacillus casei strain Shirota (LcS) ameliorated sarcopenia in SAMP8 mutant mice, a senescence-accelerated model with increased DD, by reconfiguring the microbiome and upregulating the production of short-chain fatty acids, resulting in decreased expression of apoptotic, p53 signaling, NHEJ, and inflammatory pathways in muscle tissue [108].

Additionally, early-life colonization of wild-type mice with *Lactobacillus rhamnosus* GG was associated with activation of the protective *Sirt1/Ampk/Ppargc1a* pathway, which coincided with enhanced antioxidant defenses (*Sod1* and *Sod2* upregulation) and reduced markers of DD (γH2AX) and inflammation (*Il1a, Il6, Tnf*) in the colon [109]. Furthermore, in DNA repair-deficient $Ercc1^{\Delta/-}$ mutant mice, supplementation with *Akkermansia muciniphila* mitigated age-related thinning of the colonic mucus layer and decreased the expression of pro-inflammatory genes in the colon [110]. While these findings suggest a potential mechanistic link, the precise causal contributions of microbiota-derived factors, such as short-chain fatty acids, remain to be fully elucidated [109].

Collectively, these findings suggest several potential mechanisms by which the microbiota may influence host genomic stability. Beyond the observed modulation of inflammatory responses and enhancement of antioxidant defenses, other mechanisms may include the microbiota's influence on host metabolism and nutrient absorption, affecting the availability of essential cofactors for DNA repair enzymes [111,112]. While further research is needed to fully elucidate these mechanisms and exclude artificial explanations, such as multiple-testing artifacts, the emerging evidence suggests that targeted modulation of the gut microbiota through probiotic interventions or dietary changes could be a promising strategy to promote genomic stability.

3.4. Micronutrients

Maintaining essential micronutrients within specific physiological ranges is crucial for optimal cellular function and the prevention of adverse health outcomes, while deviations from these ranges can lead be permanent detrimental outcomes [113–115]. Despite extensive research documenting the impact of micronutrient deficiencies on health [116–118], the precise extent of these optimal dose ranges and their impact on genomic stability in mice remain poorly characterized.

Most research investigating the role of micronutrients in genomic stability in mice primarily focuses on their antioxidant potential. For instance, vitamin C supplementation has been shown to exert varying effects on DNA integrity depending on environmental and genetic context, with benefits observed in Werner syndrome progeroid mutant mice ($Wrn^{\Delta hel/\Delta hel}$) and wild-type C57BL/6J mice, while vitamin C supplementation had no effect on wild-type mice under cold stress conditions [119–121]. Similarly, studies on vitamin E supplementation have yielded mixed results. In DNA repair-deficient progeroid $Xpg^{-/-}$ mutant mice, vitamin E has been associated with a reduction in the number of TRP53-

https://doi.org/10.3390/nu18020246

positive cells and an extension of neurological healthspan [122] ‡. However, other studies have reported no significant effect of vitamin E on oxidative DD in wild-type mice [123,124], although vitamin E was observed to increase both median and maximum lifespan, likely through enhanced resilience mechanisms [124]. Adding to the growing evidence that micronutrients may affect the genome, recent data show that folic acid, a vitamin B9 precursor, can mitigate radiation-induced lung injury by suppressing senescence-associated signaling [125].

Multi-micronutrient supplementation has shown promise in enhancing genomic stability and mitigating DD. Studies have reported increased long-term survival following radiation or genotoxic exposure [126,127], reduced apoptosis in *Apoe*$^{-/-}$ mutant mice on a high-fat diet [128], and lower levels of malondialdehyde and 8-OHdG oxidative stress markers in prematurely aging mutant mice [129].

Based on the studies reviewed, the potential benefits of optimizing micronutrient dosages beyond adequate levels remain unclear. When present at adequate levels, micronutrients appear to delay age-associated metabolic changes and reduce genomic instability. However, to what extent are these effects attributable to antioxidant activity or metabolic regulation, rather than alternative mechanisms, is currently largely unknown [130]. Beyond direct redox actions, micronutrients may indirectly influence genome integrity by modulating cellular stress responses, metabolic homeostasis, or damage tolerance pathways in a compound-specific manner. Such effects could alter either the burden of DNA damage or its downstream consequences, highlighting the need for further research in this area.

3.5. Fatty Acids

Recent work highlights the role of fatty acids, specifically omega-3 polyunsaturated fatty acids (*n*-3 PUFAs), in the context of DD and repair. Docosahexaenoic acid (DHA) is a major *n*-3 PUFA found in fish oil, which plays a pivotal role in reducing oxidative stress and enhancing genomic stability. This effect is mediated through the upregulation of antioxidant enzymes SOD1, SOD2, and catalase in the liver and heart, thereby reducing oxidative stress markers and, e.g., protecting against telomere shortening [131]. DHA also alleviates cellular senescence and ameliorates inflammation and γH2AX accumulation through improved mitochondrial homeostasis and recruitment of PARP1, a key component in the DD response, in telomerase-deficient mutant mice [132].

Additionally, maternal diets rich in *n*-3 PUFAs have been proposed to enhance homeostatic control, leading to the suppression of aberrant cell proliferation in the F1 offspring of breast cancer-prone mutant mice. This improved homeostatic regulation is associated with upregulation of pathways related to p53 signaling, DNA repair, and inflammatory responses [133]. Notably, while *n*-3 PUFAs appear beneficial in wild-type mice, a study with *Ercc1*$^{-/-}$ mutant mice demonstrated that a diet high in safflower oil, consisting of ~90% *n*-6 and *n*-9 PUFAs [134], actually shortened lifespan and increased γH2AX in vitro [135], suggesting a potential hormetic or PUFA-specific effect on DD.

Extra virgin olive oil (EVOO), a rich source of monounsaturated fatty acids, has been associated with enhanced genome stability by counteracting hypomethylation induced by environmental carcinogens such as dimethylbenz[a]anthracene and trifluoroacetic acid. This protection may help suppress hypomethylation-driven LINE-1 retrotransposon activity, a class of mutagenic non-coding DNA [136,137]. The current number of mechanistic studies is, however, limited, and further research is needed to characterize the involved molecular compounds and validate these effects more broadly.

In conclusion, fatty acids, particularly *n*-3 PUFAs and monounsaturated fatty acids, exhibit potential in promoting genomic stability and reducing DD, in contrast to *n*-6 and *n*-9 PUFAs, which might be able to increase DD. These effects are likely achieved through

https://doi.org/10.3390/nu18020246

oxidative stress reduction, telomere preservation, and cellular senescence alleviation. However, the varied impact of different PUFAs on DD pathways highlights the complexity and potential specificity of these interactions, necessitating further research to fully understand these mechanisms in relation to genome stability.

3.6. Hormones

Diet influences many somatic processes, including hormone levels. The importance of hormones in somatic functions has long been recognized, and there is growing evidence that hormone regulation through supplementation can play a role in maintaining genomic stability and mitigating age-related decline. For example, supplementation with dehydroepiandrosterone (DHEA), a steroid hormone precursor and ligand of PPARα, PXR, and CAR [138], delays the age-associated decline in oocyte cohesin levels and reduces the level of γH2AX foci in aged wild-type C57BL/6J mice [139]. This improved chromosomal stability correlates with decreased oocyte apoptosis and amelioration of follicle count, ovarian aging, and fertility decline [139].

Melatonin, a sleep–wake cycle synchronizing hormone and potent antioxidant whose production diminishes with aging, shows promising effects on DNA repair mechanisms in a supplementation time-dependent manner. In aged wild-type Swiss albino mice, eighteen months of melatonin supplementation starting at three months of age increased lifespan, reduced DD markers, and increased the levels of APE1 and OGG1 repair enzymes, indicating an enhanced DNA repair capacity [140]. This effect may be attributed to melatonin's ability to modulate circadian rhythms and sleep patterns, which also influence cellular repair processes [141,142]. However, it is unknown how well this treatment would translate to other mouse models, as Swiss mice exhibit a 94% reduction in pineal gland melatonin levels, but only a 25% reduction in plasma when compared to wild-type C3H/HENHSD mice [143], complicating the interpretation of these findings.

3.7. Nicotinamide Adenine Dinucleotide Precursors

One process closely regulated by the circadian rhythm is the synthesis of nicotinamide adenine dinucleotide (NAD+), a vital coenzyme that plays a critical role in numerous cellular processes, including energy metabolism, DNA repair, and epigenetic regulation. However, with aging, NAD+ levels decline due to several factors, including senescence-associated CD38 activation, increased consumption by poly(ADP-ribose) polymerases (PARPs) in response to DD, and declining biosynthesis efficiency [144–146]. To counteract this age-related decline, supplementation with precursors such as nicotinamide (NA), nicotinamide mononucleotide (NMN), and nicotinamide riboside (NR) has been proposed. These precursors boost NAD+ availability and could thus enhance cellular repair and overall cellular health. Importantly, reported health benefits of NAD+ precursors can reflect both NAD+-dependent DD signaling and/or repair and indirect effects via improved mitochondrial function, redox homeostasis, and inflammatory signaling that may reduce the upstream burden of DD.

One of the key consumers of NAD+ is sirtuins, a class of NAD+-dependent deacetylases important for various processes, including metabolism, inflammation, and apoptosis [147–150]. Supplementation with NAD+ precursors have, likely due to its central role across various cellular pathways, shown promise in various disease models. In a mouse model of alcohol-associated liver disease, NA lowered the expression of DD marker genes (e.g., *Rec8* and *E2f1*) while upregulating *Sirt1* [151]. Likewise, in a D-galactose-induced aging model, NMN improved locomotor activity and spatial memory, attenuated oxidative stress, neuroinflammation, and apoptosis, and preserved intestinal barrier integrity. Notably, these benefits were abolished by pharmacological SIRT1 inhibition, underscoring the

https://doi.org/10.3390/nu18020246

importance of SIRT1 [152]. In Alzheimer's disease models, NR supplementation has been reported to effectively decrease microglia and astrocyte activation and reduce neuroinflammation, senescence markers, and apoptosis in hippocampal neurons, while also promoting mitophagy, synaptic function, and cognition [153–155]. Complementing these findings, NR modulates brain region-specific redox and metabolic networks, enhancing mitochondrial pathways in the cerebral cortex and neurotransmitter regulation in the hippocampus [156]. In the cardiovascular system of *Snhg12*$^{-/-}$ mutant mice, a model of atherosclerotic lesion formation characterized by DD and senescence, NR significantly abrogated γH2AX foci formation and related senescence markers, an effect that may reflect reduced damage accumulation and/or altered damage signaling [157]. Some of these beneficial effects extend to DNA-repair-deficient models of accelerated aging like *Csb*$^{-/-}$ and *Ercc1*$^{\Delta/-}$ mutant mice, where NR supplementation sustains SIRT1 activity, maintains mitochondrial function, and partially ameliorates their progeroid phenotypes [158,159], despite their inherently lowered DNA repair capacity, suggesting that these health benefits likely arise from mechanisms distinct from direct enhancement of repair.

NR has also demonstrated potential in improving genomic stability in *Tert*$^{-/-}$ mutant models by preserving telomere length and attenuating 53BP1-associated DD signaling. This leads to enhanced mitochondrial function and reduced systemic inflammation, ultimately mitigating hematopoietic myeloid skewing [160] ‡. Another NAD+ supplement, NMN, has also shown beneficial effects in *Tert*$^{-/-}$ mice, as it reduced liver fibrosis, an effect that appears to be partially dependent on SIRT1 activation [161] ‡. Additionally, NMN can rejuvenate mitochondrial function in aged oocytes of healthy wild-type mice, resulting in improved redox homeostasis, reduced endogenous γH2AX foci, and normalized spindle and chromosome structure [162,163].

These studies, along with others that supplement NAD+ precursors through injection [164–169], collectively highlight the broad-ranging benefits of NAD+ precursors in counteracting age-related cellular decline. While direct stimulation of NAD$^+$-dependent DNA repair pathways may contribute, reductions in DD markers are likely mediated indirectly through improved mitochondrial function and the consequent reduction in endogenous damage burden. Distinguishing direct repair enhancement from secondary protective effects in vivo remains an important objective for future research. Overall, by supporting metabolic health and enhancing cellular resilience against DD, NAD+ precursors show promise as therapeutic agents for promoting longevity and mitigating the effects of aging and diseases associated with genomic instability.

3.8. Plant Derivatives

A substantial number of plant-derived compounds have been reported to enhance genomic stability. However, many of these compounds have not been comprehensively studied in relation to DD in mice. Nonetheless, a large proportion is reported to exhibit common biological effects like enhanced mitochondrial function, reduced inflammation, or the induction of cellular stress responses, thereby promoting genomic stability, immune function, and fertility [170–189] ‡.

Additionally, some plant derivatives have demonstrated protective effects against exogenous sources of DD. For example, theaflavins [190], carotenoids [191], and several plant extracts and compound derivates [192–198] ‡ have been shown to possess radioprotective properties, mitigating DD and related effects induced by UVB and gamma radiation. Furthermore, theaflavins [199] and Shoutai pills [200] have also been reported to confer protection against DD induced by chemotherapy, as evidenced by reduced γH2AX levels in wild-type mice. Some plant-derived substances have also shown efficacy in mitigating genomic insults induced by injury [201,202], exposure to genotoxic chemicals [203,204],

https://doi.org/10.3390/nu18020246

or iron-induced oxidative stress [205]. Other compounds have exhibited anticarcinogenic properties in cancer-prone contexts [206,207] ‡ or in carcinogen-related causes of cancer [208,209], highlighting the potential of plant derivatives not only to prevent DD but also to mitigate its long-term consequences across various contexts of genomic stress.

While many studies are fragmentary and the efficacy and precise mechanisms of many of these plant-derived substances in DD and repair are incompletely understood, the consistency in their downstream effects, e.g., enhanced cellular resilience and improved DNA repair, lends credibility to their potential therapeutic value. Further investigation into these shared mechanisms could reveal broader applications for DNA repair and cellular health, potentially leading to the development of novel therapeutic strategies based on these natural compounds.

3.9. Synthetic Drugs

Natural compounds have frequently inspired the development of synthetic drugs, which, in some cases, also exhibit potential in enhancing genomic stability and modulating the effects of natural aging. These synthetic compounds exert their influence through mechanisms similar to their natural counterparts, including the regulation of energy metabolism, resilience, and inflammation.

For instance, the oral administration of the antioxidant butylated hydroxyanisole, as well as the antioxidant inducer oltipraz, have been demonstrated to reduce endogenous single-strand DD in the liver during aging of wild-type Swiss-Webster mice, likely through the preservation of glutathione levels [210]. Similarly, metformin, a widely used antidiabetic drug, has been found to decrease ROS production, upregulate antioxidant enzymes, and inhibit γH2AX and cellular senescence in various disease models [211–214].

Beyond general antioxidant and metabolic effects, several synthetic compounds have demonstrated specific interactions with distinct cellular processes that contribute to genomic stability and the modulation of aging [215–218] ‡. For instance, the small-molecule DDO1002, an NRF2–KEAP1 PPI inhibitor, lowered intracellular ROS and reduced the DD marker γH2AX, delayed cellular senescence, and improved regenerative capacity in wild-type C57BL/6J aged or irradiated hematopoietic stem cells [218]. Another example is aspirin and its nitric oxide-donating derivative, which mitigate microsatellite instability in a Lynch syndrome mouse model deficient in mismatch repair (MMR), leading to increased lifespan through the modulation of stress-related signaling pathways [219]. Low-dose aspirin likewise showed a tendency toward extended lifespan in DNA repair-deficient $Xpg^{-/-}$ mutant mice (p = 0.056) [159]. Exogenous protection has also been reported. The fatty acid oxidation inhibitor meldonium reduces mitochondrial DD and improves cognitive function in aged wild-type mice subjected to LPS-induced inflammation [220]. The senolytic compound ABT-263, a Bcl-2/Bcl-xL inhibitor, selectively eliminated doxorubicin-induced senescent retinal pigment epithelial cells and alleviated retinal degeneration in wild-type mice, while reducing CDKN1A (p21) and CDKN2A (p16) protein levels, suggesting mitigation of DD-associated senescence [221].

In mutant models with deficient DNA repair accelerated aging, synthetic compounds have also demonstrated significant benefits. In $Ercc1^{\Delta/-}$ mice, treatment with the HSP90 inhibitor and senolytic agent 17-DMAG reduced *Cdkn2a* expression and cellular senescence [222] ‡. Additionally, the compound UCM-13207 has been found to extend lifespan and improve healthspan in HGPS models by reducing nuclear levels of progerin, thereby decreasing senescence and the γH2AX DD markers associated with it [223]. Interestingly, since progerin levels also gradually increase during natural aging, it may be worthwhile to validate this treatment in wild-type models.

https://doi.org/10.3390/nu18020246

While these findings are promising, most of these substances have primarily been studied in specific contexts characterized by heightened DD or impaired repair capacity. Further research is needed to fully elucidate the potential of these compounds in mitigating genome instability-driven aging across broader contexts and conditions.

3.10. Miscellaneous Compounds and Interventions

A variety of substances, not classified under the earlier categories used in this study, along with combinations of previously discussed interventions [224,225], have shown potential in enhancing genomic stability. Many of these compounds, like hydrolyzed chicken extract ‡ and royal jelly, modulate ROS homeostasis similarly to other treatments previously examined [226,227]. This modulation can result in a decrease in DD markers, like γH2AX and 8-OHdG, following genomic insults [227–230], while some of these interventions also prolong the lifespan of wild-type and *Atm*-deficient mutant mice [226,231,232]. However, the relationship between these substances and genome stability in mice has often been explored in only a single study, limiting the generalizability of these findings beyond their specific experimental conditions. For example, spermidine has recently been recognized as a pro-longevity drug that protects wild-type C57BL/6J mice against the genotoxic and mutagenic compound 4-nitroquinoline 1-oxide, resulting in a slowdown of oral carcinoma development and a reduction in DD, as measured by γH2AX and comet assay tail moment [233].

Another compound, taurine, a semi-essential amino sulfonic acid, has recently been identified to influence aging. Circulating taurine levels decline with age in mice, monkeys, and humans, and supplementation was shown to reduce DD, cellular senescence, and mitochondrial dysfunction while extending lifespan in various organisms, including wild-type mice [234].

Another relatively well-documented substance is pyrroloquinoline quinone (PQQ), a vitamin-like biofactor that has shown to exert genome-protective effects in various situations of increased genomic instability [235]. $Bmi^{-/-}$ mutant mice exhibit increased oxidative damage, reduced cell proliferation, increased cell senescence, and compromised collagen synthesis due to enhanced matrix metalloproteinase activity. PQQ supplementation alleviated these pathological changes and reduced oxidative damage and DD, as indicated by decreased γH2AX markers [236,237]. In osteoporosis-prone orchiectomy mice, PQQ lowered the DD-related markers γH2AX, TRP53, CHK2, and NFκB p65 [238]. Similarly, in natural aging-related osteoporosis in wild-type mice, PQQ supplementation reduced oxidative stress, osteocyte senescence, and DD (8-OHdG immunostaining) while preventing bone loss. This involved stabilization of MCM3 and activation of the Keap1-Nrf2 axis, which strengthened antioxidant defenses and reduced DD in osteoblasts [239]. In a model of osteoarthritis induced by anterior cruciate ligament transection, PQQ treatment reduced DD, inflammation, and senescence in articular cartilage compared to sham-operated controls [240], suggesting a potential role in genomic stability and longevity.

In conclusion, various compounds, such as royal jelly and PQQ, show promise in enhancing genomic stability and reducing DD markers. While these interventions have demonstrated benefits under specific experimental conditions, the limited number of studies in relation to natural aging calls for further research to validate their broader applicability. Expanding research in this area could pave the way for novel therapeutic strategies aimed at preserving genome integrity and promoting healthy aging.

4. Discussion

Aging is affected by various factors. One of these is dietary consumption, which influences homeostasis by modulating energy balance, metabolic fitness, and overall health.

https://doi.org/10.3390/nu18020246

Alterations to these processes, e.g., by excessive food intake [26], are closely linked to aging and age-related diseases, with DD being a significant mediator, as shown by DNA repair-deficient syndromes and progeroid mouse models. In this review, we highlighted and assessed the evidence of known nutritional interventions that improve genomic stability and healthy aging in mice. Many interventions discussed here, particularly CR/DR and their mimetics, act on more than one mechanistic layer (e.g., different DNA repair processes, metabolism, and/or antioxidant systems; see also Figure 2), complicating causal interpretation when relying solely on DD markers or lifespan readouts. Moreover, while some dietary interventions have been studied for decades, others are supported by only a limited number of small studies, and relatively few directly assess DD or DNA repair. In Figure 3, we outline the relationship between DNA damage, response signaling, and repair, and their effects on resilience; summarize the relative fidelity and specificity of common biomarkers; and provide a qualitative contextual overview of the discussed literature. Interventions were positioned based on the amount and consistency of available data, and on how the reported outcomes relate to genomic stability (DD markers and/or repair readouts). As such, Figure 3 should be viewed as a guide to where evidence is stronger and where important gaps remain.

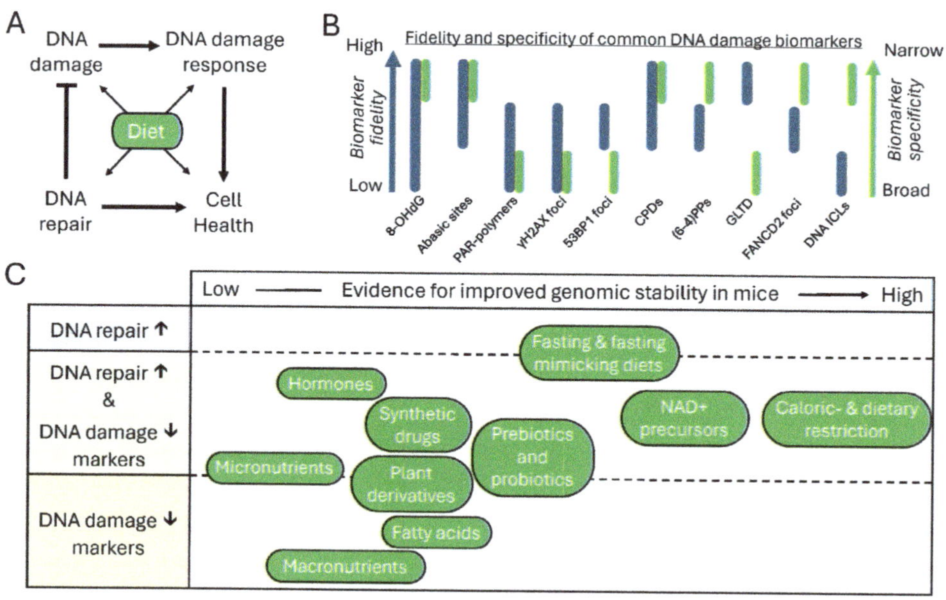

Figure 3. Schematic representation of consumable interventions and their impact on DNA damage and repair. (**A**) Simplified schematic depicting the relationships between DNA damage burden, DNA repair, DNA damage response signaling, and cellular health, which all could be affected by dietary interventions. Note that by altering metabolism, diet could influence DNA damage bidirectionally. (**B**) Relative technique-dependent detection fidelity (blue) and biomarker specificity (green) of commonly used DNA damage markers. Bar ranges reflect variability among measurement techniques and biomarker specificity (also see details on biomarker specificity and accuracy/reliability of the detection method in Table 1). (**C**) Interventions are categorized into three groups: those that increase DNA repair (**top**), those that reduce DNA damage (**bottom**), and those that have dual effects (**middle**). The horizontal positioning of interventions reflects the strength of evidence supporting their effects, with those on the right, such as CR/DR, being more strongly supported by evidence than those on the left, which in contrast mostly consisted of interventions based on a few studies, sometimes using only a single marker.

https://doi.org/10.3390/nu18020246

Limitations of this study include the lack of a formal quality assessment, as usually indicated in systematic reviews. Instead, our semi-systematic search resulted in a broad overview of the literature, for which we acknowledge a potential bias due to high heterogeneity between studies (i.e., due to varying mouse strains, tissues, intervention lengths, and markers) and/or a small number of studies per compound, making reproducibility unclear. Such compounds/interventions with limited studies are therefore also more depicted on the left side of Figure 3. Concomitantly, tissue-specific effects, strain variability, or sex differences are not discussed or only marginally indicated, due to the limited number of studies identified for several dietary interventions, particularly plant derivatives and synthetic drugs, which often assessed only a single or less specific biomarker, limiting generalizability. However, we do refer to such reviews with a focus on the most robust health- and lifespan-extending intervention: calorie restriction [34,44,48]. Moreover, this review was intended to reveal interventions that could enhance genomic stability and to serve as guide for future longevity research. As such, we revealed many connections of nutrition-based interventions affecting genome integrity for further exploration.

The restriction of diet (CR/DR), which is known to robustly delay aging in a wide range of organisms separated by large evolutionary distances, from mice to non-human primates, indicating that its underlying molecular mechanism is strongly conserved, is emerging as a genuine, potent modulator of DD, repair, and response processes in various organisms [14,45,51,241]. Besides extending lifespan and improving genomic stability through the above-indicated mechanisms, CR (mimetics) influence multiple age-related nodes, including epigenetic integrity, autophagy, and activation of cellular stress responses [242–245]. Thus, genome maintenance appears to be part of a coordinated resilience program aiming to promote cellular and organismal survival at the expense of growth.

Beyond model systems, CR and related strategies such as intermittent fasting are being explored in oncology and neurodegeneration, with early trials indicating feasibility and acceptable safety. However, efficacy in humans remains inconclusive, potentially reflecting adherence challenges, mismatches with standard-of-care regimens, or biological differences [245–249]. Species-specific physiological features, such as higher mass-specific metabolic rates, shorter lifespans, and accelerated molecular turnover in mice, are likely to shape both damage accumulation and responsiveness to intervention. These differences suggest that dietary interventions that robustly extend lifespan or reduce DD in mice may require careful adjustment in timing, duration, or intensity to achieve benefits in humans.

Interestingly, many of the interventions discussed here act on a subset of mechanisms employed by CR/DR, hence operating as partial mimetics without necessitating reduced food intake [250]. NAD^+ precursors such as NMN and NR, for example, activate sirtuins and improve mitochondrial function, recapitulating some CR/DR-associated benefits; however, current evidence suggests that their effects on genomic stability are largely indirect, arising from improved metabolic homeostasis, reduced inflammation, and enhanced cellular stress resilience rather than from direct stimulation of DNA repair [251,252]. Another emerging class of metabolic modulators includes GLP-1R and GIPR agonists, such as semaglutide and tirzepatide, which reduce appetite, lower body weight, and counteract metabolic diseases like diabetes. While their primary mechanisms involve metabolic regulation, their potential effects on genomic stability and aging remain underexplored. Given their strong influence on energy balance and cellular stress pathways, future studies should assess whether these compounds also contribute to DD mitigation or repair processes, potentially offering novel avenues for aging interventions.

However, while some interventions demonstrate promising results, their effects are often less pronounced or process-specific. To remedy this, future research should focus on exploring combinations of dissimilar interventions to identify optimal strategies for miti-

https://doi.org/10.3390/nu18020246

gating DD and promoting longevity [253,254]. Another aspect that should be considered is that basal genotoxic exposure, energy expenditure, and cell division rates vary between tissues, leading to non-uniform aging that might influence the organ-specific efficacy of these interventions.

Currently, much of the research in this field is rather fragmented or inconsistent, with highly variable techniques like the comet assay and frequent reliance on RNA expression data without confirming protein levels or functional impact on DNA repair. Establishing rigorous markers for assessing DD and genome instability, such as γH2AX foci, 53BP1, or RAD51 foci, and novel nanopore-based structural analysis for DNA damage [255], along with standardized protocols, would greatly enhance study reproducibility and comparability. Without such consistency, drawing reliable conclusions about the effectiveness of nutritional interventions remains challenging.

Beyond methodological inconsistencies, another challenge lies in testing these findings in a real-world setting. Laboratory experiments often focus on endogenous or supraphysiological levels of exogenous DD, while real-world conditions present additional challenges from environmental stressors. Future studies should incorporate realistic environmental insults to genome stability to better assess the efficacy of interventions. Moreover, the issue of survival bias in publishing needs consideration, as positive results are much more likely to be published, skewing the perceived efficacy of interventions. Potential translation to humans is additionally complicated because some interventions are mentally exhaustive (CR/DR), expensive (synthetic diet to limit specific amino acids), or prone to interfere with social aspects of life (fasting). In contrast, other interventions like NAD+ precursors or oral medication are quite feasible and are being actively trialed in humans [256–258].

One key area of debate in this context is the role of oxidative stress and antioxidants in genomic stability. While many studies focus on the antioxidative properties of a substance, evidence that ROS at physiological levels causes genomic damage [259–261], or that antioxidants are beneficial protectors of the genome [262–264], is heavily debated. Moreover, studies in humans have often yielded negative results, with various meta-analyses even suggesting a likely increase in disease incidence [265,266]. While the exact reasons for this are unknown, dosage and context might be an important factor, highlighting the limited ability of in vitro antioxidant assays to predict in vivo efficacy [267]. For example, while physiological levels of vitamin C behave largely as an antioxidant in vivo, pharmacological dosing can shift toward prooxidant activity via Fenton chemistry. Moreover, although the increase in oxidative DD and engagement of DNA repair pathways can be beneficial in some situations (e.g., cancer treatment), it does show the importance of situational awareness and balanced application of these and similar types of compounds [268,269]. Additionally, the genome-protective effects of many so-called "antioxidative" compounds extend beyond simple ROS scavenging, as they often also modulate stress resilience pathways and energy metabolism to improve cellular function, longevity, and genomic maintenance [270–272].

Alternatively, compounds that boost endogenous antioxidant systems (e.g., as associated with fasting and DR) might result in a stronger and more adjusted response than the artificial administration of exogenous antioxidants. The optimal timing and duration of interventions targeting ROS and genomic stability also warrant consideration. While some approaches may require lifelong implementation (e.g., ROS scavengers), there is a growing interest in compounds that potentiate long-term effects to improve efficacy and reduce costs. Elucidating these aspects will therefore be crucial for developing targeted therapeutic applications.

https://doi.org/10.3390/nu18020246

5. Conclusions

In conclusion, the modulation of genomic instability by consumable interventions holds considerable promise, but future research should broaden their focus beyond antioxidant mechanisms and extend the scope of investigation to include the effects of these interventions on the natural aging process. Moreover, combinatory approaches may yield synergistic benefits, leading to a deeper understanding of the underlying mechanisms and the development of more comprehensive strategies for promoting genomic stability and healthy aging.

Supplementary Materials: The following supporting information can be downloaded at: https://www.mdpi.com/article/10.3390/nu18020246/s1, File S1: Keywords and search query; File S2: PubMed references search 1 (till March 2023); File S3: PubMed references search 2 (2023–2025).

Author Contributions: I.v.G. collected, analyzed, and graded relevant scientific literature, and drafted the manuscript. J.H.J.H. and W.P.V. provided feedback and support throughout the writing process. Additionally, W.P.V. contributed to the analysis and grading of scientific papers that were ambiguous in relation to the selection criteria. All authors have read and agreed to the published version of the manuscript.

Funding: This research was funded by ONCODE, supported by the Dutch Cancer Society. J.H.J.H. was additionally supported by the National Institute of Health (NIH)/National Institute of Aging (NIA) (AG17242), the European Research Council Advanced Grant Dam2Age, and the Deutsche Forschungsgemeinschaft (DFG, German Research Foundation—Project-ID 73111208—SFB 829). J.H.J.H. and W.P.V. were supported by Memorabel (ZonMW 733050810), BBoL (NWO-ENW 737.016.015), and the European Joint Programme on Rare Diseases (TC-NER RD20-113). W.P.V. was supported by the Regiodeal Foodvalley (162135) and the ADPS Longevity Research Award.

Data Availability Statement: The original contributions presented in this study are included in the article/Supplementary Material. Further inquiries can be directed to the corresponding author.

Acknowledgments: Generative AI tools were used for minor improvements to grammar and sentence structure, but not for data acquisition or analysis. The authors reviewed and edited AI-generated changes and take full responsibility for the content of this publication.

Conflicts of Interest: The authors declare no conflict of interest.

Abbreviations

The following abbreviations are used in this manuscript:

DD	DNA damage
BER	Base excision repair
NER	Nucleotide excision repair
TCR	Transcription-coupled repair
HR	Homologous recombination
NHEJ	Non-homologous end joining
DR	Dietary restriction
CR	Caloric restriction
IGF1	Insulin-like growth factor
ICL	Interstrand crosslink
DSB	Double-strand break
8-OHdG	8-Hydroxyguanosine
UDS	Unscheduled DNA synthesis
GG-NER	Global genome nucleotide excision repair
XLR	Crosslink repair
GLTD	Gene length-dependent transcriptional decline

https://doi.org/10.3390/nu18020246

HSCs	Hematopoietic stem cells
ROS	Reactive oxygen species
GI	Glycemic index
HGPS	Hutchinson–Gilford progeria syndrome
PUFAs	Polyunsaturated fatty acids
DHA	Docosahexaenoic acid
EVOO	Extra virgin olive oil
DHEA	Dehydroepiandrosterone
NAD	Nicotinamide adenine dinucleotide
PARP	Poly ADP-ribose polymerase
NA	Nicotinamide
NMN	Nicotinamide mononucleotide
NR	Nicotinamide riboside
MMR	Mismatch repair
PQQ	Pyrroloquinoline quinone

References

1. Judge, A.; Dodd, M.S. Metabolism. *Essays Biochem.* **2020**, *64*, 607–647. [CrossRef] [PubMed]
2. Li, B.; Tang, X.; Le, G. Dietary Habits and Metabolic Health. *Nutrients* **2023**, *15*, 3975. [CrossRef] [PubMed]
3. Clemente-Suárez, V.J.; Beltrán-Velasco, A.I.; Redondo-Flórez, L.; Martín-Rodríguez, A.; Tornero-Aguilera, J.F. Global Impacts of Western Diet and Its Effects on Metabolism and Health: A Narrative Review. *Nutrients* **2023**, *15*, 2749. [CrossRef] [PubMed]
4. Papadaki, A.; Nolen-Doerr, E.; Mantzoros, C.S. The Effect of the Mediterranean Diet on Metabolic Health: A Systematic Review and Meta-Analysis of Controlled Trials in Adults. *Nutrients* **2020**, *12*, 3342. [CrossRef]
5. Fernández-Verdejo, R.; Moya-Osorio, J.L.; Fuentes-López, E.; Galgani, J.E. Metabolic health and its association with lifestyle habits according to nutritional status in Chile: A cross-sectional study from the National Health Survey 2016–2017. *PLoS ONE* **2020**, *15*, e0236451. [CrossRef]
6. Barzilai, N.; Huffman, D.M.; Muzumdar, R.H.; Bartke, A. The Critical Role of Metabolic Pathways in Aging. *Diabetes* **2012**, *61*, 1315–1322. [CrossRef]
7. Hamrick, M.W.; Stranahan, A.M. Metabolic regulation of aging and age-related disease. *Ageing Res. Rev.* **2020**, *64*, 101175. [CrossRef]
8. Abdellatif, M.; Rainer, P.P.; Sedej, S.; Kroemer, G. Hallmarks of cardiovascular ageing. *Nat. Rev. Cardiol.* **2023**, *20*, 754–777. [CrossRef]
9. Wilson, D.M.; Cookson, M.R.; Van Den Bosch, L.; Zetterberg, H.; Holtzman, D.M.; Dewachter, I. Hallmarks of neurodegenerative diseases. *Cell* **2023**, *186*, 693–714. [CrossRef]
10. Hanahan, D.; Weinberg, R.A. Hallmarks of Cancer: The Next Generation. *Cell* **2011**, *144*, 646–674. [CrossRef]
11. Hoeijmakers, J.H.J. DNA Damage, Aging, and Cancer. *N. Engl. J. Med.* **2009**, *361*, 1475–1485. [CrossRef] [PubMed]
12. Schumacher, B.; Pothof, J.; Vijg, J.; Hoeijmakers, J.H.J. The central role of DNA damage in the ageing process. *Nature* **2021**, *592*, 695–703. [CrossRef]
13. Niedernhofer, L.J.; Gurkar, A.U.; Wang, Y.; Vijg, J.; Hoeijmakers, J.H.J.; Robbins, P.D. Nuclear Genomic Instability and Aging. *Annu. Rev. Biochem.* **2018**, *87*, 295–322. [CrossRef] [PubMed]
14. Gyenis, A.; Chang, J.; Demmers, J.J.P.G.; Bruens, S.T.; Barnhoorn, S.; Brandt, R.M.C.; Baar, M.P.; Raseta, M.; Derks, K.W.J.; Hoeijmakers, J.H.J.; et al. Genome-wide RNA polymerase stalling shapes the transcriptome during aging. *Nat. Genet.* **2023**, *55*, 268–279. [CrossRef] [PubMed]
15. Chatterjee, N.; Walker, G.C. Mechanisms of DNA damage, repair, and mutagenesis. *Env. Mol. Mutagen.* **2017**, *58*, 235–263. [CrossRef]
16. Willers, H.; Kachnic, L.A.; Luo, C.M.; Li, L.; Purschke, M.; Borgmann, K.; Held, K.D.; Powell, S.N. Biomarkers and Mechanisms of FANCD2 Function. *BioMed Res. Int.* **2008**, *2008*, 821529. [CrossRef]
17. Wu, J.H.; Jones, N.J. Assessment of DNA Interstrand Crosslinks Using the Modified Alkaline Comet Assay. In *Genetic Toxicology*; Parry, J.M., Parry, E.M., Eds.; Methods in Molecular Biology; Springer: New York, NY, USA, 2012; Volume 817, pp. 165–181. Available online: https://link.springer.com/10.1007/978-1-61779-421-6_9 (accessed on 7 October 2024).
18. Alexander, J.L.; Orr-Weaver, T.L. Replication fork instability and the consequences of fork collisions from rereplication. *Genes Dev.* **2016**, *30*, 2241–2252. [CrossRef]
19. Abbotts, R.; Wilson, D.M. Coordination of DNA single strand break repair. *Free Radic. Biol. Med.* **2017**, *107*, 228–244. [CrossRef]
20. Lu, Y.; Liu, Y.; Yang, C. Evaluating In Vitro DNA Damage Using Comet Assay. *J. Vis. Exp.* **2017**, *128*, 56450.

https://doi.org/10.3390/nu18020246

21. Gupta, A.; Hunt, C.R.; Chakraborty, S.; Pandita, R.K.; Yordy, J.; Ramnarain, D.B.; Horikoshi, N.; Pandita, T.K. Role of 53BP1 in the Regulation of DNA Double-Strand Break Repair Pathway Choice. *Radiat. Res.* **2014**, *181*, 1–8. [CrossRef]
22. Sarkaria, J.N.; Bush, C.; Eady, J.J.; Peacock, J.H.; Steel, G.G.; Yarnold, J.R. Comparison between pulsed-field gel electrophoresis and the comet assay as predictive assays for radiosensitivity in fibroblasts. *Radiat. Res.* **1998**, *150*, 17–22. [CrossRef] [PubMed]
23. May, S.; Hirsch, C.; Rippl, A.; Bürkle, A.; Wick, P. Assessing Genotoxicity of Ten Different Engineered Nanomaterials by the Novel Semi-Automated FADU Assay and the Alkaline Comet Assay. *Nanomaterials* **2022**, *12*, 220. [CrossRef] [PubMed]
24. Chao, M.R.; Evans, M.D.; Hu, C.W.; Ji, Y.; Møller, P.; Rossner, P.; Cooke, M.S. Biomarkers of nucleic acid oxidation—A summary state-of-the-art. *Redox Biol.* **2021**, *42*, 101872. [CrossRef] [PubMed]
25. Vermeij, W.P.; Hoeijmakers, J.H.; Pothof, J. Aging: Not all DNA damage is equal. *Curr. Opin. Genet. Dev.* **2014**, *26*, 124–130. [CrossRef]
26. López-Otín, C.; Galluzzi, L.; Freije, J.M.P.; Madeo, F.; Kroemer, G. Metabolic Control of Longevity. *Cell* **2016**, *166*, 802–821. [CrossRef]
27. Kaźmierczak-Barańska, J.; Boguszewska, K.; Karwowski, B.T. Nutrition Can Help DNA Repair in the Case of Aging. *Nutrients* **2020**, *12*, 3364. [CrossRef]
28. Malesza, I.J.; Malesza, M.; Walkowiak, J.; Mussin, N.; Walkowiak, D.; Aringazina, R.; Bartkowiak-Wieczorek, J.; Mądry, E. High-Fat, Western-Style Diet, Systemic Inflammation, and Gut Microbiota: A Narrative Review. *Cells* **2021**, *10*, 3164. [CrossRef]
29. Nehme, J.; Yang, D.; Altulea, A.; Varela-Eirin, M.; Wang, L.; Hu, S.; Wu, Y.; Togo, J.; Niu, C.; Speakman, J.R.; et al. High dietary protein and fat contents exacerbate hepatic senescence and SASP in mice. *FEBS J.* **2023**, *290*, 1340–1347. [CrossRef]
30. Van Galen, I.; Birkisdóttir, M.B.; Ozinga, R.A.; Brandt, R.M.C.; Barnhoorn, S.; Imholz, S.; van Oostrom, C.T.; van der Marel, R.W.G.N.; Smit, K.; Rijksen, Y.M.A.; et al. High protein intake causes gene-length-dependent transcriptional decline, shortens lifespan and accelerates ageing in progeroid DNA repair-deficient mice. *npj Metab. Health Dis.* **2025**, *3*, 20. [CrossRef]
31. Gu, D.; Andreev, K.; Dupre, M.E.; United Nations Population Division, New York, USA; Department of Population Health Sciences & Department of Sociology, Duke University, North Carolina, USA. Major Trends in Population Growth Around the World. *China CDC Wkly.* **2021**, *3*, 604–613. [CrossRef]
32. Gilleard, C. Suffering: The darker side of ageing. *J. Aging Stud.* **2018**, *44*, 28–33. [CrossRef]
33. Scott, A.J.; Ellison, M.; Sinclair, D.A. The economic value of targeting aging. *Nat. Aging* **2021**, *1*, 616–623. [CrossRef]
34. Speakman, J.R.; Mitchell, S.E. Caloric restriction. *Mol. Asp. Med.* **2011**, *32*, 159–221. [CrossRef] [PubMed]
35. Green, C.L.; Lamming, D.W.; Fontana, L. Molecular mechanisms of dietary restriction promoting health and longevity. *Nat. Rev. Mol. Cell Biol.* **2022**, *23*, 56–73. [CrossRef] [PubMed]
36. Lee, M.B.; Hill, C.M.; Bitto, A.; Kaeberlein, M. Antiaging diets: Separating fact from fiction. *Science* **2021**, *374*, eabe7365. [CrossRef] [PubMed]
37. Cerqueira, F.M.; Kowaltowski, A.J. Commonly adopted caloric restriction protocols often involve malnutrition. *Ageing Res. Rev.* **2010**, *9*, 424–430. [CrossRef]
38. Lanza, I.R.; Zabielski, P.; Klaus, K.A.; Morse, D.M.; Heppelmann, C.J.; Bergen, H.R., 3rd; Dasari, S.; Walrand, S.; Short, K.R.; Johnson, M.L.; et al. Chronic caloric restriction preserves mitochondrial function in senescence without increasing mitochondrial biogenesis. *Cell Metab.* **2012**, *16*, 777–788. [CrossRef]
39. Lee, C.K.; Klopp, R.G.; Weindruch, R.; Prolla, T.A. Gene expression profile of aging and its retardation by caloric restriction. *Science* **1999**, *285*, 1390–1393. [CrossRef]
40. Guo, Z.M.; Yang, H.; Hamilton, M.L.; VanRemmen, H.; Richardson, A. Effects of age and food restriction on oxidative DNA damage and antioxidant enzyme activities in the mouse aorta. *Mech. Ageing Dev.* **2001**, *122*, 1771–1786. [CrossRef]
41. Sohal, R.S.; Agarwal, S.; Candas, M.; Forster, M.J.; Lal, H. Effect of age and caloric restriction on DNA oxidative damage in different tissues of C57BL/6 mice. *Mech. Ageing Dev.* **1994**, *76*, 215–224. [CrossRef]
42. Benfato, I.D.; Quintanilha, A.C.S.; Henrique, J.S.; Souza, M.A.; Dos Anjos Rosário, B.; Beserra-Filho, J.I.A.; Ribeiro, A.M.; Maluf, L.L.S.; de Oliveira, C.A.M. Long-term calorie restriction prevented memory impairment in middle-aged male mice and increased a marker of DNA oxidative stress in hippocampal dentate gyrus. *Neurobiol. Learn. Mem.* **2024**, *209*, 107902. [CrossRef]
43. Qu, B.; Halliwell, B.; Ong, C.N.; Lee, B.L.; Li, Q.T. Caloric restriction prevents oxidative damage induced by the carcinogen clofibrate in mouse liver. *FEBS Lett.* **2000**, *473*, 85–88. [CrossRef] [PubMed]
44. Swindell, W.R. Dietary restriction in rats and mice: A meta-analysis and review of the evidence for genotype-dependent effects on lifespan. *Ageing Res. Rev.* **2012**, *11*, 254–270. [CrossRef] [PubMed]
45. Vermeij, W.P.; Dollé, M.E.T.; Reiling, E.; Jaarsma, D.; Payan-Gomez, C.; Bombardieri, C.R.; Wu, H.; Roks, A.J.M.; Botter, S.M.; van der Eerden, B.C.; et al. Restricted diet delays accelerated ageing and genomic stress in DNA-repair-deficient mice. *Nature* **2016**, *537*, 427–431. [CrossRef] [PubMed]
46. Birkisdóttir, M.B.; Van't Sant, L.J.; Brandt, R.M.C.; Barnhoorn, S.; Hoeijmakers, J.H.J.; Vermeij, W.P.; Jaarsma, D. Purkinje-cell-specific DNA repair-deficient mice reveal that dietary restriction protects neurons by cell-intrinsic preservation of genomic health. *Front. Aging Neurosci.* **2022**, *14*, 1095801. [CrossRef]

https://doi.org/10.3390/nu18020246

47. He, Y.; Yang, W.; Huang, L.; Mever, M.A.; Ramautar, R.; Harms, A.; Rijksen, Y.; Brandt, R.M.; Barnhoorn, S.; Smit, K.; et al. Metabolomic analysis of dietary-restriction-induced attenuation of sarcopenia in prematurely aging DNA repair-deficient mice. *J. Cachexia Sarcopenia Muscle* **2024**, *15*, 868–882. [CrossRef]
48. Mitchell, S.J.; Mitchell, J.R. Sexual dimorphism in the response to dietary restriction in mice: A systematic review of the literature. *NHA* **2022**, *7*, 87–120. [CrossRef]
49. Vermeij, W.P.; Alyodawi, K.; Van Galen, I.; Von Der Heide, J.L.; Birkisdóttir, M.B.; Sant, L.J.V.; Ozinga, R.A.; Komninos, D.S.; Smit, K.; Rijksen, Y.M.; et al. Improved health by combining dietary restriction and promoting muscle growth in DNA repair-deficient progeroid mice. *J. Cachexia Sarcopenia Muscle* **2024**, *15*, 2361–2374. [CrossRef]
50. Stefens, S.J.M.; Van Der Linden, J.; Heredia-Genestar, J.M.; Brandt, R.M.C.; Barnhoorn, S.; Nieuwenhuizen-Bakker, I.; van Vliet, N. Dietary Restriction Mitigates Vascular Aging, Modulates the CGAS—STING Pathway and Reverses Macrophage-Like VSMC Phenotypes in Progeroid DNA -Repair-Deficient ERCC1$^{\Delta/-}$ Mice. *Aging Cell* **2025**, *24*, e70062. [CrossRef]
51. Ke, Z.; Firsanov, D.; Spencer, B.; Seluanov, A.; Gorbunova, V. Short-term calorie restriction enhances DNA repair by non-homologous end joining in mice. *npj Aging Mech. Dis.* **2020**, *6*, 9. [CrossRef]
52. Cabelof, D.C.; Yanamadala, S.; Raffoul, J.J.; Guo, Z.; Soofi, A.; Heydari, A.R. Caloric restriction promotes genomic stability by induction of base excision repair and reversal of its age-related decline. *DNA Repair* **2003**, *2*, 295–307. [CrossRef] [PubMed]
53. Stuart, J.A.; Karahalil, B.; Hogue, B.A.; Souza-Pinto, N.C.; Bohr, V.A. Mitochondrial and nuclear DNA base excision repair are affected differently by caloric restriction. *FASEB J.* **2004**, *18*, 595–597. [CrossRef] [PubMed]
54. Swindell, W.R. Gene expression profiling of long-lived dwarf mice: Longevity-associated genes and relationships with diet, gender and aging. *BMC Genom.* **2007**, *8*, 353. [CrossRef] [PubMed]
55. Swift, L.P.; Lagerholm, B.C.; Henderson, L.R.; Ratnaweera, M.; Baddock, H.T.; Sengerova, B.; Lee, S.; Cruz-Migoni, A.; Waithe, D.; Renz, C.; et al. SNM1A is crucial for efficient repair of complex DNA breaks in human cells. *Nat. Commun.* **2024**, *15*, 5392. [CrossRef]
56. Van't Sant, L.J.; Birkisdóttir, M.B.; Ozinga, R.A.; Gyenis, Á.; Hoeijmakers, J.H.J.; Vermeij, W.P.; Jaarsma, D. Gene expression changes in cerebellum induced by dietary restriction. *Front. Mol. Neurosci.* **2023**, *16*, 1185665. [CrossRef]
57. Lee, C.K.; Allison, D.B.; Brand, J.; Weindruch, R.; Prolla, T.A. Transcriptional profiles associated with aging and middle age-onset caloric restriction in mouse hearts. *Proc. Natl. Acad. Sci. USA* **2002**, *99*, 14988–14993. [CrossRef]
58. Swer, P.B.; Kharbuli, B.; Syiem, D.; Sharma, R. Age-related decline in the expression of BRG1, ATM and ATR are partially reversed by dietary restriction in the livers of female mice. *Biogerontology* **2024**, *25*, 1025–1037. [CrossRef]
59. Fu, C.S.; Harris, S.B.; Wilhelmi, P.; Walford, R.L. Lack of effect of age and dietary restriction on DNA single-stranded breaks in brain, liver, and kidney of (C3H x C57BL/10)F1 mice. *J. Gerontol.* **1991**, *46*, B78–B80. [CrossRef]
60. Kelly, C.M.; Latimer, J.J. Unscheduled DNA Synthesis: A Functional Assay for Global Genomic Nucleotide Excision Repair. In *Molecular Toxicology Protocols*; Humana Press: Totowa, NJ, USA, 2004; pp. 303–320. Available online: http://link.springer.com/10.1385/1-59259-840-4:303 (accessed on 6 August 2024).
61. Lipman, J.M.; Turturro, A.; Hart, R.W. The influence of dietary restriction on DNA repair in rodents: A preliminary study. *Mech. Ageing Dev.* **1989**, *48*, 135–143. [CrossRef]
62. Srivastava, V.; Tilley, R.; Miller, S.; Hart, R.; Busbee, D. Effects of aging and dietary restriction on DNA polymerases: Gene expression, enzyme fidelity, and DNA excision repair. *Exp. Gerontol.* **1992**, *27*, 593–613. [CrossRef]
63. Srivastava, V.K.; Busbee, D.L. Decreased fidelity of DNA polymerases and decreased DNA excision repair in aging mice: Effects of caloric restriction. *Biochem. Biophys. Res. Commun.* **1992**, *182*, 712–721. [CrossRef] [PubMed]
64. Tang, D.; Wu, J.; Wang, Y.; Cui, H.; Tao, Z.; Lei, L.; Zhou, Z.; Tao, S. Dietary Restriction Attenuates Inflammation and Protects Mouse Skin from High-Dose Ultraviolet B Irradiation. *Rejuvenation Res.* **2022**, *25*, 149–157. [CrossRef] [PubMed]
65. Qiu, R.; Qiu, X.; Su, M.; Sun, M.; Wang, Y.; Wu, J.; Wang, H.; Tang, D.; Tao, S. Dietary Restriction Delays But Cannot Heal Irradiation-Induced Hair Graying by Preserving Hair Follicle Stem Cells in Quiescence. *Rejuvenation Res.* **2023**, *26*, 242–252. [CrossRef] [PubMed]
66. Birkisdóttir, M.B.; Jaarsma, D.; Brandt, R.M.C.; Barnhoorn, S.; van Vliet, N.; Imholz, S.; van Oostrom, C.T.; Nagarajah, B.; Fernández, E.P.; Roks, A.J.M.; et al. Unlike dietary restriction, rapamycin fails to extend lifespan and reduce transcription stress in progeroid DNA repair-deficient mice. *Aging Cell* **2021**, *20*, e13302. [CrossRef]
67. Yamaza, H.; Komatsu, T.; Wakita, S.; Kijogi, C.; Park, S.; Hayashi, H.; Chiba, T.; Mori, R.; Furuyama, T.; Mori, N.; et al. FoxO1 is involved in the antineoplastic effect of calorie restriction. *Aging Cell* **2010**, *9*, 372–382. [CrossRef]
68. Garcia, A.M.; Busuttil, R.A.; Calder, R.B.; Dollé, M.E.T.; Diaz, V.; McMahan, C.A.; Bartke, A.; Nelson, J.; Reddick, R.; Vijg, J. Effect of Ames dwarfism and caloric restriction on spontaneous DNA mutation frequency in different mouse tissues. *Mech. Ageing Dev.* **2008**, *129*, 528–533. [CrossRef]
69. He, D.; Uehara, Y.; Furuya, M.; Ikehata, H.; Komura, J.-I.; Yamauchi, K.; Kakinuma, S.; Shang, Y.; Shimada, Y.; Ootsuyama, A.; et al. Effects of calorie restriction on the age-dependent accumulation of mutations in the small intestine of lacZ-transgenic mice. *Mech. Ageing Dev.* **2011**, *132*, 117–122. [CrossRef]

70. Li, D.; Chen, S.; Li, Q.; Chen, L.; Zhang, H.; Li, H.; Yu, D.; Zhang, R.; Niu, Y.; Lu, S.; et al. Caloric restriction attenuates C57BL/6J mouse lung injury and extra-pulmonary toxicity induced by real ambient particulate matter exposure. *Part. Fibre Toxicol.* **2020**, *17*, 22. [CrossRef]
71. Ishaq, A.; Schröder, J.; Edwards, N.; von Zglinicki, T.; Saretzki, G. Dietary Restriction Ameliorates Age-Related Increase in DNA Damage, Senescence and Inflammation in Mouse Adipose Tissuey. *J. Nutr. Health Aging* **2018**, *22*, 555–561. [CrossRef]
72. Hallam, D.; Wan, T.; Saretzki, G. Dietary restriction mitigates age-related accumulation of DNA damage, but not all changes in mouse corneal epithelium. *Exp. Gerontol.* **2015**, *67*, 72–79. [CrossRef]
73. Zhang, Z.; Epstein, A.; Schaefer, C.; Abdulraouf, A.; Jiang, W.; Zhou, W.; Cao, J. Spatiotemporal profiling reveals the impact of caloric restriction in the aging mammalian brain. *Cell Rep.* **2025**, *44*, 116165. [CrossRef] [PubMed]
74. Yu, C.; Qiu, X.; Tao, S.; Wu, Y.; He, S.; Wang, Q.; Tang, D.; Wang, Y. The impact of dietary restriction on transcriptional profiles of hematopoietic stem cells in aged female mice. *Biogerontology* **2025**, *26*, 122. [CrossRef] [PubMed]
75. Tao, S.; Wang, Y.; Wu, J.; Zeng, T.; Cui, H.; Tao, Z.; Lei, L.; Yu, L.; Liu, A.; Wang, H.; et al. Long-term mid-onset dietary restriction rejuvenates hematopoietic stem cells and improves regeneration capacity of total bone marrow from aged mice. *Aging Cell* **2020**, *19*, e13241. [CrossRef]
76. Ishaq, A.; Dufour, D.; Cameron, K.; von Zglinicki, T.; Saretzki, G. Metabolic memory of dietary restriction ameliorates DNA damage and adipocyte size in mouse visceral adipose tissue. *Exp. Gerontol.* **2018**, *113*, 228–236. [CrossRef] [PubMed]
77. Mackieh, R.; Al-Bakkar, N.; Kfoury, M.; Okdeh, N.; Pietra, H.; Roufayel, R.; Legros, C.; Fajloun, Z.; Sabatier, J.-M. Unlocking the Benefits of Fasting: A Review of its Impact on VariousBiological Systems and Human Health. *CMC* **2024**, *31*, 1781–1803. [CrossRef]
78. Boccardi, V.; Pigliautile, M.; Guazzarini, A.G.; Mecocci, P. The Potential of Fasting-Mimicking Diet as a Preventive and Curative Strategy for Alzheimer's Disease. *Biomolecules* **2023**, *13*, 1133. [CrossRef]
79. Wang, R.; Lv, X.; Xu, W.; Li, X.; Tang, X.; Huang, H.; Yang, M.; Ma, S.; Wang, N.; Niu, Y. Effects of the periodic fasting-mimicking diet on health, lifespan, and multiple diseases: A narrative review and clinical implications. *Nutr. Rev.* **2024**, *83*, e412–e426. [CrossRef]
80. Di Francesco, A.; Di Germanio, C.; Bernier, M.; De Cabo, R. A time to fast. *Science* **2018**, *362*, 770–775. [CrossRef]
81. Li, C.; Zhang, H.; Wu, H.; Li, R.; Wen, D.; Tang, Y.; Gao, Z.; Xu, R.; Lu, S.; Wei, Q.; et al. Intermittent fasting reverses the declining quality of aged oocytes. *Free Radic. Biol. Med.* **2023**, *195*, 74–88. [CrossRef]
82. Raffaghello, L.; Lee, C.; Safdie, F.M.; Wei, M.; Madia, F.; Bianchi, G.; Longo, V.D. Starvation-dependent differential stress resistance protects normal but not cancer cells against high-dose chemotherapy. *Proc. Natl. Acad. Sci. USA* **2008**, *105*, 8215–8220. [CrossRef]
83. Tinkum, K.L.; Stemler, K.M.; White, L.S.; Loza, A.J.; Jeter-Jones, S.; Michalski, B.M.; Kuzmicki, C.; Pless, R.; Stappenbeck, T.S.; Piwnica-Worms, D.; et al. Fasting protects mice from lethal DNA damage by promoting small intestinal epithelial stem cell survival. *Proc. Natl. Acad. Sci. USA* **2015**, *112*, E7148–E7154. [CrossRef] [PubMed]
84. De Cabo, R.; Mattson, M.P. Effects of Intermittent Fasting on Health, Aging, and Disease. *N. Engl. J. Med.* **2019**, *381*, 2541–2551. [CrossRef] [PubMed]
85. Rizkalla, S.W.; Bellisle, F.; Slama, G. Health benefits of low glycaemic index foods, such as pulses, in diabetic patients and healthy individuals. *Br. J. Nutr.* **2002**, *88*, 255–262. [CrossRef] [PubMed]
86. Folmer, V.; Soares, J.C.M.; Rocha, J.B.T. Oxidative stress in mice is dependent on the free glucose content of the diet. *Int. J. Biochem. Cell Biol.* **2002**, *34*, 1279–1285. [CrossRef]
87. Hanssen, N.M.J.; Kraakman, M.J.; Flynn, M.C.; Nagareddy, P.R.; Schalkwijk, C.G.; Murphy, A.J. Postprandial Glucose Spikes, an Important Contributor to Cardiovascular Disease in Diabetes? *Front. Cardiovasc. Med.* **2020**, *7*, 570553. [CrossRef]
88. 88; Nankervis, S.A.; Mitchell, J.M.; Charchar, F.J.; McGlynn, M.A.; Lewandowski, P.A. Consumption of a low glycaemic index diet in late life extends lifespan of Balb/c mice with differential effects on DNA damage. *Longev. Heal.* **2013**, *2*, 4. [CrossRef]
89. Hill, C.M.; Albarado, D.C.; Coco, L.G.; Spann, R.A.; Khan, M.S.; Qualls-Creekmore, E.; Burk, D.H.; Burke, S.J.; Collier, J.J.; Yu, S.; et al. FGF21 is required for protein restriction to extend lifespan and improve metabolic health in male mice. *Nat. Commun.* **2022**, *13*, 1897. [CrossRef]
90. Yu, D.; Richardson, N.E.; Green, C.L.; Spicer, A.B.; Murphy, M.E.; Flores, V.; Jang, C.; Kasza, I.; Nikodemova, M.; Wakai, M.H.; et al. The adverse metabolic effects of branched-chain amino acids are mediated by isoleucine and valine. *Cell Metab.* **2021**, *33*, 905–922.e6. [CrossRef]
91. Zhang, Y.; Jelleschitz, J.; Grune, T.; Chen, W.; Zhao, Y.; Jia, M.; Wang, Y.; Liu, Z.; Höhn, A. Methionine restriction—Association with redox homeostasis and implications on aging and diseases. *Redox Biol.* **2022**, *57*, 102464. [CrossRef]
92. Bárcena, C.; Quirós, P.M.; Durand, S.; Mayoral, P.; Rodríguez, F.; Caravia, X.M.; Mariño, G.; Garabaya, C.; Fernández-García, M.T.; Kroemer, G.; et al. Methionine Restriction Extends Lifespan in Progeroid Mice and Alters Lipid and Bile Acid Metabolism. *Cell Rep.* **2018**, *24*, 2392–2403. [CrossRef]

https://doi.org/10.3390/nu18020246

93. Solon-Biet, S.M.; McMahon, A.C.; Ballard, J.W.O.; Ruohonen, K.; Wu, L.E.; Cogger, V.C.; Warren, A.; Huang, X.; Pichaud, N.; Melvin, R.G.; et al. The Ratio of Macronutrients, Not Caloric Intake, Dictates Cardiometabolic Health, Aging, and Longevity in Ad Libitum-Fed Mice. *Cell Metab.* **2014**, *19*, 418–430. [CrossRef]
94. Solon-Biet, S.M.; Mitchell, S.J.; Coogan, S.C.P.; Cogger, V.C.; Gokarn, R.; McMahon, A.C.; Raubenheimer, D.; de Cabo, R.; Simpson, S.J.; Le Couteur, D.G. Dietary Protein to Carbohydrate Ratio and Caloric Restriction: Comparing Metabolic Outcomes in Mice. *Cell Rep.* **2015**, *11*, 1529–1534. [CrossRef] [PubMed]
95. Kimura, Y.; Sumiyoshi, M.; Kobayashi, T. Whey peptides prevent chronic ultraviolet B radiation-induced skin aging in melanin-possessing male hairless mice. *J. Nutr.* **2014**, *144*, 27–32. [CrossRef] [PubMed]
96. Osorio, M.J.; Mitchell, S.E.; Hambly, C.; Allison, D.B.; Speakman, J.R. Not feeling the heat? Effects of dietary protein on satiation and satiety in mice are not due to its impact on body temperature. *Appetite* **2024**, *200*, 107421. [CrossRef]
97. Guo, X.; Su, F.; Gao, Y.; Tang, L.; Yu, X.; Zi, J.; Zhou, Y.; Wang, H.; Xue, J.; Wang, X. Effects of dietary restriction on genome stability are sex and feeding regimen dependent. *Food Funct.* **2023**, *14*, 471–488. [CrossRef] [PubMed]
98. Forster, M.J.; Morris, P.; Sohal, R.S. Genotype and age influence the effect of caloric intake on mortality in mice. *FASEB J.* **2003**, *17*, 690–692. [CrossRef]
99. Conlon, M.; Bird, A. The Impact of Diet and Lifestyle on Gut Microbiota and Human Health. *Nutrients* **2014**, *7*, 17–44. [CrossRef]
100. Lopez-Legarrea, P.; Fuller, N.R.; Zulet, M.A.; Martinez, J.A.; Caterson, I.D. The Influence of Mediterranean Carbohydrate High Protein Diets on Gut Microbiota Composition in the Treatment of Obesity Associated Inflammatory State. *Asia Pac. J. Clin. Nutr.* **2014**, *23*, 360–368.
101. Danneskiold-Samsøe, N.B.; Dias De Freitas Queiroz Barros, H.; Santos, R.; Bicas, J.L.; Cazarin, C.B.B.; Madsen, L.; Kristiansen, K.; Pastore, G.M.; Brix, S.; Júnior, M.R.M. Interplay between food and gut microbiota in health and disease. *Food Res. Int.* **2019**, *115*, 23–31. [CrossRef]
102. Langille, M.G.; Meehan, C.J.; Koenig, J.E.; Dhanani, A.S.; Rose, R.A.; Howlett, S.E.; Beiko, R.G. Microbial shifts in the aging mouse gut. *Microbiome* **2014**, *2*, 50. [CrossRef]
103. Fransen, F.; Van Beek, A.A.; Borghuis, T.; Aidy, S.E.; Hugenholtz, F.; van der Gaast-de Jongh, C.; Savelkoul, H.F.J.; De Jonge, M.I.; Boekschoten, M.V.; Smidt, H.; et al. Aged Gut Microbiota Contributes to Systemical Inflammaging after Transfer to Germ-Free Mice. *Front. Immunol.* **2017**, *8*, 1385. [CrossRef] [PubMed]
104. Guedj, A.; Volman, Y.; Geiger-Maor, A.; Bolik, J.; Schumacher, N.; Künzel, S.; Baines, J.F.; Nevo, Y.; Elgavish, S.; Galun, E.; et al. Gut microbiota shape "inflamm-ageing" cytokines and account for age-dependent decline in DNA damage repair. *Gut* **2020**, *69*, 1064–1075. [CrossRef] [PubMed]
105. Xu, H.; Li, O.; Kim, D.; Yang, F.; Bao, Z. Age-Related Gut Microbiota Transplantation Disrupts Myocardial Energy Homeostasis and Induces Oxidative Damage. *J. Nutr.* **2024**, *154*, 1189–1199. [CrossRef] [PubMed]
106. Li, T.; Yang, S.; Liu, X.; Li, Y.; Gu, Z.; Jiang, Z. Dietary neoagarotetraose extends lifespan and impedes brain aging in mice via regulation of microbiota-gut-brain axis. *J. Adv. Res.* **2023**, *52*, 119–134. [CrossRef]
107. Kim, H.; Shin, J.; Kim, S.; Kim, S.; Cho, B.; Park, S.J.; Park, G.; Shin, H.; Park, M.S.; Kim, J. Bifidobacterium bifidum BGN4 and Bifidobacterium longum BORI promotes neuronal rejuvenation in aged mice. *Biochem. Biophys. Res. Commun.* **2022**, *603*, 41–48. [CrossRef]
108. Chen, L.H.; Chang, S.S.; Chang, H.Y.; Wu, C.H.; Pan, C.H.; Chang, C.C.; Chan, C.; Huang, H. Probiotic supplementation attenuates age-related sarcopenia via the gut-muscle axis in SAMP8 mice. *J. Cachexia Sarcopenia Muscle* **2022**, *13*, 515–531. [CrossRef]
109. Liu, T.; Song, X.; An, Y.; Wu, X.; Zhang, W.; Li, J. *Lactobacillus rhamnosus* GG Colonization in Early Life Ameliorates Inflammaging of Offspring by Activating SIRT1/AMPK/PGC-1α Pathway. *Oxid. Med. Cell Longev.* **2021**, *2021*, 3328505. [CrossRef]
110. Van Der Lugt, B.; Van Beek, A.A.; Aalvink, S.; Meijer, B.; Sovran, B.; Vermeij, W.P.; Brandt, R.M.C.; de Vos, W.M.; Savelkoul, H.F.J.; Steegenga, W.T.; et al. Akkermansia muciniphila ameliorates the age-related decline in colonic mucus thickness and attenuates immune activation in accelerated aging Ercc1−/Δ7 mice. *Immun. Ageing* **2019**, *16*, 6. [CrossRef]
111. Barone, M.; D'Amico, F.; Brigidi, P.; Turroni, S. Gut microbiome–micronutrient interaction: The key to controlling the bioavailability of minerals and vitamins? *BioFactors* **2022**, *48*, 307–314. [CrossRef]
112. Fenech, M.F.; Bull, C.F.; Van Klinken, B.J.W. Protective Effects of Micronutrient Supplements, Phytochemicals and Phytochemical-Rich Beverages and Foods Against DNA Damage in Humans: A Systematic Review of Randomized Controlled Trials and Prospective Studies. *Adv. Nutr.* **2023**, *14*, 1337–1358. [CrossRef]
113. van Dijk, M.; Dijk, F.J.; Hartog, A.; van Norren, K.; Verlaan, S.; van Helvoort, A. Reduced dietary intake of micronutrients with antioxidant properties negatively impacts muscle health in aged mice. *J. Cachexia Sarcopenia Muscle* **2018**, *9*, 146–159. [CrossRef]
114. Alamy, M.; Bengelloun, W.A. Malnutrition and brain development: An analysis of the effects of inadequate diet during different stages of life in rat. *Neurosci. Biobehav. Rev.* **2012**, *36*, 1463–1480. [CrossRef] [PubMed]
115. Chultemsuren, M.; Song, S.J.; Han, K.H.; Shin, J.A. Iron Overload Accelerates Aging-Associated Kidney Injury in Mice: Implications for Iron Supplementation in the Elderly. *Nutrients* **2025**, *17*, 2580. [CrossRef] [PubMed]

https://doi.org/10.3390/nu18020246

116. Zhang, X.; Wang, Y.; Zhao, R.; Hu, X.; Zhang, B.; Lv, X.; Guo, Z.; Zhang, Z.; Yuan, J.; Chu, X.; et al. Folic Acid Supplementation Suppresses Sleep Deprivation-Induced Telomere Dysfunction and Senescence-Associated Secretory Phenotype (SASP). *Oxid. Med. Cell Longev.* **2019**, *2019*, 4569614.
117. Yang, R.; Chen, J.; Zhang, J.; Qin, R.; Wang, R.; Qiu, Y. 1,25-Dihydroxyvitamin D protects against age-related osteoporosis by a novel VDR-Ezh2-p16 signal axis. *Aging Cell* **2020**, *19*, e13095. [CrossRef] [PubMed]
118. Shenkin, A. Micronutrients in health and disease. *Postgrad. Med. J.* **2006**, *82*, 559–567. [CrossRef]
119. Lebel, M.; Massip, L.; Garand, C.; Thorin, E. Ascorbate improves metabolic abnormalities in Wrn mutant mice but not the free radical scavenger catechin. *Ann. N. Y. Acad. Sci.* **2010**, *1197*, 40–44. [CrossRef]
120. Massie, H.R.; Aiello, V.R.; Doherty, T.J. Dietary Vitamin C Improves the Survival of Mice. *Gerontology* **1984**, *30*, 371–375. [CrossRef]
121. Selman, C.; McLaren, J.S.; Meyer, C.; Duncan, J.S.; Redman, P.; Collins, A.R.; Duthie, G.G.; Speakman, J.R. Life-long vitamin C supplementation in combination with cold exposure does not affect oxidative damage or lifespan in mice, but decreases expression of antioxidant protection genes. *Mech. Ageing Dev.* **2006**, *127*, 897–904. [CrossRef]
122. La Fata, G.; van Vliet, N.; Barnhoorn, S.; Brandt, R.M.C.; Etheve, S.; Chenal, E. Vitamin E Supplementation Reduces Cellular Loss in the Brain of a Premature Aging Mouse Model. *J. Prev. Alzheimers Dis.* **2017**, *4*, 226–235.
123. Kagan, V.E.; Kisin, E.R.; Kawai, K.; Serinkan, B.F.; Osipov, A.N.; Serbinova, E.A. Toward mechanism-based antioxidant interventions: Lessons from natural antioxidants. *Ann. N. Y. Acad. Sci.* **2002**, *959*, 188–198. [CrossRef] [PubMed]
124. Selman, C.; McLaren, J.S.; Mayer, C.; Duncan, J.S.; Collins, A.R.; Duthie, G.G.; Redman, P.; Speakman, J.R. Lifelong alpha-tocopherol supplementation increases the median life span of C57BL/6 mice in the cold but has only minor effects on oxidative damage. *Rejuvenation Res.* **2008**, *11*, 83–96. [CrossRef] [PubMed]
125. Zhong, L.; Guo, X.; Yang, Y.; Jian, D.; Peng, Y.; Lu, X. Folic Acid Protects Against Radiation-Induced Lung Injury by Suppressing Senescence of Lung Epithelial Cells. *Mol. Carcinog.* **2025**, *64*, 1913–1925. [CrossRef] [PubMed]
126. Epperly, M.W.; Wang, H.; Jones, J.A.; Dixon, T.; Montesinos, C.A.; Greenberger, J.S. Antioxidant-chemoprevention diet ameliorates late effects of total-body irradiation and supplements radioprotection by MnSOD-plasmid liposome administration. *Radiat. Res.* **2011**, *175*, 759–765. [CrossRef]
127. Barkallah, M.; Slima, A.B.; Elleuch, F.; Fendri, I.; Pichon, C.; Abdelkafi, S.; Baril, P. Protective Role of Spirulina platensis Against Bifenthrin-Induced Reprotoxicity in Adult Male Mice by Reversing Expression of Altered Histological, Biochemical, and Molecular Markers Including MicroRNAs. *Biomolecules* **2020**, *10*, 753. [CrossRef]
128. Veurink, G.; Liu, D.; Taddei, K.; Perry, G.; Smith, M.A.; Robertson, T.A. Reduction of inclusion body pathology in ApoE-deficient mice fed a combination of antioxidants. *Free Radic. Biol. Med.* **2003**, *34*, 1070–1077. [CrossRef]
129. Alvarado, C.; Alvarez, P.; Puerto, M.; Gausserès, N.; Jiménez, L.; De la Fuente, M. Dietary supplementation with antioxidants improves functions and decreases oxidative stress of leukocytes from prematurely aging mice. *Nutrition* **2006**, *22*, 767–777. [CrossRef]
130. Varela-López, A.; Romero-Márquez, J.M.; Navarro-Hortal, M.D.; Ramirez-Tortosa, C.L.; Battino, M.; Forbes-Hernández, T.Y.; Quiles, J.L. Dietary antioxidants and lifespan: Relevance of environmental conditions, diet, and genotype of experimental models. *Exp. Gerontol.* **2023**, *178*, 112221. [CrossRef]
131. Chen, J.; Wei, Y.; Chen, X.; Jiao, J.; Zhang, Y. Polyunsaturated fatty acids ameliorate aging via redox-telomere-antioncogene axis. *Oncotarget* **2017**, *8*, 7301–7314. [CrossRef]
132. Wu, S.; Wu, Y.; Chen, J.; Zhuang, P.; Zhang, Y.; Jiao, J. Lifelong docosahexaenoic acid intervention ameliorates aging in the telomere-DNA-mitochondria axis in telomerase-deficient mice. *J. Nutr. Biochem.* **2023**, *112*, 109202. [CrossRef]
133. Abbas, A.; Witte, T.; Patterson WL3rd Fahrmann, J.F.; Guo, K.; Hur, J.; Hardman, W.E.; Georgel, P.T. Epigenetic Reprogramming Mediated by Maternal Diet Rich in Omega-3 Fatty Acids Protects From Breast Cancer Development in F1 Offspring. *Front. Cell Dev. Biol.* **2021**, *9*, 682593. [CrossRef] [PubMed]
134. Ghareeb, S.A.; Hasan, S.S.; Ali, S.H.S.; Ahmad, N.S. Comparative analysis of safflower (*Carthamus tinctorius* L.) genotypes based seed oil characteristics. *Appl. Ecol. Environ. Res.* **2020**, *18*, 7587–7605. [CrossRef]
135. Czerwińska, J.; Nowak, M.; Wojtczak, P.; Dziuban-Lech, D.; Cieśla, J.M.; Kołata, D.; Gajewska, B.; Barańczyk-Kuźma, A.; Robinson, A.R.; Shane, H.L.; et al. ERCC1-deficient cells and mice are hypersensitive to lipid peroxidation. *Free Radic. Biol. Med.* **2018**, *124*, 79–96. [CrossRef] [PubMed]
136. Szabo, L.; Molnar, R.; Tomesz, A.; Deutsch, A.; Darago, R.; Varjas, T.; Ritter, Z.; Szentpeteri, J.L.; Andreidesz, K.; Mathe, D.; et al. Olive Oil Improves While Trans Fatty Acids Further Aggravate the Hypomethylation of LINE-1 Retrotransposon DNA in an Environmental Carcinogen Model. *Nutrients* **2022**, *14*, 908. [CrossRef]
137. Fabiani, R.; Vella, N.; Rosignoli, P. Epigenetic Modifications Induced by Olive Oil and Its Phenolic Compounds: A Systematic Review. *Molecules* **2021**, *26*, 273. [CrossRef]
138. Prough, R.A.; Clark, B.J.; Klinge, C.M. Novel mechanisms for DHEA action. *J. Mol. Endocrinol.* **2016**, *56*, R139–R155. [CrossRef]
139. Chu, N.; Gui, Y.; Qiu, X.; Zhang, N.; Li, L.; Li, D.; Tang, W.; Gober, H.-J.; Zhang, B.; Wang, L. The effect of DHEA on apoptosis and cohesin levels in oocytes in aged mice. *Biosci. Trends* **2017**, *11*, 427–438. [CrossRef]

140. Damiani, A.P.; Strapazzon, G.; de Oliveira Sardinha, T.T.; Rohr, P.; Gajski, G.; de Pinho, R.A.; de Andrade, V.M. Melatonin supplementation over different time periods until ageing modulates genotoxic parameters in mice. *Mutagenesis* **2020**, *35*, 465–478. [CrossRef]
141. Ruby, C.L.; Major, R.J.; Hinrichsen, R.D. Regulation of tissue regeneration by the circadian clock. *Eur. J. Neurosci.* **2021**, *53*, 3576–3597. [CrossRef]
142. Kolinjivadi, A.M.; Chong, S.T.; Ngeow, J. Molecular connections between circadian rhythm and genome maintenance pathways. *Endocr.-Relat. Cancer* **2021**, *28*, R55–R66. [CrossRef]
143. Gómez-Corvera, A.; Cerrillo, I.; Molinero, P.; Naranjo, M.C.; Lardone, P.J.; Sanchez-Hidalgo, M.; Carrascosa-Salmoral, M.P.; Medrano-Campillo, P.; Guerrero, J.M.; Rubio, A. Evidence of immune system melatonin production by two pineal melatonin deficient mice, C57BL/6 and Swiss strains. *J. Pineal Res.* **2009**, *47*, 15–22. [CrossRef] [PubMed]
144. Camacho-Pereira, J.; Tarragó, M.G.; Chini, C.C.S.; Nin, V.; Escande, C.; Warner, G.M.; Puranik, A.S.; Schoon, R.A.; Reid, J.M.; Galina, A.; et al. CD38 Dictates Age-Related NAD Decline and Mitochondrial Dysfunction through an SIRT3-Dependent Mechanism. *Cell Metab.* **2016**, *23*, 1127–1139. [CrossRef] [PubMed]
145. Fang, E.F.; Scheibye-Knudsen, M.; Brace, L.E.; Kassahun, H.; SenGupta, T.; Nilsen, H.; Mitchell, J.R.; Croteau, D.L.; Bohr, V.A. Defective Mitophagy in XPA via PARP-1 Hyperactivation and NAD+/SIRT1 Reduction. *Cell* **2014**, *157*, 882–896. [CrossRef] [PubMed]
146. McReynolds, M.R.; Chellappa, K.; Baur, J.A. Age-related NAD+ decline. *Exp. Gerontol.* **2020**, *134*, 110888. [CrossRef]
147. Yang, Y.; Liu, Y.; Wang, Y.; Chao, Y.; Zhang, J.; Jia, Y.; Tie, J.; Hu, D. Regulation of SIRT1 and Its Roles in Inflammation. *Front. Immunol.* **2022**, *13*, 831168. [CrossRef]
148. Cantó, C.; Auwerx, J. Targeting Sirtuin 1 to Improve Metabolism: All You Need Is NAD+? *Pharmacol. Rev.* **2012**, *64*, 166–187. [CrossRef]
149. Zhang, Q.; Siyuan, Z.; Xing, C.; Ruxiu, L. SIRT3 regulates mitochondrial function: A promising star target for cardiovascular disease therapy. *Biomed. Pharmacother.* **2024**, *170*, 116004. [CrossRef]
150. Haigis, M.C.; Sinclair, D.A. Mammalian Sirtuins: Biological Insights and Disease Relevance. *Annu. Rev. Pathol. Mech. Dis.* **2010**, *5*, 253–295. [CrossRef]
151. Gold, N.M.; Ding, Q.; Yang, Y.; Pu, S.; Cao, W.; Ge, X.; Yang, P.; Okeke, M.N.; Nisar, A.; Pan, Y.; et al. Therapeutic potential of nicotinamide and ABT263 in alcohol-associated liver disease through targeting cellular senescence. *MedComm* **2025**, *6*, e70086. [CrossRef]
152. Lin, Y.; Wang, Y.; Yang, X.; Ding, Z.; Hu, M.; Huang, X.; Zhang, Q.; Yu, Y. NMN reverses D-galactose-induced neurodegeneration and enhances the intestinal barrier of mice by activating the Sirt1 pathway. *Front. Pharmacol.* **2025**, *16*, 1545585. [CrossRef]
153. Hou, Y.; Lautrup, S.; Cordonnier, S.; Wang, Y.; Croteau, D.L.; Zavala, E.; Zhang, Y.; Moritoh, K.; O'connell, J.F.; Baptiste, B.A.; et al. NAD(+) supplementation normalizes key Alzheimer's features and DNA damage responses in a new AD mouse model with introduced DNA repair deficiency. *Proc. Natl. Acad. Sci. USA* **2018**, *115*, E1876–E1885. [CrossRef]
154. Hou, Y.; Wei, Y.; Lautrup, S.; Yang, B.; Wang, Y.; Cordonnier, S. NAD(+) supplementation reduces neuroinflammation and cell senescence in a transgenic mouse model of Alzheimer's disease via cGAS-STING. *Proc. Natl. Acad. Sci. USA* **2021**, *118*, e2011226118. [CrossRef]
155. Larrick, J.W.; Mendelsohn, A.R. Modulation of cGAS-STING Pathway by Nicotinamide Riboside in Alzheimer's Disease. *Rejuvenation Res.* **2021**, *24*, 397–402. [CrossRef] [PubMed]
156. Marmolejo-Garza, A.; Chatre, L.; Croteau, D.L.; Herron-Bedoya, A.; Luu, M.D.A.; Bernay, B.; Pontin, J.; Bohr, V.A.; Boddeke, E.; Dolga, A.M. Nicotinamide riboside modulates the reactive species interactome, bioenergetic status and proteomic landscape in a brain-region-specific manner. *Neurobiol. Dis.* **2024**, *200*, 106645. [CrossRef] [PubMed]
157. Haemmig, S.; Yang, D.; Sun, X.; Das, D.; Ghaffari, S.; Molinaro, R.; Chen, L.; Deng, Y.; Freeman, D.; Moullan, N.; et al. Long noncoding RNA SNHG12 integrates a DNA-PK-mediated DNA damage response and vascular senescence. *Sci. Transl. Med.* **2020**, *12*, eaaw1868. [CrossRef] [PubMed]
158. Scheibye-Knudsen, M.; Mitchell, S.J.; Fang, E.F.; Iyama, T.; Ward, T.; Wang, J.; Dunn, C.A.; Singh, N.; Veith, S.; Hasan-Olive, M.; et al. A high-fat diet and NAD(+) activate Sirt1 to rescue premature aging in cockayne syndrome. *Cell Metab.* **2014**, *20*, 840–855. [CrossRef]
159. Birkisdóttir, M.B.; van Galen, I.; Brandt, R.M.C.; Barnhoorn, S.; van Vliet, N.; van Dijk, C. The use of progeroid DNA repair-deficient mice for assessing anti-aging compounds, illustrating the benefits of nicotinamide riboside. *Front. Aging* **2022**, *3*, 1005322.
160. Stock, A.J.; Ayyar, S.; Kashyap, A.; Wang, Y.; Yanai, H.; Starost, M.F.; Tanaka-Yano, M.; Bodogai, M.; Sun, C.; Wang, Y.; et al. Boosting NAD ameliorates hematopoietic impairment linked to short telomeres in vivo. *Geroscience* **2023**, *45*, 2213–2228. [CrossRef]

161. Amano, H.; Chaudhury, A.; Rodriguez-Aguayo, C.; Lu, L.; Akhanov, V.; Catic, A.; Popov, Y.V.; Verdin, E.; Johnson, H.; Stossi, F.; et al. Telomere Dysfunction Induces Sirtuin Repression that Drives Telomere-Dependent Disease. *Cell Metab.* **2019**, *29*, 1274–1290.e9. [CrossRef]
162. Miao, Y.; Cui, Z.; Gao, Q.; Rui, R.; Xiong, B. Nicotinamide Mononucleotide Supplementation Reverses the Declining Quality of Maternally Aged Oocytes. *Cell Rep.* **2020**, *32*, 107987. [CrossRef]
163. Ramírez-Martín, N.; Buigues, A.; Rodríguez-Varela, C.; Martínez, J.; Blázquez-Simón, P.; Rodríguez-Hernández, C.; Pellicer, N.; Pellicer, A.; Escribá, M.J.; Herraiz, S. Nicotinamide mononucleotide supplementation improves oocyte developmental competence in different ovarian damage conditions. *Am. J. Obstet. Gynecol.* **2025**, *233*, 112.e1–112.e20. [CrossRef] [PubMed]
164. Wang, Z.; Zhao, X.; Zhou, Z.; Wang, F.; Zhang, X.; Tse, G.; Li, G.; Liu, Y.; Liu, T. Protective effects of nicotinamide mononucleotide on radiation-related cardiac injury. *Eur. Heart J.* **2023**, *44*, ehad655.2691. [CrossRef]
165. Zhao, X.; Zhang, M.; Wang, J.; Ji, K.; Wang, Y.; Sun, X.; Xu, C.; Wang, Q.; He, N.; Song, H.; et al. NMN ameliorated radiation induced damage in NRF2-deficient cell and mice via regulating SIRT6 and SIRT7. *Free Radic. Biol. Med.* **2022**, *193*, 342–353. [CrossRef] [PubMed]
166. Wong, W.; Crane, E.D.; Zhang, H.; Li, J.; Day, T.A.; Green, A.E.; Menzies, K.J.; Crane, J.D. Pgc-1α controls epidermal stem cell fate and skin repair by sustaining NAD(+) homeostasis during aging. *Mol. Metab.* **2022**, *65*, 101575. [CrossRef] [PubMed]
167. Fragola, G.; Mabb, A.M.; Taylor-Blake, B.; Niehaus, J.K.; Chronister, W.D.; Mao, H.; Simon, J.M.; Yuan, H.; Li, Z.; McConnell, M.J.; et al. Deletion of Topoisomerase 1 in excitatory neurons causes genomic instability and early onset neurodegeneration. *Nat. Commun.* **2020**, *11*, 1962. [CrossRef]
168. Jia, Y.; Kang, X.; Tan, L.; Ren, Y.; Qu, L.; Tang, J.; Liu, G.; Wang, S.; Xiong, Z.; Yang, L. Nicotinamide Mononucleotide Attenuates Renal Interstitial Fibrosis After AKI by Suppressing Tubular DNA Damage and Senescence. *Front. Physiol.* **2021**, *12*, 649547. [CrossRef]
169. Adams, J.D.; Mukherjee, S.K.; Klaidman, L.K.; Chang, M.L.; Yasharel, R. Apoptosis and oxidative stress in the aging brain. *Ann. N. Y. Acad. Sci.* **1996**, *786*, 135–151. [CrossRef]
170. Del Mar Rivas-Chacón, L.; Yanes-Díaz, J.; de Lucas, B.; Riestra-Ayora, J.I.; Madrid-García, R.; Sanz-Fernández, R.; Sánchez-Rodríguez, C. Preventive Effect of Cocoa Flavonoids via Suppression of Oxidative Stress-Induced Apoptosis in Auditory Senescent Cells. *Antioxidants* **2022**, *11*, 1450. [CrossRef]
171. Mao, X.; Hou, Y.; Fang, C.; Ma, K.; Zhang, S.; Guo, Z.; Kang, N.; Niu, K.; Shen, X.; Li, Y.; et al. Bazi Bushen mitigates epigenetic aging and extends healthspan in naturally aging mice. *Biomed. Pharmacother.* **2023**, *160*, 114384. [CrossRef]
172. Hua, K.F.; Chao, A.C.; Lin, T.Y.; Chen, W.T.; Lee, Y.C.; Hsu, W.H.; Lee, S.-L.; Wang, H.-M.; Yang, D.-I.; Ju, T.-C. Ginsenoside compound K reduces the progression of Huntington's disease via the inhibition of oxidative stress and overactivation of the ATM/AMPK pathway. *J. Ginseng Res.* **2022**, *46*, 572–584. [CrossRef]
173. Chávez-Hurtado, P.; González-Castañeda, R.E.; Beas-Zarate, C.; Flores-Soto, M.E.; Viveros-Paredes, J.M. β-Caryophyllene Reduces DNA Oxidation and the Overexpression of Glial Fibrillary Acidic Protein in the Prefrontal Cortex and Hippocampus of d-Galactose-Induced Aged BALB/c Mice. *J. Med. Food* **2020**, *23*, 515–522. [CrossRef]
174. Ma, W.; Wei, S.; Peng, W.; Sun, T.; Huang, J.; Yu, R. Antioxidant Effect of Polygonatum sibiricum Polysaccharides in D-Galactose-Induced Heart Aging Mice. *Biomed. Res. Int.* **2021**, *2021*, 6688855. [CrossRef]
175. He, X.; Wang, Y.; Wu, M.; Wei, J.; Sun, X.; Wang, A.; Hu, G.; Jia, J. Secoisolariciresinol Diglucoside Improves Ovarian Reserve in Aging Mouse by Inhibiting Oxidative Stress. *Front. Mol. Biosci.* **2021**, *8*, 806412. [CrossRef] [PubMed]
176. Chen, Q.; Xin, G.; Li, S.; Dong, Y.; Yu, X.; Wan, C.; Wei, Z.; Zhu, Y.; Zhang, K.; Wang, Y.; et al. Berberine-mediated REDD1 down-regulation ameliorates senescence of retinal pigment epithelium by interrupting the ROS-DDR positive feedback loop. *Phytomedicine* **2022**, *104*, 154181. [CrossRef] [PubMed]
177. Sharma, R.; Kumar, R.; Sharma, A.; Goel, A.; Padwad, Y. Long-term consumption of green tea EGCG enhances murine health span by mitigating multiple aspects of cellular senescence in mitotic and post-mitotic tissues, gut dysbiosis, and immunosenescence. *J. Nutr. Biochem.* **2022**, *107*, 109068. [CrossRef] [PubMed]
178. Lane, S.L.; Parks, J.C.; Russ, J.E.; Khan, S.A.; Schoolcraft, W.B.; Yuan, Y.; Katz-Jaffe, M.G. Increased Systemic Antioxidant Power Ameliorates the Aging-Related Reduction in Oocyte Competence in Mice. *Int. J. Mol. Sci.* **2021**, *22*, 13019. [CrossRef]
179. Trentin, G.A.; Moody, J.; Torous, D.K.; Thompson, L.U.; Heddle, J.A. The influence of dietary flaxseed and other grains, fruits and vegetables on the frequency of spontaneous chromosomal damage in mice. *Mutat. Res.* **2004**, *551*, 213–222. [CrossRef]
180. Wei, J.; Zhang, G.; Zhang, X.; Xu, D.; Gao, J.; Fan, J.; Zhou, Z. Anthocyanins from Black Chokeberry (Aroniamelanocarpa Elliot) Delayed Aging-Related Degenerative Changes of Brain. *J. Agric. Food Chem.* **2017**, *65*, 5973–5984. [CrossRef]
181. Barros, D.; Amaral, O.B.; Izquierdo, I.; Geracitano, L.; do Carmo Bassols Raseira, M.; Henriques, A.T.; Ramirez, M.R. Behavioral and genoprotective effects of Vaccinium berries intake in mice. *Pharmacol. Biochem. Behav.* **2006**, *84*, 229–234. [CrossRef]
182. Giridharan, V.V.; Karupppagounder, V.; Arumugam, S.; Nakamura, Y.; Guha, A.; Barichello, T.; Quevedo, J.; Watanabe, K.; Konishi, T.; Thandavarayan, R.A. 3,4-Dihydroxybenzalacetone (DBL) Prevents Aging-Induced Myocardial Changes in Senescence-Accelerated Mouse-Prone 8 (SAMP8) Mice. *Cells* **2020**, *9*, 597. [CrossRef]

https://doi.org/10.3390/nu18020246

183. Liu, G.S.; Zhang, Z.S.; Yang, B.; He, W. Resveratrol attenuates oxidative damage and ameliorates cognitive impairment in the brain of senescence-accelerated mice. *Life Sci.* **2012**, *91*, 872–877. [CrossRef] [PubMed]
184. Wong, Y.T.; Gruber, J.; Jenner, A.M.; Ng, M.P.E.; Ruan, R.; Tay, F.E.H. Elevation of oxidative-damage biomarkers during aging in F2 hybrid mice: Protection by chronic oral intake of resveratrol. *Free Radic. Biol. Med.* **2009**, *46*, 799–809. [CrossRef] [PubMed]
185. Pal, K.; Raghuram, G.V.; Dsouza, J.; Shinde, S.; Jadhav, V.; Shaikh, A.; Rane, B.; Tandel, H.; Kondhalkar, D.; Chaudhary, S.; et al. A pro-oxidant combination of resveratrol and copper down-regulates multiple biological hallmarks of ageing and neurodegeneration in mice. *Sci. Rep.* **2022**, *12*, 17209. [CrossRef] [PubMed]
186. Heredia-Molina, R.F.; Riestra-Ayora, J.I.; Vasallo, I.J.T.; Sanz-Fernández, R.; Sánchez-Rodríguez, C. Sirtuins mediate the reduction of age-related oxidative damage in the cochlea under a cocoa-rich diet. *GeroScience* **2025**. Available online: https://link.springer.com/10.1007/s11357-025-01847-8 (accessed on 19 November 2025).
187. Umeda, T.; Sakai, A.; Uekado, R.; Shigemori, K.; Nakajima, R.; Yamana, K. Simply crushed Zizyphi spinosi semen prevents neurodegenerative diseases and reverses age-related cognitive decline in mice. *eLife* **2024**, *13*, RP100737. [CrossRef]
188. Chen, K.; Qin, C.; Ji, C.; Yu, Y.; Wu, Y.; Xu, L.; Jiang, Y.; Zou, G. Astragalus polysaccharide alleviates oxidative stress and senescence in chondrocytes in osteoarthritis via GCN2/ATF4/TXN axis. *Int. J. Biol. Macromol.* **2025**, *310*, 143285. [CrossRef]
189. Yang, L.; Lai, X.; Jin, S.; Wang, H.; Lin, F.; Jin, X.; Chen, Y.; Wang, R.; Huang, Y.; Zhang, Y.; et al. Exploring the anti-ovarian aging mechanism of He's Yangchao formula: Insights from multi-omics analysis in naturally aged mice. *Phytomedicine* **2024**, *134*, 155961. [CrossRef]
190. Han, X.; Zhang, J.; Xue, X.; Zhao, Y.; Lu, L.; Cui, M.; Miao, W.; Fan, S. Theaflavin ameliorates ionizing radiation-induced hematopoietic injury via the NRF2 pathway. *Free Radic. Biol. Med.* **2017**, *113*, 59–70. [CrossRef]
191. Firdous, A.P.; Sindhu, E.R.; Ramnath, V.; Kuttan, R. Amelioration of radiation-induced damages in mice by carotenoid meso-zeaxanthin. *Int. J. Radiat. Biol.* **2013**, *89*, 171–181. [CrossRef]
192. Rastogi, L.; Feroz, S.; Pandey, B.N.; Jagtap, A.; Mishra, K.P. Protection against radiation-induced oxidative damage by an ethanolic extract of *Nigella sativa* L. *Int. J. Radiat. Biol.* **2010**, *86*, 719–731. [CrossRef]
193. Truong, V.L.; Rarison, R.H.G.; Jeong, W.S. Protective Effects of Orange Sweet Pepper Juices Prepared by High-Speed Blender and Low-Speed Masticating Juicer against UVB-induced Skin Damage in SKH-1 Hairless Mice. *Molecules* **2022**, *27*, 6394. [CrossRef]
194. Kim, Y.H.; Cho, A.; Kwon, S.A.; Kim, M.; Song, M.; Han, H.W.; Shin, E.-J.; Park, E.; Lee, S.-M. Potential Photoprotective Effect of Dietary Corn Silk Extract on Ultraviolet B-Induced Skin Damage. *Molecules* **2019**, *24*, 2587. [CrossRef] [PubMed]
195. Liu, S.; Sui, Q.; Zou, J.; Zhao, Y.; Chang, X. Protective effects of hawthorn (*Crataegus pinnatifida*) polyphenol extract against UVB-induced skin damage by modulating the p53 mitochondrial pathway in vitro and in vivo. *J. Food Biochem.* **2019**, *43*, e12708. [CrossRef] [PubMed]
196. Parrado, C.; Nicolas, J.; Juarranz, A.; Gonzalez, S. The role of the aqueous extract Polypodium leucotomos in photoprotection. *Photochem. Photobiol. Sci.* **2020**, *19*, 831–843. [CrossRef] [PubMed]
197. Zattra, E.; Coleman, C.; Arad, S.; Helms, E.; Levine, D.; Bord, E.; Guillaume, A.; El-Hajahmad, M.; Zwart, E.; van Steeg, H.; et al. Polypodium leucotomos extract decreases UV-induced Cox-2 expression and inflammation, enhances DNA repair, and decreases mutagenesis in hairless mice. *Am. J. Pathol.* **2009**, *175*, 1952–1961. [CrossRef]
198. Geng, R.; Kang, S.G.; Huang, K.; Tong, T. Dietary supplementation with α-ionone alleviates chronic UVB exposure-induced skin photoaging in mice. *Food Funct.* **2024**, *15*, 1884–1898. [CrossRef]
199. Chen, Q.; Xu, Z.; Li, X.; Du, D.; Wu, T.; Zhou, S.; Yan, W.; Wu, M.; Jin, Y.; Zhang, J.; et al. Epigallocatechin gallate and theaflavins independently alleviate cyclophosphamide-induced ovarian damage by inhibiting the overactivation of primordial follicles and follicular atresia. *Phytomedicine* **2021**, *92*, 153752. [CrossRef]
200. Zhang, Y.; Tan, R.; Wang, L.; Shi, X.; Li, Y.; Zhong, X.; He, X.; Xiong, B. Shoutai pills improve the quality of oocytes exposed to the chemotherapeutic drug Hydroxyurea. *Aging* **2020**, *12*, 8473–8483. [CrossRef]
201. Chen, Y.H.; Chen, Y.C.; Chin, Y.T.; Wang, C.C.; Hwang, L.L.; Yang, L.Y.; Lu, D.Y. 2,3,5,4′-tetrahydroxystilbene-2-O-beta-D-glucoside protects against neuronal cell death and traumatic brain injury-induced pathophysiology. *Aging* **2022**, *14*, 2607–2627. [CrossRef]
202. Jie, L.; Shi, X.; Kang, J.; Fu, H.; Yu, L.; Tian, D.; Mei, W.; Yin, S. Protocatechuic aldehyde attenuates chondrocyte senescence via the regulation of PTEN-induced kinase 1/Parkin-mediated mitochondrial autophagy. *Int. J. Immunopathol. Pharmacol.* **2024**, *38*, 03946320241271724. [CrossRef]
203. Yu, W.; Zhao, J.; Li, W.; Zheng, Y.; Zhu, J.; Liu, J.; Liu, R.; Wang, Z.; Wang, X.; Hai, C. 2,3,5,4′-Tetrahydroxystilbene-2-O-β-d-glucoside alleviated the acute hepatotoxicity and DNA damage in diethylnitrosamine-contaminated mice. *Life Sci.* **2020**, *243*, 117274. [CrossRef]
204. Bouchab, H.; Ishaq, A.; El Kebbaj, R.; Nasser, B.; Saretzki, G. Protective effect of argan oil on DNA damage in vivo and in vitro. *Biomarkers* **2021**, *26*, 425–433. [CrossRef] [PubMed]
205. Bouchab, H.; Ishaq, A.; Limami, Y.; Saretzki, G.; Nasser, B.; El Kebbaj, R. Antioxidant Effects of Cactus Seed Oil against Iron-Induced Oxidative Stress in Mouse Liver, Brain and Kidney. *Molecules* **2024**, *29*, 4463. [CrossRef]

https://doi.org/10.3390/nu18020246

206. Pettan-Brewer, C.; Morton, J.; Mangalindan, R.; Ladiges, W. Curcumin suppresses intestinal polyps in APC Min mice fed a high fat diet. *Pathobiol. Aging Age Relat. Dis.* **2011**, *1*, 7013. [CrossRef]
207. Matsuno, Y.; Atsumi, Y.; Alauddin, M.; Rana, M.M.; Fujimori, H.; Hyodo, M.; Shimizu, A.; Ikuta, T.; Tani, H.; Torigoe, H.; et al. Resveratrol and its Related Polyphenols Contribute to the Maintenance of Genome Stability. *Sci. Rep.* **2020**, *10*, 5388. [CrossRef] [PubMed]
208. Mishra, P.K.; Raghuram, G.V.; Bhargava, A.; Ahirwar, A.; Samarth, R.; Upadhyaya, R. In vitro and in vivo evaluation of the anticarcinogenic and cancer chemopreventive potential of a flavonoid-rich fraction from a traditional Indian herb Selaginella bryopteris. *Br. J. Nutr.* **2011**, *106*, 1154–1168. [CrossRef] [PubMed]
209. Ganguly, C.; De, S.; Das, S. Prevention of carcinogen-induced mouse skin papilloma by whole fruit aqueous extract of Momordica charantia. *Eur. J. Cancer Prev.* **2000**, *9*, 283–288. [CrossRef]
210. Lawson, T.; Stohs, S. Changes in endogenous DNA damage in aging mice in response to butylated hydroxyanisole and oltipraz. *Mech. Ageing Dev.* **1985**, *30*, 179–185. [CrossRef]
211. Park, S.K.; Shin, O.S. Metformin alleviates ageing cellular phenotypes in Hutchinson-Gilford progeria syndrome dermal fibroblasts. *Exp. Dermatol.* **2017**, *26*, 889–895. [CrossRef]
212. Kim, H.; Yu, M.R.; Lee, H.; Kwon, S.H.; Jeon, J.S.; Han, D.C.; Noh, H. Metformin inhibits chronic kidney disease-induced DNA damage and senescence of mesenchymal stem cells. *Aging Cell* **2021**, *20*, e13317. [CrossRef]
213. Kretschmer, T.; Turnwald, E.M.; Thiele, A.; Kallage, C.; Neweling, L.; Kammerer, M.; Janoschek, R.; Zentis, P.; Handwerk, M.; Wohlfarth, M.; et al. Maternal body composition and the placental-fetal unit under maternal high-fat feeding partially improve by metformin treatment or lifestyle interventions during pregnancy in a mouse model. *Placenta* **2025**, *171*, 91–101. [CrossRef]
214. Zhu, J.; Zhu, M.; Zhao, H.; Lin, Y.; Han, X.; Tan, A.; Wang, Y.; Ma, Y.; Li, J.; Liu, Z. Metformin alleviates cadmium-induced reproductive toxicity by enhancing mitochondrial biosynthesis and epigenetic modifications in female mice. *Toxicol. Appl. Pharmacol.* **2025**, *500*, 117390. [CrossRef] [PubMed]
215. Xing, J.; Chen, K.; Gao, S.; Pousse, M.; Ying, Y.; Wang, B.; Chen, L.; Wang, C.; Wang, L.; Hu, W.; et al. Protein phosphatase 2A activators reverse age-related behavioral changes by targeting neural cell senescence. *Aging Cell* **2023**, *22*, e13780. [CrossRef] [PubMed]
216. Bernardes de Jesus, B.; Schneeberger, K.; Vera, E.; Tejera, A.; Harley, C.B.; Blasco, M.A. The telomerase activator TA-65 elongates short telomeres and increases health span of adult/old mice without increasing cancer incidence. *Aging Cell* **2011**, *10*, 604–621. [CrossRef] [PubMed]
217. Oe, Y.; Kim, Y.C.; Sidorenko, V.S.; Zhang, H.; Kanoo, S.; Lopez, N.; Goodluck, H.A.; Crespo-Masip, M.; Vallon, V. SGLT2 inhibitor dapagliflozin protects the kidney in a murine model of Balkan nephropathy. *Am. J. Physiol. Ren. Physiol.* **2024**, *326*, F227–F240. [CrossRef]
218. Li, Y.; Wu, A.; Jin, X.; Shen, H.; Zhao, C.; Yi, X.; Nie, H.; Wang, M.; Yin, S.; Zuo, H.; et al. DDO1002, an NRF2–KEAP1 inhibitor, improves hematopoietic stem cell aging and stress response. *Life Med.* **2024**, *3*, lnae043. [CrossRef]
219. McIlhatton, M.A.; Tyler, J.; Kerepesi, L.A.; Bocker-Edmonston, T.; Kucherlapati, M.H.; Edelmann, W.; Kucherlapati, R.; Kopelovich, L.; Fishel, R. Aspirin and low-dose nitric oxide-donating aspirin increase life span in a Lynch syndrome mouse model. *Cancer Prev. Res.* **2011**, *4*, 684–693. [CrossRef]
220. Shaforostova, E.A.; Gureev, A.P.; Volodina, D.E.; Popov, V.N. Neuroprotective effect of mildronate and L-carnitine on the cognitive parameters of aged mice and mice with LPS-induced inflammation. *Metab. Brain Dis.* **2022**, *37*, 2497–2510. [CrossRef]
221. Ryu, W.; Park, C.W.; Kim, J.; Lee, H.; Chung, H. The Bcl-2/Bcl-xL Inhibitor ABT-263 Attenuates Retinal Degeneration by Selectively Inducing Apoptosis in Senescent Retinal Pigment Epithelial Cells. *Mol. Cells* **2023**, *46*, 420–429. [CrossRef]
222. Fuhrmann-Stroissnigg, H.; Ling, Y.Y.; Zhao, J.; McGowan, S.J.; Zhu, Y.; Brooks, R.W.; Grassi, D.; Gregg, S.Q.; Stripay, J.L.; Dorronsoro, A.; et al. Identification of HSP90 inhibitors as a novel class of senolytics. *Nat. Commun.* **2017**, *8*, 422. [CrossRef]
223. Marcos-Ramiro, B.; Gil-Ordóñez, A.; Marín-Ramos, N.I.; Ortega-Nogales, F.J.; Balabasquer, M.; Gonzalo, P.; Khiar-Fernández, N.; Rolas, L.; Barkaway, A.; Nourshargh, S.; et al. Isoprenylcysteine Carboxylmethyltransferase-Based Therapy for Hutchinson-Gilford Progeria Syndrome. *ACS Cent. Sci.* **2021**, *7*, 1300–1310. [CrossRef]
224. Lemon, J.A.; Rollo, C.D.; Boreham, D.R. Elevated DNA damage in a mouse model of oxidative stress: Impacts of ionizing radiation and a protective dietary supplement. *Mutagenesis* **2008**, *23*, 473–482. [CrossRef] [PubMed]
225. Kulala, D.S.; Prasad, K.; Reddy, P.S.; Maruthiyodan, S.; Joshi, M.B.; Satyamoorthy, K.; Guruprasad, K.P. Understanding the effects of Abhraka Bhasma on genotoxicity and its DNA repair potential in mouse model. *J. Ayurveda Integr. Med.* **2022**, *14*, 100598. [CrossRef] [PubMed]
226. Inoue Sichiro Koya-Miyata, S.; Ushio, S.; Iwaki, K.; Ikeda, M.; Kurimoto, M. Royal Jelly prolongs the life span of C3H/HeJ mice: Correlation with reduced DNA damage. *Exp. Gerontol.* **2003**, *38*, 965–969.
227. Chou, M.Y.; Chen, Y.J.; Lin, L.H.; Nakao, Y.; Lim, A.L.; Wang, M.F.; Yong, S.M. Protective Effects of Hydrolyzed Chicken Extract (Probeptigen®/Cmi-168) on Memory Retention and Brain Oxidative Stress in Senescence-Accelerated Mice. *Nutrients* **2019**, *11*, 1870. [CrossRef] [PubMed]

228. Gudkov, S.V.; Shtarkman, I.N.; Smirnova, V.S.; Chernikov, A.V.; Bruskov, V.I. Guanosine and inosine display antioxidant activity, protect DNA in vitro from oxidative damage induced by reactive oxygen species, and serve as radioprotectors in mice. *Radiat. Res.* **2006**, *165*, 538–545. [CrossRef]
229. Chen, L.; Wang, G.; Wang, Q.; Liu, Q.; Sun, Q.; Chen, L. N-acetylcysteine prevents orchiectomy-induced osteoporosis by inhibiting oxidative stress and osteocyte senescence. *Am. J. Transl. Res.* **2019**, *11*, 4337–4347.
230. Loi, M.; Valenti, F.; Medici, G.; Mottolese, N.; Candini, G.; Bove, A.M.; Trebbi, F.; Pincigher, L.; Fato, R.; Bergamini, C.; et al. Beneficial Antioxidant Effects of Coenzyme Q10 in In Vitro and In Vivo Models of CDKL5 Deficiency Disorder. *Int. J. Mol. Sci.* **2025**, *26*, 2204. [CrossRef]
231. Kumar, P.; Osahon, O.W.; Sekhar, R.V. GlyNAC (Glycine and N-Acetylcysteine) Supplementation in Mice Increases Length of Life by Correcting Glutathione Deficiency, Oxidative Stress, Mitochondrial Dysfunction, Abnormalities in Mitophagy and Nutrient Sensing, and Genomic Damage. *Nutrients* **2022**, *14*, 1114. [CrossRef]
232. Schubert, R.; Erker, L.; Barlow, C.; Yakushiji, H.; Larson, D.; Russo, A.; Mitchell, J.B.; Wynshaw-Boris, A. Cancer chemoprevention by the antioxidant tempol in Atm-deficient mice. *Hum. Mol. Genet.* **2004**, *13*, 1793–1802. [CrossRef]
233. Coeli-Lacchini, F.B.; Da Silva, G.; Belentani, M.; Alves, J.S.F.; Ushida, T.R.; Lunardelli, G.T.; Garcia, C.B.; Silva, T.A.; Lopes, N.P.; Leopoldino, A.M. Spermidine Suppresses Oral Carcinogenesis through Autophagy Induction, DNA Damage Repair, and Oxidative Stress Reduction. *Am. J. Pathol.* **2023**, *193*, 2172–2181. [CrossRef]
234. Singh, P.; Gollapalli, K.; Mangiola, S.; Schranner, D.; Yusuf, M.A.; Chamoli, M.; Shi, S.L.; Bastos, B.L.; Nair, T.; Riermeier, A.; et al. Taurine deficiency as a driver of aging. *Science* **2023**, *380*, eabn9257. [CrossRef] [PubMed]
235. Jonscher, K.R.; Chowanadisai, W.; Rucker, R.B. Pyrroloquinoline-Quinone Is More Than an Antioxidant: A Vitamin-like Accessory Factor Important in Health and Disease Prevention. *Biomolecules* **2021**, *11*, 1441. [CrossRef]
236. Li, J.; Liu, M.; Liang, S.; Yu, Y.; Gu, M. Repression of the Antioxidant Pyrroloquinoline Quinone in Skin Aging Induced by Bmi-1 Deficiency. *Biomed. Res. Int.* **2022**, *2022*, 1732438. [CrossRef] [PubMed]
237. Huang, Y.; Chen, N.; Miao, D. Biological effects of pyrroloquinoline quinone on liver damage in Bmi-1 knockout mice. *Exp. Ther. Med.* **2015**, *10*, 451–458. [CrossRef]
238. Wu, X.; Li, J.; Zhang, H.; Wang, H.; Yin, G.; Miao, D. Pyrroloquinoline quinone prevents testosterone deficiency-induced osteoporosis by stimulating osteoblastic bone formation and inhibiting osteoclastic bone resorption. *Am. J. Transl. Res.* **2017**, *9*, 1230–1242.
239. Li, J.; Zhang, J.; Xue, Q.; Liu, B.; Qin, R.; Li, Y.; Qiu, Y.; Wang, R.; Goltzman, D.; Miao, D.; et al. Pyrroloquinoline quinone alleviates natural aging-related osteoporosis via a novel MCM3-Keap1-Nrf2 axis-mediated stress response and Fbn1 upregulation. *Aging Cell* **2023**, *22*, e13912. [CrossRef] [PubMed]
240. Qin, R.; Sun, J.; Wu, J.; Chen, L. Pyrroloquinoline quinone prevents knee osteoarthritis by inhibiting oxidative stress and chondrocyte senescence. *Am. J. Transl. Res.* **2019**, *11*, 1460–1472.
241. Haley-Zitlin, V.; Richardson, A. Effect of dietary restriction on DNA repair and DNA damage. *Mutat. Res./DNAging* **1993**, *295*, 237–245. [CrossRef]
242. Heydari, A.R.; Unnikrishnan, A.; Lucente, L.V.; Richardson, A. Caloric restriction and genomic stability. *Nucleic Acids Res.* **2007**, *35*, 7485–7496. [CrossRef]
243. López-Lluch, G.; Hunt, N.; Jones, B.; Zhu, M.; Jamieson, H.; Hilmer, S.; Cascajo, M.V.; Allard, J.; Ingram, D.K.; Navas, P.; et al. Calorie restriction induces mitochondrial biogenesis and bioenergetic efficiency. *Proc. Natl. Acad. Sci. USA* **2006**, *103*, 1768–1773. [CrossRef]
244. Yu, B.P.; Chung, H.Y. Stress Resistance by Caloric Restriction for Longevity. *Ann. N. Y. Acad. Sci.* **2001**, *928*, 39–47. [CrossRef] [PubMed]
245. Trisal, A.; Singh, A.K. Mechanisms and early efficacy data of caloric restriction and caloric restriction mimetics in neurodegenerative disease. *Neuroscience* **2025**, *567*, 235–248. [CrossRef] [PubMed]
246. De-Leon-Covarrubias, U.E.; Perez-Trujillo, J.J.; Villa-Cedillo, S.A.; Martinez-Perez, A.G.; Montes-de-Oca-Saucedo, C.R.; Loera-Arias Mde, J.; Garcia-Garcia, A.; Saucedo-Cardenas, O.; Montes-De-Oca-Luna, R. Unlocking the Potential: Caloric Restriction, Caloric Restriction Mimetics, and Their Impact on Cancer Prevention and Treatment. *Metabolites* **2024**, *14*, 418. [CrossRef] [PubMed]
247. Maes, J.; Durieux, V.; Liebmann, M.; Salmon, M.; Preiser, J.C. Impact of intermittent fasting on patients with cancer undergoing chemotherapy and/or targeted therapies: A systematic review of the literature. *Support. Care Cancer* **2025**, *33*, 863. [CrossRef]
248. Elias, A.; Padinjakara, N.; Lautenschlager, N.T. Effects of intermittent fasting on cognitive health and Alzheimer's disease. *Nutr. Rev.* **2023**, *81*, 1225–1233. [CrossRef]
249. Tagliafico, L.; Nencioni, A.; Monacelli, F. Fasting and Cognitive Impairment. *Nutrients* **2023**, *15*, 5108. [CrossRef]
250. Hofer, S.J.; Davinelli, S.; Bergmann, M.; Scapagnini, G.; Madeo, F. Caloric Restriction Mimetics in Nutrition and Clinical Trials. *Front. Nutr.* **2021**, *8*, 717343. [CrossRef]

https://doi.org/10.3390/nu18020246

251. Membrez, M.; Migliavacca, E.; Christen, S.; Yaku, K.; Trieu, J.; Lee, A.K.; Morandini, F.; Giner, M.P.; Stiner, J.; Makarov, M.V.; et al. Trigonelline is an NAD+ precursor that improves muscle function during ageing and is reduced in human sarcopenia. *Nat. Metab.* **2024**, *6*, 433–447. [CrossRef]
252. Khan, N.A.; Auranen, M.; Paetau, I.; Pirinen, E.; Euro, L.; Forsström, S.; Pasila, L.; Velagapudi, V.; Carroll, C.J.; Auwerx, J.; et al. Effective treatment of mitochondrial myopathy by nicotinamide riboside, a vitamin B3. *EMBO Mol. Med.* **2014**, *6*, 721–731. [CrossRef]
253. Partridge, L.; Fuentealba, M.; Kennedy, B.K. The quest to slow ageing through drug discovery. *Nat. Rev. Drug Discov.* **2020**, *19*, 513–532. [CrossRef]
254. Parkhitko, A.A.; Filine, E.; Tatar, M. Combinatorial interventions in aging. *Nat. Aging* **2023**, *3*, 1187–1200. [CrossRef]
255. Zhang, J.; Wang, Y.; Wang, Y.; Zhang, P.; Chen, H.Y.; Huang, S. Discrimination between Different DNA Lesions by Monitoring Single-Molecule Polymerase Stalling Kinetics during Nanopore Sequencing. *Nano Lett.* **2022**, *22*, 5561–5569. [CrossRef] [PubMed]
256. Brakedal, B.; Dölle, C.; Riemer, F.; Ma, Y.; Nido, G.S.; Skeie, G.O.; Craven, A.R.; Schwarzlmüller, T.; Brekke, N.; Diab, J.; et al. The NADPARK study: A randomized phase I trial of nicotinamide riboside supplementation in Parkinson's disease. *Cell Metab.* **2022**, *34*, 396–407.e6. [CrossRef] [PubMed]
257. Guarente, L.; Sinclair, D.A.; Kroemer, G. Human trials exploring anti-aging medicines. *Cell Metab.* **2024**, *36*, 354–376. [CrossRef] [PubMed]
258. Presterud, R.; Deng, W.H.; Wennerström, A.B.; Burgers, T.; Gajera, B.; Mattsson, K.; Solberg, A.; Fang, E.F.; Nieminen, A.I.; Stray-Pedersen, A.; et al. Long-Term Nicotinamide Riboside Use Improves Coordination and Eye Movements in Ataxia Telangiectasia. *Mov. Disord.* **2024**, *39*, 360–369. [CrossRef]
259. Van Soest, D.M.K.; Polderman, P.E.; Den Toom, W.T.F.; Keijer, J.P.; Van Roosmalen, M.J.; Leyten, T.M.F.; Lehmann, J.; Zwakenberg, S.; De Henau, S.; van Boxtel, R.; et al. Mitochondrial H2O2 release does not directly cause damage to chromosomal DNA. *Nat. Commun.* **2024**, *15*, 2725. [CrossRef]
260. Sharma, V.; Collins, L.B.; Chen Thuei Herr, N.; Takeda, S.; Sun, W.; Swenberg, J.A.; Nakamura, J. Oxidative stress at low levels can induce clustered DNA lesions leading to NHEJ mediated mutations. *Oncotarget* **2016**, *7*, 25377–25390. [CrossRef]
261. Li, T.S.; Marbán, E. Physiological Levels of Reactive Oxygen Species Are Required to Maintain Genomic Stability in Stem Cells. *Stem Cells* **2010**, *28*, 1178–1185. [CrossRef]
262. Sakellariou, G.K.; Pearson, T.; Lightfoot, A.P.; Nye, G.A.; Wells, N.; Giakoumaki, I.I.; Griffiths, R.D.; McArdle, A.; Jackson, M.J. Long-term administration of the mitochondria-targeted antioxidant mitoquinone mesylate fails to attenuate age-related oxidative damage or rescue the loss of muscle mass and function associated with aging of skeletal muscle. *FASEB J.* **2016**, *30*, 3771–3785. [CrossRef]
263. Bast, A.; Haenen, G.R.M.M. Ten misconceptions about antioxidants. *Trends Pharmacol. Sci.* **2013**, *34*, 430–436. [CrossRef]
264. Lu, L.Y.; Ou, N.; Lu, Q.B. Antioxidant Induces DNA Damage, Cell Death and Mutagenicity in Human Lung and Skin Normal Cells. *Sci. Rep.* **2013**, *3*, 3169. [CrossRef] [PubMed]
265. Sadowska-Bartosz, I.; Bartosz, G. Effect of Antioxidants Supplementation on Aging and Longevity. *BioMed Res. Int.* **2014**, *2014*, 404680. [CrossRef]
266. Milisav, I.; Ribarič, S.; Poljsak, B. Antioxidant Vitamins and Ageing. In *Biochemistry and Cell Biology of Ageing: Part I Biomedical Science [Internet]*; Harris, J.R., Korolchuk, V.I., Eds.; Subcellular Biochemistry; Springer: Singapore, 2018; Volume 90, pp. 1–23. Available online: http://link.springer.com/10.1007/978-981-13-2835-0_1 (accessed on 3 February 2025).
267. Gulcin, İ. Antioxidants: A comprehensive review. *Arch. Toxicol.* **2025**, *99*, 1893–1997. [CrossRef]
268. Arczewska, K.D.; Piekiełko-Witkowska, A. The Influence of Micronutrients and Environmental Factors on Thyroid DNA Integrity. *Nutrients* **2025**, *17*, 2065. [CrossRef]
269. Wang, X.; He, J.; Sun, M.; Wang, S.; Qu, J.; Shi, H.; Rao, B. High-dose vitamin C as a metabolic treatment of cancer: A new dimension in the era of adjuvant and intensive therapy. *Clin. Transl. Oncol.* **2025**, *27*, 1366–1382. [CrossRef]
270. Borsoi, F.T.; Neri-Numa, I.A.; De Oliveira, W.Q.; De Araújo, F.F.; Pastore, G.M. Dietary polyphenols and their relationship to the modulation of non-communicable chronic diseases and epigenetic mechanisms: A mini-review. *Food Chem. Mol. Sci.* **2023**, *6*, 100155. [CrossRef]
271. Brabson, J.P.; Leesang, T.; Mohammad, S.; Cimmino, L. Epigenetic Regulation of Genomic Stability by Vitamin C. *Front. Genet.* **2021**, *12*, 675780. [CrossRef]
272. Speciale, A.; Chirafisi, J.; Saija, A.; Cimino, F. Nutritional Antioxidants and Adaptive Cell Responses: An Update. *CMM* **2011**, *11*, 770–789. [CrossRef]

https://doi.org/10.3390/nu18020246

nutrients

MDPI

Review

From Evidence to Practice: A Narrative Framework for Integrating the Mediterranean Diet into Inflammatory Bowel Disease Management

Riya Gautam Naik [1,2], Sarah A. Purcell [2,3,4], Stephanie L. Gold [5], Victoria Christiansen [6], Leah D. D'Aloisio [1], Maitreyi Raman [7] and Natasha Haskey [1,*]

1 Department of Biology, Irving K. Barber Faculty of Science, University of British Columbia Okanagan, Kelowna, BC V1V 1V7, Canada; riyagn@student.ubc.ca (R.G.N.); leahdaloisio@hotmail.com (L.D.D.)
2 Centre for Chronic Disease Prevention and Management, Southern Medical Program, Faculty of Medicine, University of British Columbia, Kelowna, BC V1V 1V7, Canada; sarah.purcell@ubc.ca
3 Division of Endocrinology, Department of Medicine, University of British Columbia, Vancouver, BC V5Z 1M9, Canada
4 School of Health and Exercise Sciences, Faculty of Health and Social Development, University of British Columbia Okanagan, Kelowna, BC V1V 1V7, Canada
5 The Henry D. Janowitz Division of Gastroenterology, Icahn School of Medicine at Mount Sinai, New York, NY 10029, USA; stephanie.gold@mountsinai.org
6 Gastroenterology Clinic, Red Deer Regional Hospital, Department of Nutrition Services, Alberta Health Services, Red Deer, AB T4N 4E7, Canada; victoria.christiansen@albertahealthservices.ca
7 Division of Gastroenterology and Hepatology, Department of Medicine, Cumming School of Medicine, University of Calgary, Calgary, AB T2N 1N4, Canada; mkothand@ucalgary.ca
* Correspondence: natasha.haskey@ubc.ca

Abstract: Emerging evidence underscores the pivotal role of diet in preventing and managing inflammatory bowel disease (IBD). As our comprehension of the microbiome's role in IBD expands, dietary modifications are increasingly recognized as potential adjuncts or primary therapeutic strategies. Key components of the Mediterranean diet (MD)—including microbiota-accessible carbohydrates, omega-3 fatty acids, polyphenols, and antioxidants—have demonstrated promise in enhancing gut microbiota diversity and reducing intestinal inflammation, making it a practical approach for managing IBD. Moreover, the MD offers additional benefits considering the rising prevalence of comorbid chronic inflammatory conditions such as diabetes, cardiovascular disease, and obesity in IBD patients. The purpose of this narrative review was to provide an overview of the feasibility and clinical outcomes of the MD and offer evidence-based guidance for researchers and practitioners on how to adapt the MD to patients with IBD. According to several cross-sectional and interventional studies, the MD is feasible for patients with IBD and confers several benefits, such as reduced inflammation, improved disease activity, and enhanced quality of life, with a strong adherence rate and minimal adverse effects. To facilitate knowledge translation, we provide a practical framework for integrating the MD as a nutritional therapy for IBD, including specific recommendations and messaging that researchers, practitioners, and patients can use. By synthesizing current evidence and offering actionable insights, the aim is to facilitate the integration of the MD into IBD management, with the potential to improve patient outcomes.

Keywords: Mediterranean diet; ulcerative colitis; Crohn's disease; nutrition therapy

1. Introduction

Inflammatory bowel disease (IBD), which includes Crohn's disease (CD) and ulcerative colitis (UC), is a chronic, debilitating inflammatory condition affecting the gastrointestinal tract.

Its relapsing and remitting pattern, characterized by symptoms such as diarrhea, abdominal pain, rectal bleeding, and weight loss, negatively impacts patients' morbidity and quality of life [1]. While advancements in treatments have provided relief for some, a "therapeutic ceiling" has been reached, as 30–40% of patients do not respond or lose response to biological therapies [2,3]. This challenge has ignited growing interest among patients and clinicians in non-pharmacological strategies, particularly dietary interventions, which promise to reshape the gut microbiota, restore microbial balance, and reduce intestinal inflammation.

The increasing global prevalence of IBD, particularly in newly industrialized regions such as South America, Eastern Europe, South Asia, and Africa, as well as among immigrants transitioning from developing to developed countries, highlights the critical role of environmental factors in the pathophysiology of the disease [4]. The increase in IBD cases among ethnic groups and nationalities, where it was previously uncommon, is closely linked to the adoption of the Western lifestyle [5]. This results in alterations in environmental factors, including better hygiene standards, lifestyle shifts, changes in nutritional patterns, and modifications in food products, including increased quantities of xenobiotics in food [6]. The Western diet of today is characterized by a high consumption of refined sugars, refined carbohydrates, sodium, animal proteins, and ultra-processed foods, which contrasts sharply with the traditional diets of previous generations [7]. Growing evidence highlights the detrimental impact of this modern dietary pattern on the gut microbiome [8]. Alterations in the microbiota compromise intestinal barrier integrity, allowing antigenic microbial and diet-derived components to translocate into the underlying mucosa [7]. This triggers an abnormal immune response and perpetuates a cycle of inflammation, further linking dietary factors to the onset and worsening of chronic conditions such as IBD [8].

The Mediterranean diet (MD) is a whole-food, plant-based dietary approach recommended for patients with IBD [9]. Its core elements include high consumption of olive oil and plant-based foods such as vegetables, fruits, whole grains, legumes, nuts, and seeds, moderate intake of fish, seafood, and dairy, low-to-moderate alcohol consumption (primarily red wine), and limited intake of red meat and processed foods [10]. The MD emphasizes unprocessed, anti-inflammatory foods, promoting a diet rich in microbiota-accessible carbohydrates, lean protein, and omega-3 fatty acids [10]. Due to its established benefits in enhancing gut microbiota diversity, composition, and function, as well as its anti-inflammatory properties—both in healthy individuals and emerging studies in IBD [11–14]—the best practice guidelines recommend that all patients with IBD should be encouraged to adopt the MD for its potential to improve gut health and manage inflammation [9].

Several studies support the importance of diet in the management of IBD, with a growing number of solid food diets for patients with IBD [15,16]. A comprehensive comparison of these approaches is beyond the scope of this review; however, exclusive enteral nutrition, the Crohn's disease exclusion diet (CDED), the specific carbohydrate diet (SCD), and the low fermentable oligosaccharides, disaccharides, monosaccharides, and polyol (FODMAP) diet show promise for improving the management of IBD [17]. Exclusion diets have been the primary focus for managing IBD, with few studies exploring the benefits of inclusion diets, such as the MD [15,18,19]. This shift in perspective emphasizes incorporating nutrient-rich, health-promoting foods rather than focusing on elimination. This narrative review critically examines the unique attributes and potential benefits of the MD in IBD management. By synthesizing the existing literature, this review aims to highlight the MD's effects on IBD outcomes and offer practical guidance for integrating this dietary approach in to clinical practice.

2. Methods

To enhance the rigor of this narrative review, a literature search was conducted in PubMed from inception until 4 June 2024 to identify English-language articles involving human participants. To identify relevant articles, we combined IBD-related terms ((Inflammatory Bowel Diseases[mh] OR "inflammatory bowel disease*" [Title/Abstract] OR IBD[Title/Abstract] OR Crohn*[Title/Abstract] OR "ulcerative colitis" [Title/Abstract])) with MD-related terms ("Mediterranean diet" [Title/Abstract] OR Mediterranean diet [mh]). The reference lists of articles identified on PubMed were also reviewed to identify other potentially relevant articles. Both observational and interventional studies were included.

3. The Mechanisms for Diet in Inflammatory Bowel Disease

The bacteriome in IBD is altered and is characterized by the loss of beneficial microbes, expansion of pathobionts, and reduced microbial diversity [20]. It is well established that patients with IBD have reduced levels of beneficial anaerobic microbes, including *Faecalibacterium prausnitzii, Roseburia, Bacteroides, Suterella, Bifidobacterium,* and *Lachnospiraceae* [20]. These microbes play a critical role in breaking down microbiota-accessible carbohydrates (MACs) to produce short-chain fatty acids (SCFAs) like butyrate, acetate, and propionate. SCFAs are highly relevant in IBD due to their ability to modulate immune responses and maintain intestinal homeostasis [21]. They reprogram the metabolism of innate immune cells like macrophages, monocytes, and neutrophils, promoting anti-inflammatory phenotypes and reducing pro-inflammatory cytokine production. SCFAs inhibit histone deacetylases (HDACs), leading to epigenetic suppression of pro-inflammatory genes, and they downregulate nuclear factor-kappa B (NF-κB) signaling, a central driver of inflammation in IBD [21,22]. Additionally, SCFAs strengthen the intestinal barrier by enhancing epithelial cell function, mucin production, and tight junction integrity, preventing microbial translocation and excessive immune activation [21]. The alterations in SCFAs in IBD, often linked to microbial dysbiosis and low MAC intake, contribute to disease pathogenesis, highlighting their therapeutic potential [23,24].

In contrast, patients with IBD have an overgrowth of bacteria such as *Escherichia, Clostridioides difficile, Salmonella, Enterobacteriaceae,* and *Proteobacteria* [20]. These microbes can disrupt gut homeostasis by producing pro-inflammatory metabolites, such as lipopolysaccharides (LPS), that stimulate the innate immune system via toll-like receptors (TLRs) [22]. This microbial dysbiosis, marked by an imbalance of protective and harmful microbes, compromises the intestinal barrier. Increased permeability allows the translocation of bacteria and dietary antigens into the underlying mucosa, triggering abnormal immune activation and perpetuating chronic inflammation [23]. For instance, emulsifiers and other components of processed foods common in the Western diet can exacerbate this process by destabilizing the mucus layer and promoting immune activation [24].

The Western dietary pattern's role in the development of chronic diseases, such as IBD, is well established [25]. Several reviews and large cohort studies have consistently shown that the Western dietary pattern plays a significant role in the etiology of IBD [26–30]. These studies consistently highlight an increased risk of developing IBD among individuals with a high consumption of animal fats (omega-6 fatty acids), red and processed meat, sugar, refined grains, and ultra-processed foods [26,30]. In contrast, high fiber and fruit intakes are inversely associated with IBD risk [29]. The positive link between fat consumption, particularly trans fatty acids and omega-6 fatty acids, is most predominant in UC [31], while fish consumption is associated with a reduced risk of CD [32]. Western dietary patterns show an overall decrease in abundance in *Bifidobacterium, Lactobacillus,* and *Eubacterium,* while increasing the abundance of pathobionts such as *Clostridium bolteae, Ruminoccocus obeum, Ruminococcus gnavus,* and

Blautia hydrogenotrophica [25]. The mucolytic nature of microbes combined with low fiber intake results in these bacteria using the mucus layer as their primary food source, leading to erosion of the epithelial barrier, gut permeability, and intestinal inflammation [33].

Adopting dietary patterns, such as the MD, has been shown to foster a health-associated microbiome and mitigate intestinal inflammation in patients with IBD [12,34]. The MD, rich in fiber, antioxidants, omega-3 fatty acids, polyphenols, and plant-based proteins, provides substrates for beneficial microbes, enhancing SCFA production and promoting a balanced gut microbiota and balancing inflammation [34]. Polyphenols, for example, exert prebiotic-like effects by selectively enriching commensal bacteria, while omega-3 fatty acids modulate inflammatory pathways by altering the composition of gut microbiota and reducing pro-inflammatory cytokines through the production of specialized pro-resolving mediators (SPMs) [35,36].

While preclinical evidence provides mechanistic insights on how the components of the MD influence intestinal epithelial barrier function and can alter immune function, clinical studies show moderate improvements in clinical markers, inflammation, and quality of life in IBD patients adhering to this diet [34]. These findings highlight the potential of the MD as a therapeutic dietary strategy. Additionally, dietary interventions can induce microbiota shifts, potentially resulting in significant and stable changes that contribute to improved disease outcomes [37]. However, substantial variation between studies underscores the need for further research into diet-microbiota interactions. Robust and consistent methodologies are essential to better understand these mechanisms, refine dietary strategies, and develop personalized treatment approaches for IBD patients.

4. The Mediterranean Diet in IBD: Transforming Clinical Biomarkers and Patient Outcomes

In the past five years, several studies have investigated the impact of dietary interventions, particularly the MD, in adults with IBD (Table 1). Chicco et al. (2020) conducted a six-month single-arm prospective MD intervention involving patients with UC ($n = 84$) or CD ($n = 58$) [38]. The study demonstrated significant improvements in obesity-related parameters, including body mass index (BMI) and waist circumference, and a reduction in liver steatosis assessed using abdominal ultrasound. Additionally, the intervention normalized C-reactive protein (CRP) and fecal calprotectin (FCP) levels, which are key biomarkers of inflammation and suggest reduced inflammatory burden, thereby improving disease control. Lewis et al. (2021) conducted a randomized control trial comparing the MD to the specific carbohydrate diet in patients with CD [13]. The study found no significant differences in remission rates or biomarker responses between the two diet interventions. The comparable symptomatic outcomes observed between the treatment groups may be attributed to similarities in the study diets, specifically that both were prepared using fresh ingredients. The study suggested that the MD may be preferable due to its greater ease of adherence and its broader health benefits, which extend beyond IBD management [13]. Haskey et al. (2023) examined MD versus a Canadian Habitual Diet in UC patients, with 40% of the MD group reporting improvement in the Simple Clinical Colitis Activity Index, maintenance or improvement of FCP, and alterations in microbiome composition [12]. These findings further emphasize the role of the MD in stabilizing inflammatory biomarkers and enhancing gut health, which are critical for maintaining disease remission and improving long-term outcomes. Dogan et al. (2024) investigated the MD, the MD with resveratrol supplementation, or the MD with curcumin supplementation in UC patients [39]. Improvements in waist/hip circumference, CRP, erythrocyte sedimentation rate, bowel movement frequency, MD adherence, and quality of life scores improved across all groups. However, supplementation with resveratrol or curcumin did not appear to amplify the effects of the MD. Although most studies have shown favorable results, Strauss et al. [40] and Zhang et al. [41] reported no significant changes in FCP and short-chain fatty acids in participants following an MD intervention.

Table 1. Intervention studies that assess the effect of the Mediterranean diet on clinical biomarkers in inflammatory bowel disease.

Author, Year	Study Design	Population	Diet Intervention	Outcomes	Results	Limitations
Chicco et al., 2020 [38]	Single arm intervention study	$n = 142$ adults with active IBD ($n = 84$ UC; $n = 58$ CD) Disease activity assessed through the Crohn's disease activity index for CD and partial Mayo score for UC	Six months of MD adherence Nutritional counseling provided by a nutritionist: ≥2 vegetable servings per meal, 1–2 fruit servings per meal, and 1–2 bread/cereals servings per meal, and olive oil at every meal alongside ≥2 legume servings weekly, ≥2 fish/seafood servings weekly, 2–4 egg servings weekly, and 2 poultry servings weekly and 2 dairy foods servings daily while limiting red meat and sweets to <2 servings per week. Patient adherence was assessed using 24 h recall during nutritional interviews after 6 months	Nutritional status, presence/severity of liver steatosis, therapy response Anthropometric measures: weight, BMI, visceral fat, lean body mass, fat body mass, waist circumference (measured with bioelectrical impedance analysis) Serum lipid profile and lipid function (chemical analysis) Hepatic steatosis (abdominal ultrasound exam) Quality of life (Inflammatory Bowel Disease Questionnaire)	In UC patients: ↓ BMI ($p = 0.002$) ↓ Waist circumference ($p = 0.037$) ↓ N of patients with elevated CRP ($p = 0.013$) ↓ N of patients with FCP > 250 mg/kg ($p = 0.049$) ↑ Quality of life ($p < 0.001$) In CD patients: ↓ BMI ($p = 0.023$) ↓ Waist circumference ($p = 0.040$) ↓ N of patients with elevated CRP ($p = 0.035$) ↓ N of patients with FCP > 250 mg/kg ($p = 0.035$) ↑ Quality of life ($p < 0.001$)	The lack of a control group, therefore improvements may have occurred independent of the diet. Participants were in clinical remission or affected by mild disease which might lead to overestimated effect of the dietary intervention on disease activity and QoL. Researchers did not use any specific score to quantify adherence to diet, and this was mainly based on patients' dietary recall.
Zhang et al., 2020 [41]	Randomized controlled trial	Adults ($n = 40$) with luminal CD in remission (Harvey Bradshaw Index < 5)	Two diet groups were studied: Patients that habitually consume a diversified diet pattern [DD] [higher plant-based and lower red and processed meat-based diet] compared to patients following a non-diversified diet pattern [NDD] + MD intervention for 12 weeks Adherence was assessed by 3-day weighted food records	To compare microbiota composition and function between patients in the DD group with patients in the NDD group following a 12-week structured dietary intervention based on principles from the MD	No difference in microbial beta-diversity between the two groups was observed ($p = 0.43$) The NDD + MD group demonstrated an increase in *Faecalibacterium*. No association of diet with fecal SCFAs or FCP.	No significant changes in FCP levels observed at week 12, likely due to the clinically and biochemically quiescent baseline disease state. Researchers did not use any specific score to quantify adherence to diet, and this was mainly based on patients' dietary recall.
Lewis et al., 2021 [13]	Randomized control trial	Adults ($n = 93$, 63% women) with active CD with mild to moderate CD symptoms (short CD Activity Index Score > 175 and < 400)	Participants randomly received either the SCD or the MD for the first 6 weeks (prepared meals consisting of breakfast, lunch, dinner, and 2 snacks) After the first 6 weeks, participants were instructed on food purchase and preparation that aligned with MD Participants completed a 24 h recall at baseline, weeks 6 and 12. These data were used to assign an alternate MD score	Primary outcome: Symptomatic remission at week 6 without increasing CD medication Secondary outcome: changes in FCP and CRP	Symptomatic remission in participants at week 6 ($p = 0.77$) and week 12 ($p = 0.87$) was not superior in SCD as compared to MD Among those with an elevated FCP at screening, FCP response was achieved in 8/23 participants (34.8%) with SCD and 4/13 participants (30.8%) with MD ($p = 0.83$) Among those with elevated CRP at screening, CRP response was achieved in only 2/37 participants (5.4%) with SCD and 1/28 participant (3.6%) with MD ($p = 0.68$) from screening to week 6	The study was not designed to assess endoscopic healing. Symptomatic remission was common, few patients achieved combined symptomatic remission and resolution of inflammation. This study included patients with longstanding disease, many of whom had been treated with biologics, which limits generalizability.

Table 1. *Cont.*

Author, Year	Study Design	Population	Diet Intervention	Outcomes	Results	Limitations
Haskey et al., 2023 [12]	Randomized controlled trial	Adults (n = 28) with mild-moderate UC in remission (partial Mayo score 0–2)	Two intervention diets were used, the Canadian Habitual Diet and the MD, for 12 weeks The MD group received sessions from dietitians to help adapt to the MD (based on the MD pyramid) The Canadian Habitual Diet group followed their habitual diet MD adherence was assessed using the MD serving score (MDSS)	Assessing whether MD intervention could reduce SCCAI, FCP levels, and microbiome changes	40% of MD intervention group reported minor improvements in the SCCAI scores, 27% achieved clinical response, whereas 1% reported a decrease in 1-point SCCAI score At week 12, 75% [9/12] of participants in the CHD had an FCP > 100 µg/g vs. 20% [3/15] of participants in the MD group The MD induced alterations in microbial species known to be protective in UC (*Alistipes finegoldii* and *Flavonifractor plautii*), as well as the production of short-chain fatty acids (*Ruminococcus bromii*)	A 12-week follow-up may limit insights into long-term MD effects on disease activity. Results are not generalizable to active IBD patients, as only adults in clinical remission were studied. The small sample size may reduce the study's statistical power.
Strauss and Haskey et al., 2023 [40]	Randomized open-label trial	Adults (n = 40) with active UC (partial Mayo score > 2)	Participants were assigned to MD + low sulfur diet or habitual diet Adherence assessed by the MDS	Improvement in total Mayo score and partial Mayo score	No changes in MDS or FCP were observed within or between groups Marginal improvements in partial Mayo score (median 2.0) were observed from baseline and week 8 in participants following the intervention diet ($p = 0.003$); however, this also occurred in the habitual diet ($p = 0.007$) Valerate (SCFA) and glycochenodeoxycholic acid (bile acid) were significantly different between groups at baseline and week 8 ($p = 0.05$ and $p = 0.02$, respectively)	Despite a significant decrease in sulfur intake in the MD intervention from baseline to week 8, this did not translate into a reduced FCP. The study sample was heterogeneous in disease activity, reflected by the wide range of partial Mayo scores and total Mayo scores at baseline. Baseline MDS did not differ between intervention groups, nor did it change over time within the intervention group, underscoring the need to assign participants to dietary interventions distinct from their baseline diet.
Dogan et al., 2024 [39]	Three-arm intervention study	Adults (n = 46) with mild-to-moderate UC determined by a gastroenterologist	Participants were randomly assigned into three groups: MD, MD + resveratrol (1600 mg/day), MD + curcumin (500 mg/day) for 8 weeks Bi-weekly MD education with dietitian Patient adherence was assessed using the MD adherence scale (MEDAS) with 14 items scored as either 0 or 1	Truelove–Witts Index of disease activity, serum inflammatory markers, and quality of life (measured by Short Form-36)	Significant improvement post intervention was observed within groups for waist and hip circumference, bowel movements, CRP, erythrocyte sedimentation rate and an increase in quality-of-life scores ($p < 0.05$)	Absence of clinical biomarkers (e.g., fecal calprotectin, cytokine data, and endoscopic imaging). The study was limited to individuals with mild-to-moderate active disease, which restricts the generalizability of the findings to individuals in remission or with severe active disease.

Abbreviations: ↑: higher; ↓: lower; IBD: inflammatory bowel disease; UC: Ulcerative colitis; CD: Crohn's disease; MD: Mediterranean diet; BMI: body mass index; CRP: C-reactive Protein; FCP: Fecal calprotectin; SCD: Specific carbohydrate diet; SCCAI: Simple Clinical Colitis Activity Index.

Collectively, these studies highlight the potential of the MD to improve clinical outcomes and enhance quality of life in patients with IBD, with minimal reported adverse effects. The normalization of CRP and FCP levels across several trials underscores the diet's ability to reduce systemic and intestinal inflammation, a critical goal in IBD management. These findings suggest that incorporating the MD as part of an integrated treatment approach could enhance disease control, improve patient outcomes, and potentially reduce the burden of pharmacologic therapies. However, the absence of control groups in some studies and the variability in study designs limit the ability to attribute these benefits solely to the MD. Rigorous, large-scale, randomized controlled trials with well-defined control diets are essential to validate these promising outcomes and to elucidate the precise mechanisms by which the MD exerts its therapeutic effects in IBD. Such research will further solidify the MD's role as a cornerstone of holistic IBD management.

5. Mediterranean Diet Adherence: A Path to Better Health in IBD

The health benefits of the Mediterranean diet (MD) are well established. However, there are concerns regarding the successful adoption of its principles in regions outside of the Mediterranean. While potential barriers to the practical implementation of the MD in IBD are acknowledged, to our knowledge, no published reports specifically address these challenges. Despite these gaps, valuable insights can be gained by translating knowledge from other chronic conditions where similar barriers have been successfully addressed [42,43]. For example, limited understanding of the MD's precise composition is common among patients and practitioners, highlighting the need for patient education on its specific components and associated health benefits. To improve acceptability, offering tasting sessions, food demonstrations, alternative meal ideas, and easy-to-prepare recipes could help.

Cultural identity plays a significant role in shaping food choices, often leading to resistance to adopting dietary patterns that diverge from cultural norms [44]. This presents important considerations for how the MD should be presented to non-Mediterranean populations. To facilitate its adoption, advice should be tailored to align with diverse cultural eating habits and traditional food views. Additionally, there is a perception that the MD is expensive. Providing budgeting tips and low-cost recipe ideas could help address financial concerns [43]. Furthermore, the availability of MD components in colder climates is often questioned, as the diet is traditionally associated with salads and fresh fruits. To address this, offering practical information on which foods are in season to purchase and providing alternative sources of fruits and vegetables (e.g., frozen or canned) will make the diet more feasible for individuals living in colder regions [42]. Concerns about weight gain from consuming olive oil and nuts are common, but research has shown that these components do not promote adiposity [45,46]. Education on the health benefits of replacing saturated fats with monounsaturated and polyunsaturated fats could help address these misconceptions.

While these factors—such as cultural identity, perceived costs, and ingredient availability—pose challenges to adopting the MD in IBD, recent studies demonstrate that high adherence to the MD is achievable within the IBD population (Table 2).

Papada et al. (2019) reported that higher adherence to the MD in patients with CD was associated with reduced disease activity ($p < 0.001$) and inflammation ($p = 0.027$) [47]. Similarly, Godny et al. (2020) observed that UC patients post-pouch surgery with higher MD adherence ($p < 0.05$) had lower FCP levels ($p < 0.05$) during an eight-year follow-up and lower rates of pouchitis [48]. Naqvi et al. (2021) reported a positive association between leafy green vegetables and a reduced FCP and an omega-6:omega-3 ratio of 8:1 was associated with normalized CRP. However, no specific relationships with MD adherence were observed [49]. Fiorindi et al. (2021) and Celik et al. (2023) found that higher MD adherence was associated with lower disease activity scores and improved mental health outcomes in both CD and UC [50,51]. A randomized trial by Haskey et al. (2022) demonstrated that a structured MD intervention in patients with UC improved diet quality (p = 0.007), and patients could successfully adhere to the MD [52]. Despite these promising findings, several limitations should be acknowledged. Studies have utilized varying symptom scoring systems, biomarkers, and MD adherence tools, which complicate direct comparisons, and the duration of dietary assessments varies widely. Additionally, the reliance on self-reported dietary data introduces potential inaccuracies, such as misreporting and bias, underscoring the need for future research in this area.

Table 2. Summary of research studies evaluating adherence to the Mediterranean diet and its impact on inflammatory bowel disease clinical aspects.

Author, Year	Population	Primary Objective	Diet Assessment Methods	MED Diet Assessment/Adherence	Results
Papada et al., 2019 [47]	Outpatient adults with endoscopically proven CD (n = 86)	Characterize the effects of MD adherence on quality of life, disease activity, and inflammatory markers	Assignment of MedDiet scores based on 24 h recall	MedDiet score evaluated by an experienced dietitian	↑ MedDiet scores in patients with inactive CD versus patients with active CD (p = 0.005) MedDiet score was negatively correlated with Harvey–Bradshaw Index (p < 0.001) and CRP (p = 0.027)
Godny et al., 2020 [48]	UC patients who underwent pouch surgery (n = 153)	Assess changes in inflammation markers, and reduced risk of pouchitis development in patients with UC after pouch surgery	Assessment of MD adherence during a 6-month interval between 2015 and 2018 based on a food frequency questionnaire	MED score Adherence defined as MED score ≥ 5	↔ MED scores between patients with active and inactive disease (p = 0.10) Patients with <200 mcg/g fecal calprotectin had ↑ MED score versus patients with elevated fecal calprotectin (p < 0.05) ↔ pouchitis development rates in patients with high MED diet adherence versus patients with low adherence (p = 0.17)
Naqvi et al., 2021 [49]	Adults (n = 66) with CD and clinical remission (steroid-free, clinical remission with Harvey–Bradshaw Index < 5 for > 3 months)	Assess the relationship between diet and markers of inflammation	A 3-day weighted food/drink intake, reviewed by a dietitian	pMDS score modified to exclude red wine consumption	Increasing daily servings of leafy green vegetables were associated with FCP ≤ 100 µg/mg (p < 0.05) omega-6:omega-3 polyunsaturated fatty acid ratio of 8:1 was associated with CRP ≤ 5 mg/L
Fiorindi et al., 2021 [50]	Adults with IBD (n = 62 CD, n = 18 UC)	Assess level of MD adherence in IBD patients with MEDI-LITE questionnaire	MEDI-LITE questionnaire conducted via face-to-face interview	MEDI-LITE questionnaire scores > 11 deemed adherent	↔ between CD and UC patients in the MEDI-LITE scores (p = 0.543) ↑ MEDI-LITE score in remission CD patients than active CD patients (p < 0.001) No significant differences in MEDI-LITE scores were found in remission UC patients and active UC patients with pouchitis (p = 0.218)
Haskey et al., 2022 [52]	Randomized controlled trial Adults (n = 28) with mild-moderate UC in remission (partial Mayo score 0–2)	Examining the proportion of participants achieving high adherence to the MD measured by the MDSSs Changes in diet quality, quality of life, nutritional diet adequacy were also measured as secondary analysis	Two intervention diets were used, the CHD (Canadian Habitual Diet) and the MD The MD group received sessions from dietitians to help adapt to the MD (based on the MD pyramid) with MD specific recipes, 4-week meal plan, food lists The CHD group followed their habitual diet	MDSSs (> 16 points) as measured after 12 weeks deemed adherent	After 12 weeks, there was a significantly higher MDSS in the MD intervention group compared to the CHD group (p = 0.010) and improved diet quality (p = 0.007) as measured by the Healthy Eating Index. No significance in changes in quality-of-life scores in both the groups

Table 2. *Cont.*

Author, Year	Population	Primary Objective	Diet Assessment Methods	MED Diet Assessment/Adherence	Results
Celik et al., 2023 [51]	Adults diagnosed with IBD ($n = 83$; $n = 38$ UC patients; $n = 45$ CD patients)	Assess the effect of MD adherence on disease activity (Crohn's disease activity index; Mayo Score for UC) and quality of life (Short Form-36) in IBD patients	Face-to-face interviews with a dietitian to provide MEDAS scores	MEDAS scores of ≤ 6, 7–9 and ≥ 9 categorized as low, acceptable and high adherence, respectively	Low MD adherence had higher Mayo Clinic scores ($p = 0.018$) No significant differences in Crohn's disease activity index scores and BMI with MD adherence ($p > 0.05$) In UC patients, high MD adherence was associated with better scores in emotional problems ($p = 0.03$), mental health ($p = 0.03$), and overall health perception ($p < 0.01$) UC patients categorized as 'low adherence' had higher UC Mayo Clinic scores ($p = 0.018$). In CD patients, MD adherence was not correlated with any sub-dimensions of quality of life measured by the Short Form-36 ($p > 0.05$).

↔: no difference; ↑: higher; CD: Crohn's disease; IBD: Inflammatory bowel disease; MD: Mediterranean diet; UC: Ulcerative colitis; CD: Crohn's disease; BMI: body mass index; MDSS: Mediterranean diet serving score; MEDAS: Mediterranean diet adherence score; pMDS: partial Mediterranean diet score.

6. Current Gaps in Research

Future studies should address existing limitations by standardizing tools for assessing dietary adherence and symptom scoring, enabling consistent comparisons across studies. The use of digital tools, such as mobile apps for real-time tracking of adherence and symptoms, could refine dietary strategies and improve patient outcomes. These tools can offer patients personalized guidance, track dietary intake, and provide real-time feedback, ultimately enhancing adherence to the MD and improving overall patient engagement. Incorporating control groups and conducting long-term, multicenter trials with larger sample sizes would provide valuable insights into the sustained benefits of MD adherence over time, helping to establish the MD as an effective long-term nutritional therapy for IBD management.

Consideration of cultural preferences, ingredient accessibility, and socioeconomic factors are necessary to develop tailored interventions that improve adherence to the MD. Structured dietary education programs, along with guidance on ingredient substitutions, could help overcome barriers to adoption. An examination of the impact of the MD on quality of life and mental health outcomes, particularly across subgroups with differing disease activity levels, is warranted.

Finally, advanced biomarker analysis and exploration of the mechanistic pathways underlying the MD's anti-inflammatory effects would provide deeper insights into its therapeutic potential. It is equally important to focus on the variability of individual responses to the MD and the impact of confounding variables, as this will be key to advancing the field and optimizing personalized treatment strategies.

7. From Research to Practice: Bridging the Mediterranean Diet and IBD Care

The literature highlights the effectiveness of a dietary intervention rooted in the core principles of the MD, as represented by the IBD Food Pyramid (Table 3) [53]. Research indicates that the MD is generally well tolerated among patients with IBD [52,54]. However, tolerance to specific foods can vary and may need to be adjusted based on the individual's disease phenotype (Table 4 and Figure 1) [55].

Table 3. Key features of the inflammatory bowel disease food pyramid.

Guiding Principles

- Main meals consumed daily should include three components: vegetables, fruits and whole-grains. In addition, legumes, fermented dairy should be consumed, though not necessarily in every meal.
- Stock kitchens with minimally processed foods.
- Eating 3–5 x/day, smaller meals may be better tolerated when gastrointestinal symptoms are present. In some patients, structured fasting can help.
- Frequencies and serving sizes should be aligned with the individual's energy requirements.
- Mindful eating, thorough chewing, and pausing for meals are essential for individuals with IBD. Since digestion begins in the mouth, paying extra attention to these habits becomes even more crucial when the gut is inflamed to optimize digestive and absorptive functions.
- Slowly adapt your diet to make it more MD-like, pick one change every week and incorporate it gradually.

	Frequency	**Serving Size**	**Included Foods ***
Every Meal			
Extra Virgin Olive Oil	1 serving/main meal	1 tablespoon	High quality oil (see commentary about choosing quality)
Fruit	1–2 servings/main meal	½ cup or 1 medium sized piece	A variety of colors in both vegetables and fruits is strongly recommended to ensure intake of a broad range of micronutrients and phytochemicals
Vegetables	2 servings/day plus 1–2 servings/day of leafy greens	½ cup or 1 medium sized piece plus 1 cup raw	
Cereals	1–2 servings/main meal	1 cup cooked or 1 slice of bread	Includes bread, pasta, rice, oats Preferably whole grains as tolerated
Daily			
Starchy Foods (Resistant Starch)	1–2 servings/day	1 cup per day	Includes cooked, cooled reheated rice, pasta, potatoes, winter squash, yams, cassava, and taro
Dairy	2 servings/day	¾ cup yogurt or 1.5 ounces of hard cheese (cheddar) or 1 cup of milk	Yogurt (Greek yogurt, low sugar), kefir or hard cheese may be better tolerated due to lower lactose content
Nuts/Seeds	1–2 servings/day	1 ounce or 1/4 of a cup	Without sugar, fat or salt, nut/seed butters may be better tolerated
Weekly			
Legumes	3 servings/week	¾ cup (150 g) cooked	Includes beans, peas, lentils, edamame, and soy
Fatty Fish and Seafood	2 servings/week	6 ounces twice per week	Includes salmon, mackerel, tuna, trout, herring, and sardines
Eggs	1 egg/daily	1 large egg (with yolk and white)	Whole eggs, including those used for cooking and baking
White Meat	2 servings/week	4 ounces	Includes skinless chicken and turkey Choose lean poultry (e.g., breast, wing, or back portions)
Red Meat	1 serving/week	< 8 ounces per week	Includes pork, beef, and lamb

Table 3. *Cont.*

Limit		
Sweets	< 2 servings per week	Includes sugar, candies, pastries, sweetened fruit juice, and soft drinks Fruit should be eaten in place of sweets
Processed Meat	< 1 ounce (30 g) per week	Includes deli meats, ham, sausages, bacon, jerky, and hot dogs
Ultra-Processed Foods	Avoid as much as possible	Includes ice cream, chips/crisps, mass-produced bread and bread products, crackers, biscuits, cookies, instant soups
Additives	Limit	Includes maltodextrin, carrageenan, carboxymethylcellulose, polysorbate-80, titanium dioxide and sulfites, xanthan gum, aspartame, sucralose, saccharin
Alcohol (includes spirits, beer and wine)	Limit	Replace with water or herbal infusions

* Does not apply to patients with strictures, texture modification is needed.

Table 4. Modifications of fruit and vegetables based on the stage of disease.

	Active	Strictures/Ileostomy #	Remission
Fruit	Remove skin/peel Blend into smoothies Apples, bananas and canned/pureed fruit packed in water or juice Pureed fruit (e.g., applesauce, fruit coulis) Cooked/stewed fruit * Limit: dried fruit, coconut, pineapple, prunes	Follow active disease recommendations Smoothies are a great option	No restrictions, based on individual tolerance
Vegetables	Cook vegetables until fork tender and remove peels Blend greens into smoothies Consider blended soups * Limit: brussels sprouts, cabbage, cauliflower, kale, asparagus, peas, corn, artichoke	Follow active disease recommendations **plus:** Avoid skins, tough stalks and seeds as well as raw salads	No restrictions, based on individual tolerance
Whole Grains and Starchy Foods (Resistant Starch)	Focus on including soluble fiber: barley, oats, psyllium Green bananas Cook, cool, reheat pasta, rice, sweet potato, and potatoes Limit whole wheat flour, wheat bran	Avoid insoluble fiber, corn hulls, popcorn, wild rice Cook, cool, reheat pasta, rice, and potatoes	Replace refined grains with whole grains, including both insoluble and soluble fiber Cook, cool, reheat pasta, rice, and potatoes No restrictions, based on individual tolerance
Nuts and Seeds	Nut and seed butters without added sugar, salt, or fat	Ground nut and seed butters without added sugar, salt, or fat	No restrictions, based on individual tolerance
Legumes	Lentils, split pea, tempeh or tofu	Mashed or pureed beans (e.g., hummus) or tofu	No restrictions, based on individual tolerance
Dairy Products	Lower lactose, lactose-free or fermented options may be better tolerated	No restrictions, based on individual tolerance	No restrictions, based on individual tolerance
Fatty Fish, Eggs, White Meat, and Red Meat	Focus on fish, skinless poultry and eggs while limiting red meat	Stewed, fork tender meat Avoid tougher cuts of meat, unless slow-cooking or stewing (e.g., chuck, brisket, or round, chicken wings), sausages with casing.	No restrictions, based on individual tolerance

Strictures are narrowing in the intestine. * Based on individual tolerance as tolerance may vary.

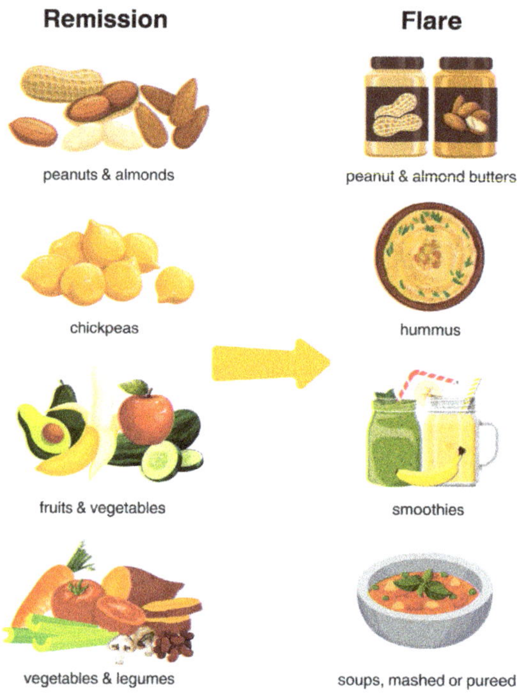
Remission
Flare
peanuts & almonds
peanut & almond butters
chickpeas
hummus
fruits & vegetables
smoothies
vegetables & legumes
soups, mashed or pureed

Figure 1. Visual comparison of dietary choices during remission versus active disease. This comparison highlights the practical implications tailored to different phases of IBD. During remission, patients can focus on nutrient-dense, whole foods such as nuts, legumes, fruits, and vegetables, consumed as tolerated. These choices support gut health, reduce inflammation, and promote overall well-being. During active disease, to ease digestion and minimize discomfort, the texture of foods can be modified—such as opting for cooked, peeled, or blended versions of fruits and vegetables and avoiding high-fiber, hard-to-digest items like nuts or raw legumes (Visual created by Leah D. D'Aloisio).

Comorbid conditions, such as cardiovascular disease, colon cancer, diabetes, and living with overweightare rising in IBD and may require special consideration in treatment planning [56]. The presence of comorbidities often requires a more holistic approach to patient care, with physicians needing to balance the management of multiple health issues simultaneously. A multidisciplinary approach involving specialists from different fields is essential for optimizing patient outcomes. Managing IBD in the context of comorbidities highlights the increased complexity of treatment and the need for personalized care strategies to ensure both diseases are addressed effectively. Collaboration with a registered dietitian specializing in IBD can help patients tailor the MD to their needs, ensuring nutritional recommendations are appropriately implemented and nutrient deficiencies are avoided.

To address implementation challenges, we present key recommendations and strategies for counseling patients with IBD on adopting the MD more effectively. Affordability, availability, and personal dietary preferences should be considered, as these factors can significantly impact adherence in diverse patient populations. We acknowledge that these recommendations are primarily based on the expert opinion of our multidisciplinary team, which includes gastroenterologists, dietitians, and scientists specializing in gastrointestinal nutrition. To the best of our knowledge, no published manuscripts have comprehensively addressed these practical recommendations for patients.

(a) Choose Extra Virgin Olive Oil (EVOO)

Messaging: "Choose good fat, not low fat"

High-quality EVOO is the primary source of dietary fat in the MD, recognized as a functional food due to its nutritional value and health benefits [57]. The health benefits are largely attributed to its high oleic acid content (65–83% monounsaturated fatty acids) and bioactive compounds like tocopherols, polyphenols, and flavonoids [58]. EVOO is distinct from other common vegetable oils (e.g., sunflower, corn, or soybeanoils), which are rich in omega-6 fatty acids and have been associated with inflammation [59,60]. Additionally, the ratio of fatty acids in EVOO confers stability against oxidative thermal degradation, particularly by reducing the formation of volatile aldehydes compared to peanut and canola oils [61]. EVOO can be heated to as high as 400 °F (deep frying occurs at 350–375 °F). For those dishes that require prolonged heat (e.g., stir-frying), avocado oil is a better option.

Patient recommendations:

Using a high-quality EVOO is important, as lower-quality olive oils lose nearly all their beneficial properties. Look for a seal of approval from the International Olive Council or North America Olive Oil Association which certifies standards for olive oil's purity and quality. High quality EVOO is typically packaged in dark bottles (amber, black, or green glass) to prevent oxidation caused by light and heat. To preserve quality, store the oil in a cool, dark place. For optimal flavor and nutritional benefits, consume the oil as soon as possible after the harvest date (generally within 18 months if unopened) and within 3 months once opened [62].

a. Use EVOO liberally in cooking (stable to 420 °F) in place of omega-6-rich vegetable oils (e.g., sunflower, corn, soybean, palm, or canola oils).
b. Drizzle EVOO on salads, vegetables, grilled fish, chicken, and pasta.
c. Use EVOO as a base for salad dressings instead of commercially prepared salad dressings.
d. Dip crusty bread in EVOO in place of butter or margarine.
e. Add citrus-infused EVOO (e.g., lemon, orange) to breakfast smoothies, oatmeal, and yogurt.
f. Add herb-infused EVOO (e.g., garlic, basil, rosemary) to salads, marinades and eggs.

(b) Fruit and Vegetables

Messaging: "The more colors the better, with fruit and vegetables being center stage".

Fruit and vegetable consumption is a cornerstone of the MD, offering health benefits due to its rich fiber content, polyphenols, antioxidants, and micronutrients. Flavonoids are a type of polyphenol found in common fruits, vegetables, nuts, cocoa, tea, grains, and herbs. They are biologically active compounds responsible for the vibrant colors in fruits and vegetables [63]. Besides flavonoids, fruits and vegetables are key sources of fiber, potassium, folate, and antioxidants such as vitamin C, α-carotene, β-carotene, β-cryptoxanthin, and lycopene. Polyphenols are also crucial as immunonutrients due to their antioxidant and anti-inflammatory properties [64]. Research suggests that polyphenols commonly found in fruit and vegetables exert their effects primarily by remodeling the gut microbiota, acting as potential prebiotics that help shape a healthier microbial composition, strengthening barrier integrity, and modulating balanced immune responses [64].

Patient recommendations:

Fruits and vegetables are the foundation of meals. Varying the types of fruit and vegetables consumed throughout the day ensures a diverse intake of nutrients and compounds, each offering unique health benefits.

a. Dark leafy greens can be used as salads, added to frittatas, eggs, smoothies, and soups.

b. Add grated vegetables, such as carrots, zucchini, spinach, and kale to pasta sauces and soups.
c. Canned tomato products are rich in lycopene (an antioxidant). A few tomato-centric recipes include shakshuka, stuffed vegetables, stews, curries, baked fish with tomatoes, and marinara sauce.
d. Load up sandwiches with vegetables.
e. Increase the nutritional value of smoothies by mixing in fruit and leafy greens.
f. Top salads with fruit.
g. Add fruit to yogurt or cereal.
h. Try baked fruit topped with oatmeal, cinnamon, and maple syrup for dessert.
i. Roast vegetables to increase flavor, drizzle with olive oil.
j. To save preparation time, consider packaged ready-to-eat fresh fruit and vegetables. Frozen and canned fruit and vegetables are budget-friendly options.
k. Choose canned vegetables packed in water and look for "no salt added" or "low sodium" options with no added sugar, preservatives. or artificial additives. Even when purchasing "no salt added" options, it is good practice to rinse them under water to remove any additives or preservatives.
l. Choose canned fruits packed in water to reduce the sugar content. Whole fruits (e.g., peaches, pears, etc.,) have generally fewer additives than "cocktails". Check for extra additives, as some products labeled "no sugar" may still contain artificial sweeteners. It is good practice to rinse them under water to remove extra sugar and preservatives.

(c) Whole Grains and Starchy Foods

Messaging: "Feed your microbes fiber, or they will feed on you".

Whole grains are essential to the MD as they are rich in vitamins, minerals, lignans, phytochemicals (phenolic acids, polyphenols, and phytosterol compounds), and fiber [65,66]. Common examples of grains include whole wheat, brown rice, oats, millets, barley, and rye. Another form of fiber is resistant starch. Resistant starch is a broad category of structurally complex starches resistant to digestive enzymes in the gastrointestinal tract, commonly found in green bananas, unprocessed whole grains, legumes, and cooked then cooled rice, pasta, or potatoes [67]. Many patients believe that they should avoid dietary fiber. Still, strong evidence suggests that dietary fiber can positively impact the gut microbiome, improve IBD symptoms, balance inflammation, and improve health-related quality of life [68]. Currently, there are no specific guidelines on the relative proportions of different dietary types of fiber to include in the diet. For patients who experience difficulty tolerating fiber or they have CD with strictures (intestinal narrowing), fiber intake can be adjusted by modifying the food textures, such as blending, mashing, or pureeing to enhance digestibility. Patient recommendations:

a. Breakfast is one of the easiest ways to increase fiber by consuming whole-grain toast or oatmeal.
b. Swap refined grains like white bread, white rice, and pasta for whole grains like brown rice, quinoa, bulgur, barley, and farro.
c. Add barley to soups to boost soluble fiber.
d. Psyllium can be sprinkled on food.
e. Cook, cool, reheat pasta, rice, and potatoes to increase resistant starch.
f. Use whole grain flours in baking (e.g., oat flour).

(d) Nuts and Seeds

Messaging: "Embrace nut and seed butters".

The MD recommends consuming nuts and seeds daily due to their high nutrient density, including unsaturated fats, protein, fiber, and polyphenols. Nut consumption is also associated with several other health benefits. For example, a recent systematic review indicates that consuming 28 g of nuts daily is associated with a reduced risk of cardiovascular disease, cancer, and overall mortality [69]. Given that patients with IBD are at risk for comorbid conditions (e.g., cardiovascular disease, colon cancer, diabetes, living withoverweights), it is imperative for people with IBD to adhere to healthy eating guidelines to prevent further deterioration in health. Additionally, the enrichment of butyrate-producing gut bacteria from nut consumption supports the hypothesis that nuts have a prebiotic effect [70]. In patients with Crohn's disease and ulcerative colitis, dietary patterns before the onset of the disease often show a decreased intake of nuts and seeds, highlighting the potential importance of emphasizing the consumption of foods for supporting gut health [71].

Whole nuts and seeds can be problematic in certain situations for individuals with IBD and may need to be consumed in a smooth nut or seed butter form. During active flare-ups, nuts and seeds may worsen intestinal symptoms such as pain, bloating, and stool frequency. In cases of stricturing disease, consuming nuts and seeds in their whole form can increase the risk of blockages. Therefore, in these patients and those who have had a recent IBD-related luminal surgery, it is recommended to enjoy these foods in their smooth butter form to prevent worsened symptoms or disease complications.

Patient recommendations:

a. Choose nuts higher in monounsaturated fats such as almonds, cashews, macadamia, hazelnuts, pistachios, pecans, and walnuts.
b. Nuts and seeds can be consumed as nut butter for easier digestion and improved tolerance. This should be favored in those with active disease, recent luminal surgery, and those with known intestinal strictures.
c. Opt for raw, unsalted nuts or nut butters without added sugars, salt, or fats.
d. A handful of raw nuts makes a healthy, nutrient-rich alternative to processed snacks.
e. Tahini (ground sesame seeds) is versatile and can be used in sauces, dressings, or drizzled over roasted vegetables or grain bowls to enhance flavor.
f. Add nuts and seeds to enhance dishes like yogurt, smoothies, oatmeal, or fruit.
g. Chia seeds expand when moistened, making them ideal for creating jams and puddings.
h. Soaking most nuts can improve their digestibility, reduce phytic acid, and enhance nutrient absorption. Soak most nuts for 4 to 12 h, or overnight, to improve their digestibility. Softer nuts, such as cashews, require a shorter soaking time, while harder nuts, like almonds, may benefit from a longer soaking period for optimal results.

(e) Legumes

Messaging: "Add legumes gradually".

Legumes are valuable protein and soluble fiber sources and contain bioactive compounds, including phytochemicals with known antitumor properties [72]. Systematic reviews and meta-analyses of prospective cohort studies have shown moderate-quality evidence that consuming legumes at a frequency of at least four 100 g servings per week can aid in preventing cardiometabolic risk factors and colorectal cancer [73]. Additionally, individuals with IBD often have an inadequate intake of legumes [74].

Patient recommendations:

a. To cook dried beans, use a 1:4 ratio of beans to water. Soak beans overnight to reduce lectins, which can interfere with nutrient absorption and cause discomfort. Discard the soaking water, rinse the beans, and cook in fresh water. Boil for 10–30 min at high heat to deactivate most lectins. Avoid slow cooking or eating raw beans, as they may not reduce lectins effectively.

b. Look for canned beans labeled low-sodium or with no salt. Rinse before serving or cooking to remove sodium that is added during processing. Rinsing canned beans can help make them more digestible.
c. Lentils may be easier to digest than other starchier legumes like black beans or chickpeas, so start with lentils if other legumes cause too much digestive distress,
d. Add legumes to the diet gradually—start with 2 to 4 tablespoons of beans or lentils at a time, then increase intake as the body adjusts.
e. Legumes lend themselves to soups, tacos, burritos, and chili, though you can also eat them independently.
f. Toss them on top of salads, purée them into a bean dip, or use them as a meat substitute in burgers, stews, and soups.
g. Beans can be roasted and used as snacks and salad toppers.

(f) Dairy Products

Messaging: "Rethinking dairy on the MD",

Dairy consumption in IBD has been controversial, with ongoing debate about whether patients with IBD should avoid milk and dairy products. Cross-sectional studies have demonstrated that the rate of intolerance to dairy among IBD patients is similar to the general population [75,76]. Moreover, a growing body of evidence indicates that dairy food consumption does not increase inflammatory biomarkers, with multiple studies documenting significant anti-inflammatory effects [75]. Dairy products are important nutritional sources that provide more calcium, protein, magnesium, potassium, zinc, and phosphorus per calorie than any other typical food in the adult diet.

Patient recommendations:

a. Replace heavy cream and processed cheese, instead, choose fermented cheeses like feta, Brie, cotija, Swiss, halloumi, ricotta, Manchego, and Parmesan.
b. Include fermented dairy (e.g., plain Greek yogurt, kefir) and limit flavored yogurts that tend to be higher in sugar, add flavorings (lemon, maple syrup, berry purees) to sweeten if needed.
c. Yogurt, kefir, and aged hard cheeses are lower-lactose options.
d. Trial lactose-free options, smaller portions spread throughout the day, if tolerance is an issue.

(g) Fatty Fish, Eggs, White Meat, and Red Meat

Messaging: "Rethink our perspective on protein".

In contrast to the Western diet, which is high in red and processed meats and linked to an increased risk of developing IBD [77], the MD emphasizes fish and shellfish as primary protein sources [40]. Although studies on the association between fish consumption and IBD risk show inconsistent results, an inverse relationship has been observed between fish intake and the risk of CD [32]. Additionally, a negative association has been noted between the consumption of omega-3 fatty acids and the incidence of UC [32]. Although the role of omega-3 fatty acids in IBD remains debated, consuming fatty fish such as salmon, mackerel, sardines, tuna, and herring—rich in omega-3 fatty acids—may provide a protective benefit against IBD [78]. Fish is also considered highly nutritious, offering antioxidant, anti-inflammatory, wound-healing, neuroprotective, cardioprotective, and hepatoprotective properties [79]. To date, there is no evidence linking egg consumption with IBD.

Patient recommendations:

a. Choose white meats (poultry without skin) instead of red meats, pork, or processed meats, sausages, cold meat, or paté.
b. Enjoy omega-3-rich fish such as tuna, sardines, and salmon, either fresh or canned.

c. Consume red meats (lamb, mutton, beef, pork, veal, goat, horse) less frequently. Opt for lean cuts and prepare in stews, stir-fries, or soups.
d. Limit intake of smoked, salted, and processed meats.
e. Eggs can be enjoyed daily and are often a well tolerated protein source.
f. Aim for moderate portions of 4 ounces per meal.

(h) Ultra-processed Foods, Sweets, and Alcohol

Messaging: "Choose minimally processed foods for better health".

Ultra-processed foods and sweets are not regularly consumed as part of the MD. Ultra-processed foods such as soft drinks, packaged snacks (sweet and savory), reconstituted meat products, and pre-prepared frozen meals primarily contain food additives, leaving little of the natural food [80]. These products are often high in saturated and trans fats, salt, high-fructose corn syrup, emulsifiers, artificial colors, and added sugars while low in phytochemicals, protein, micronutrients, and fiber [80]. Increased consumption of ultra-processed foods is associated with higher risk of IBD, with a dose–response relationship indicating a greater risk of disease flares in CD [81]. Alcohol intake has not been identified as a risk factor in IBD; however, some patients report a subjective worsening of symptoms, and some studies reporting worsening of disease activity with greater alcohol intake [82]. Patient recommendations:

a. Reduce the consumption of packaged, processed foods, and commercial sauces containing maltodextrin, carrageenan, carboxymethylcellulose, polysorbate-80, titanium dioxide, sulfites, and xanthan gum.
b. Limit sugary beverages and artificial sweeteners (e.g., aspartame, sucralose, saccharin). Replace soda and juices with water.
c. Coffee, tea, and herbal infusions (rich in flavonoids) are allowed, but they should be consumed preferably without any sweetener.
d. Avoid high-fat and sugar pastries, industrial bakery products (e.g., cakes, donuts, or cookies), and industrial desserts (e.g., puddings, custard). Save cakes and sweets for special occasions
e. Use herbs, spices, garlic, and onions to increase food palatability and reduce the use of salt in cooking.
f. Limit to low-risk alcohol consumption. Patients with IBD often report worse gastrointestinal symptoms following alcohol consumption. In the available literature, alcohol use in patients with IBD trends toward harmful effects; however, more research is needed [83].

(i) Modifying the Mediterranean diet according to the stage of the disease.

Messaging: "Tailor the Mediterranean diet to your disease stage for maximum benefit—nourish your body with the right foods at the right time!"

Certain dietary components may be challenging for some individuals to tolerate, but this varies from person to person and does not apply to everyone. All patients should be encouraged to personalize their diet to their disease stage (Table 4). For patients with strictures, limiting fibrous foods and insoluble fiber may be beneficial in reducing the risk of blockage [55,84].

8. Conclusions

In conclusion, the MD holds promise as an adjunctive approach to managing IBD. Mounting evidence supports its positive impact on clinical biomarkers and patient outcomes. Its practical nature, especially in terms of its feasibility for integration into clinical settings, makes it an attractive option for patients and healthcare providers. As a flexible, inclusive, nutrient-rich diet, the MD promotes the consumption of health-promoting foods like fruits, vegetables, whole grains, and healthy fats. This enhances patient adherence, especially compared to other more restrictive dietary approaches, such as low FODMAP or exclusive enteral nutrition, thus enhancing its effectiveness in everyday clinical practice.

Multidisciplinary teams, particularly dietitians, play a pivotal role in optimizing dietary interventions for patients with IBD. Registered dietitians (RDs) are essential for guiding patients in adopting the MD, ensuring cultural consideration and nutritional adequacy. Through proper education and support, dietitians can help manage potential challenges related to the diet's integration into treatment plans, monitor progress, and adjust strategies as necessary.

Further research is needed to deepen our understanding of the underlying mechanisms of the MD and to optimize its application in personalized nutrition treatment strategies.

Author Contributions: The authors confirm their contribution to this review as follows: study conception and design: R.G.N., N.H. and S.A.P.; data collection: R.G.N., N.H. and S.A.P.; analysis and interpretation of results: R.G.N., N.H. and S.A.P.; manuscript preparation: R.G.N., N.H., S.A.P., S.L.G., L.D.D., V.C. and M.R. All authors have read and agreed to the published version of the manuscript.

Funding: NH is supported by a Michael Smith Health Research BC Health Professional Investigator Award.

Acknowledgments: The authors would like to thank Elijah Haynes for their invaluable support in accessing and organizing research materials. Their expertise greatly facilitated the comprehensive review of the literature presented in this paper.

Conflicts of Interest: The authors declare no conflict of interest.

References

1. Benchimol, E.; Bernstein, C.N.; Bitton, A.; Murthy, S.K.; Nguyen, G.C.; Lee, K.; Cooke-Lauder, J.; Siddiq, S.; Windsor, J.W.; Carroll, M.W.; et al. The Impact of Inflammatory Bowel Disease in Canada 2018: A Scientific Report from the Canadian Gastro-Intestinal Epidemiology Consortium to Crohn's and Colitis Canada. *J. Can. Assoc. Gastroenterol.* **2019**, *2*, S1–S5. [CrossRef] [PubMed]
2. Noor, N.M. Combination therapies: The next major frontier in IBD management. *Nat. Rev. Gastroenterol. Hepatol.* **2023**, *20*, 761. [CrossRef] [PubMed]
3. Singh, S.; George, J.; Boland, B.S.; Casteele, N.; Sandborn, W.J. Primary non-response to tumor necrosis factor antagonists is associated with inferior response to second-line biologics in patients with Inflammatory bowel diseases: A systematic review and meta-analysis. *J. Crohns Colitis* **2018**, *12*, 635–643. [CrossRef] [PubMed]
4. Ananthakrishnan, A.N.; Kaplan, G.G.; Ng, S.C. Changing Global Epidemiology of Inflammatory Bowel Diseases: Sustaining Health Care Delivery Into the 21st Century. *Clin. Gastroenterol. Hepatol.* **2020**, *18*, 1252–1260. [CrossRef]
5. Zhao, M.; Feng, R.; Ben-Horin, S.; Zhuang, X.; Tian, Z.; Li, X.; Ma, R.; Mao, R.; Qiu, Y.; Chen, M. Systematic review with meta-analysis: Environmental and dietary differences of inflammatory bowel disease in Eastern and Western populations. *Aliment. Pharmacol. Ther.* **2022**, *55*, 266–276. [CrossRef]
6. Singh, N.; Bernstein, C.N. Environmental risk factors for inflammatory bowel disease. *United Eur. Gastroenterol. J.* **2022**, *10*, 1047–1053. [CrossRef]
7. Clemente-Suárez, V.J.; Beltrán-Velasco, A.I.; Redondo-Flórez, L.; Martín-Rodríguez, A.; Tornero-Aguilera, J.F. Global Impacts of Western Diet and Its Effects on Metabolism and Health: A Narrative Review. *Nutrients* **2023**, *15*, 2749. [CrossRef]
8. García-Montero, C.; Fraile-Martínez, O.; Gómez-Lahoz, A.M.; Pekarek, L.; Castellanos, A.J.; Noguerales-Fraguas, F.; Coca, S.; Guijarro, L.G.; García-Honduvilla, N.; Asúnsolo, A.; et al. Nutritional components in western diet versus mediterranean diet at the gut microbiota-immune system interplay. implications for health and disease. *Nutrients* **2021**, *13*, 699. [CrossRef]
9. Hashash, J.G.; Elkins, J.; Lewis, J.D.; Binion, D.G. AGA Clinical Practice Update on Diet and Nutritional Therapies in Patients With Inflammatory Bowel Disease: Expert Review. *Gastroenterology* **2024**, *166*, 521–532. [CrossRef]
10. Bach-Faig, A.; Berry, E.M.; Lairon, D.; Reguant, J.; Trichopoulou, A.; Dernini, S.; Medina, F.X.; Battino, M.; Belahsen, R.; Miranda, G.; et al. Mediterranean diet pyramid today. Science and cultural updates. *Public Health Nutr.* **2011**, *14*, 2274–2284. [CrossRef]
11. Turpin, W.; Dong, M.; Sasson, G.; Garay, J.A.R.; Espin-Garcia, O.; Lee, S.-H.; Neustaeter, A.; Smith, M.I.; Leibovitzh, H.; Guttman, D.S.; et al. Mediterranean-Like Dietary Pattern Associations With Gut Microbiome Composition and Subclinical Gastrointestinal Inflammation. *Gastroenterology* **2022**, *163*, 685–698. [CrossRef] [PubMed]

12. Haskey, N.; Estaki, M.; Ye, J.; Shim, R.K.; Singh, S.; A Dieleman, L.; Jacobson, K.; Gibson, D.L. A Mediterranean Diet Pattern improves intestinal inflammation concomitant with reshaping of the bacteriome in ulcerative colitis: A randomized controlled trial. *J. Crohns Colitis* **2023**, *17*, 1569–1578. [CrossRef] [PubMed]
13. Lewis, J.D.; Sandler, R.S.; Brotherton, C.; Brensinger, C.; Li, H.; Kappelman, M.D.; Daniel, S.G.; Bittinger, K.; Albenberg, L.; Valentine, J.F.; et al. A Randomized Trial Comparing the Specific Carbohydrate Diet to a Mediterranean Diet in Adults With Crohn's Disease. *Gastroenterology* **2021**, *161*, 837–852.e9. [CrossRef] [PubMed]
14. Khavandegar, A.; Heidarzadeh, A.; Angoorani, P.; Hasani-Ranjbar, S.; Ejtahed, H.-S.; Larijani, B.; Qorbani, M. Adherence to the Mediterranean diet can beneficially affect the gut microbiota composition: A systematic review. *BMC Med. Genom.* **2024**, *17*, 91. [CrossRef]
15. Limketkai, B.N.; Godoy-Brewer, G.; Parian, A.M.; Noorian, S.; Krishna, M.; Shah, N.D.; White, J.; Mullin, G.E. Dietary Interventions for the Treatment of Inflammatory Bowel Diseases: An Updated Systematic Review and Meta-analysis. *Clin. Gastroenterol. Hepatol.* **2023**, *21*, 2508–2525. [CrossRef]
16. Reznikov, E.A.; Suskind, D.L. Current Nutritional Therapies in Inflammatory Bowel Disease: Improving Clinical Remission Rates and Sustainability of Long-Term Dietary Therapies. *Nutrients* **2023**, *15*, 668. [CrossRef]
17. Aleksandrova, K.; Romero-Mosquera, B.; Hernandez, V. Diet, gut microbiome and epigenetics: Emerging links with inflammatory bowel diseases and prospects for management and prevention. *Nutrients* **2017**, *9*, 962. [CrossRef]
18. Limketkai, B.N.; Iheozor-Ejiofor, Z.; Gjuladin-Hellon, T.; Parian, A.; E Matarese, L.; Bracewell, K.; MacDonald, J.K.; Gordon, M.; E Mullin, G. Dietary interventions for induction and maintenance of remission in inflammatory bowel disease. *Cochrane Database Syst. Rev.* **2019**, *2*, CD012839. [CrossRef]
19. Limketkai, B.N.; Gordon, M.; Mutlu, E.A.; De Silva, P.S.; Lewis, J.D. Diet Therapy for Inflammatory Bowel Diseases: A Call to the Dining Table. *Inflamm. Bowel Dis.* **2020**, *26*, 510–514. [CrossRef]
20. Aldars-García, L.; Chaparro, M.; Gisbert, J.P. Systematic review: The gut microbiome and its potential clinical application in inflammatory bowel disease. *Microorganisms* **2021**, *9*, 977. [CrossRef]
21. Zheng, L.; Kelly, C.J.; Battista, K.D.; Schaefer, R.; Lanis, J.M.; Alexeev, E.E.; Wang, R.X.; Onyiah, J.C.; Kominsky, D.J.; Colgan, S.P. Microbial-Derived Butyrate Promotes Epithelial Barrier Function through IL-10 Receptor–Dependent Repression of Claudin-2. *J. Immunol.* **2017**, *199*, 2976–2984. [CrossRef] [PubMed]
22. Zhao, M.; Chu, J.; Feng, S.; Guo, C.; Xue, B.; He, K.; Li, L. Immunological mechanisms of inflammatory diseases caused by gut microbiota dysbiosis: A review. *Biomed. Pharmacother.* **2023**, *164*, 114985. [CrossRef]
23. Linares, R.; Francés, R.; Gutiérrez, A.; Juanola, O. Bacterial Translocation as Inflammatory Driver in Crohn's Disease. *Front. Cell Dev. Biol.* **2021**, *9*, 703310. [CrossRef] [PubMed]
24. Ogulur, I.; Yazici, D.; Pat, Y.; Bingöl, E.N.; Babayev, H.; Ardicli, S.; Heider, A.; Rückert, B.; Sampath, V.; Dhir, R.; et al. Mechanisms of gut epithelial barrier impairment caused by food emulsifiers polysorbate 20 and polysorbate 80. *Allergy Eur. J. Allergy Clin. Immunol.* **2023**, *78*, 2441–2455. [CrossRef] [PubMed]
25. Wagenaar, C.A.; van de Put, M.; Bisschops, M.; Walrabenstein, W.; de Jonge, C.S.; Herrema, H.; van Schaardenburg, D. The effect of dietary interventions on chronic inflammatory diseases in relation to the microbiome: A systematic review. *Nutrients* **2021**, *13*, 3208. [CrossRef]
26. Khademi, Z.; Milajerdi, A.; Larijani, B.; Esmaillzadeh, A. Dietary Intake of Total Carbohydrates, Sugar and Sugar-Sweetened Beverages, and Risk of Inflammatory Bowel Disease: A Systematic Review and Meta-Analysis of Prospective Cohort Studies. *Front. Nutr.* **2021**, *8*, 707795. [CrossRef]
27. Khorshidi, M.; Djafarian, K.; Aghayei, E.; Shab-Bidar, S. A posteriori dietary patterns and risk of inflammatory bowel disease: A meta-analysis of observational studies. *Int. J. Vitam. Nutr. Res.* **2020**, *90*, 376–384. [CrossRef]
28. Peters, V.; Bolte, L.; Schuttert, E.; Andreu-Sánchez, S.; Dijkstra, G.; Weersma, R.; Campmans-Kuijpers, M. Western and Carnivorous Dietary Patterns are Associated with Greater Likelihood of IBD Development in a Large Prospective Population-based Cohort. *J. Crohns Colitis* **2022**, *16*, 931–939. [CrossRef]
29. Milajerdi, A.; Ebrahimi-Daryani, N.; Dieleman, L.A.; Larijani, B.; Esmaillzadeh, A. Association of Dietary Fiber, Fruit, and Vegetable Consumption with Risk of Inflammatory Bowel Disease: A Systematic Review and Meta-Analysis. *Adv. Nutr.* **2021**, *12*, 735–743. [CrossRef]
30. Li, T.; Qiu, Y.; Yang, H.S.; Li, M.Y.; Zhuang, X.J.; Zhang, S.H.; Feng, R.; Chen, B.L.; He, Y.; Zeng, Z.R.; et al. Systematic review and meta-analysis: Association of a pre-illness Western dietary pattern with the risk of developing inflammatory bowel disease. *J. Dig. Dis.* **2020**, *21*, 362–371. [CrossRef]
31. Ananthakrishnan, A.N.; Khalili, H.; Konijeti, G.G.; Higuchi, L.M.; de Silva, P.; Fuchs, C.S.; Willett, W.C.; Richter, J.M.; Chan, A.T. Long-term intake of dietary fat and risk of ulcerative colitis and Crohn's disease. *Gut* **2014**, *63*, 776–784. [CrossRef] [PubMed]
32. Mozaffari, H.; Daneshzad, E.; Larijani, B.; Bellissimo, N.; Azadbakht, L. Dietary intake of fish, n-3 polyunsaturated fatty acids, and risk of inflammatory bowel disease: A systematic review and meta-analysis of observational studies. *Eur. J. Nutr.* **2020**, *59*, 1–17. [CrossRef] [PubMed]

33. Bolte, L.A.; Vich Vila, A.; Imhann, F.; Collij, V.; Gacesa, R.; Peters, V.; Wijmenga, C.; Kurilshikov, A.; Campmans-Kuijpers, M.J.E.; Fu, J.; et al. Long-term dietary patterns are associated with pro-inflammatory and anti-inflammatory features of the gut microbiome. *Gut* **2021**, *70*, 1287–1298. [CrossRef] [PubMed]
34. Deleu, S.; Becherucci, G.; Godny, L.; Mentella, M.C.; Petito, V.; Scaldaferri, F. The Key Nutrients in the Mediterranean Diet and Their Effects in Inflammatory Bowel Disease: A Narrative Review. *Nutrients* **2024**, *16*, 4201. [CrossRef]
35. Rodríguez-Daza, M.C.; Pulido-Mateos, E.C.; Lupien-Meilleur, J.; Guyonnet, D.; Desjardins, Y.; Roy, D. Polyphenol-Mediated Gut Microbiota Modulation: Toward Prebiotics and Further. *Front. Nutr.* **2021**, *8*, 689456. [CrossRef]
36. Julliard, W.A.; Myo, Y.P.A.; Perelas, A.; Jackson, P.D.; Thatcher, T.H.; Sime, P.J. Specialized pro-resolving mediators as modulators of immune responses. *Semin. Immunol.* **2022**, *59*, 101605. [CrossRef]
37. Nieva, C.; Pryor, J.; Williams, G.M.; Hoedt, E.C.; Burns, G.L.; Eslick, G.D.; Talley, N.J.; Duncanson, K.; Keely, S. The Impact of Dietary Interventions on the Microbiota in Inflammatory Bowel Disease: A Systematic Review. *J. Crohns Colitis* **2024**, *18*, 920–942. [CrossRef]
38. Chicco, F.; Magrì, S.; Cingolani, A.; Paduano, D.; Pesenti, M.; Zara, F.; Tumbarello, F.; Urru, E.; Melis, A.; Casula, L.; et al. Multidimensional Impact of Mediterranean Diet on IBD Patients. *Inflamm. Bowel Dis.* **2021**, *27*, 1–9. [CrossRef]
39. Erol Doğan, Ö.; Karaca Çelik, K.E.; Baş, M.; Alan, E.H.; Çağın, Y.F. Effects of Mediterranean Diet, Curcumin, and Resveratrol on Mild-to-Moderate Active Ulcerative Colitis: A Multicenter Randomized Clinical Trial. *Nutrients* **2024**, *16*, 1504. [CrossRef]
40. Strauss, J.C.; Haskey, N.; Ramay, H.R.; Ghosh, T.S.; Taylor, L.M.; Yousuf, M.; Ohland, C.; McCoy, K.D.; Ingram, R.J.M.; Ghosh, S.; et al. Weighted Gene Co-Expression Network Analysis Identifies a Functional Guild and Metabolite Cluster Mediating the Relationship between Mucosal Inflammation and Adherence to the Mediterranean Diet in Ulcerative Colitis. *Int. J. Mol. Sci.* **2023**, *24*, 7323. [CrossRef]
41. Zhang, Z.; Taylor, L.; Shommu, N.; Ghosh, S.; Reimer, R.; Panaccione, R.; Kaur, S.; Hyun, J.E.; Cai, C.; Deehan, E.C.; et al. A diversified dietary pattern is associated with a balanced gut microbial composition of faecalibacterium and escherichia/Shigella in patients with crohn's disease in remission. *J. Crohns Colitis* **2020**, *14*, 1547–1557. [CrossRef] [PubMed]
42. Haigh, L.; Bremner, S.; Houghton, D.; Henderson, E.; Avery, L.; Hardy, T.; Hallsworth, K.; McPherson, S.; Anstee, Q.M. Barriers and Facilitators to Mediterranean Diet Adoption by Patients With Nonalcoholic Fatty Liver Disease in Northern Europe. *Clin. Gastroenterol. Hepatol.* **2019**, *17*, 1364–1371.e3. [CrossRef] [PubMed]
43. Moore, S.E.; McEvoy, C.T.; Prior, L.; Lawton, J.; Patterson, C.C.; Kee, F.; Cupples, M.; Young, I.S.; Appleton, K.; McKinley, M.C.; et al. Barriers to adopting a Mediterranean diet in Northern European adults at high risk of developing cardiovascular disease. *J. Hum. Nutr. Diet.* **2018**, *31*, 451–462. [CrossRef]
44. Damas, O.M.; Maldonado-Contreras, A. Breaking Barriers in Dietary Research: Strategies to Diversify Recruitment in Clinical Studies and Develop Culturally Tailored Diets for Hispanic Communities Living With Inflammatory Bowel Disease. *Clin. Gastroenterol. Hepatol.* **2023**, *21*, 2169–2173. [CrossRef] [PubMed]
45. Flores-Mateo, G.; Rojas-Rueda, D.; Basora, J.; Ros, E.; Salas-Salvadó, J. Nut intake and adiposity: Meta-analysis of clinical trials. *Am. J. Clin. Nutr.* **2013**, *97*, 1346–1355. [CrossRef]
46. Santos, A.C.N.A.; Duarte de Souza, M.L.; Machado, A.M.; Kümmel Duarte, C. Olive oil and body fat: A systematic review with meta-analysis. *Food Funct.* **2023**, *14*, 5516–5536. [CrossRef]
47. Papada, E.; Amerikanou, C.; Forbes, A.; Kaliora, A.C. Adherence to Mediterranean diet in Crohn's disease. *Eur. J. Nutr.* **2020**, *59*, 1115–1121. [CrossRef]
48. Godny, L.; Reshef, L.; Pfeffer-Gik, T.; Goren, I.; Yanai, H.; Tulchinsky, H.; Gophna, U.; Dotan, I. Adherence to the Mediterranean diet is associated with decreased fecal calprotectin in patients with ulcerative colitis after pouch surgery. *Eur. J. Nutr.* **2020**, *59*, 3183–3190. [CrossRef]
49. Naqvi, S.A.; Taylor, L.M.; Panaccione, R.; Ghosh, S.; Barkema, H.W.; Hotte, N.; Shommu, N.; Kaur, S.; Reimer, R.A.; Madsen, K.L.; et al. Dietary patterns, food groups and nutrients in Crohn's disease: Associations with gut and systemic inflammation. *Sci. Rep.* **2021**, *11*, 1674. [CrossRef]
50. Fiorindi, C.; Dinu, M.; Gavazzi, E.; Scaringi, S.; Ficari, F.; Nannoni, A.; Sofi, F.; Giudici, F. Adherence to mediterranean diet in patients with inflammatory bowel disease. *Clin. Nutr. ESPEN* **2021**, *46*, 416–423. [CrossRef]
51. Çelik, K.; Güveli, H.; Erzin, Y.Z.; Kenger, E.B.; Özlü, T. The Effect of Adherence to Mediterranean Diet on Disease Activity in Patients with Inflammatory Bowel Disease. *Turk. J. Gastroenterol.* **2023**, *34*, 714–719. [CrossRef] [PubMed]
52. Haskey, N.; Shim, R.C.K.; Davidson-Hunt, A.; Ye, J.; Singh, S.; Dieleman, L.A.; Jacobson, K.; Ghosh, S.; Gibson, D.L. Dietary adherence to the Mediterranean diet pattern in a randomized clinical trial of patients with quiescent ulcerative colitis. *Front. Nutr.* **2022**, *9*, 1080156. [CrossRef] [PubMed]
53. Sasson, A.N.; Ingram, R.J.M.; Zhang, Z.; Taylor, L.M.; Ananthakrishnan, A.N.; Kaplan, G.G.; Ng, S.C.; Ghosh, S.; Raman, M. The role of precision nutrition in the modulation of microbial composition and function in people with inflammatory bowel disease. *Lancet Gastroenterol. Hepatol.* **2021**, *6*, 754–769. [CrossRef] [PubMed]

54. El Amrousy, D.; Elashry, H.; Salamah, A.; Maher, S.; Abd-Elsalam, S.M.; Hasan, S. Adherence to the Mediterranean Diet Improved Clinical Scores and Inflammatory Markers in Children with Active Inflammatory Bowel Disease: A Randomized Trial. *J. Inflamm. Res.* **2022**, *15*, 2075–2086. [CrossRef]
55. Lamb, C.A.; Kennedy, N.A.; Raine, T.; Hendy, P.A.; Smith, P.J.; Limdi, J.K.; Hayee, B.; Lomer, M.C.E.; Parkes, G.C.; Selinger, C.; et al. British Society of Gastroenterology consensus guidelines on the management of inflammatory bowel disease in adults. *Gut* **2019**, *68* (Suppl. S3), s1–s106. [CrossRef]
56. Windsor, J.W.; Kaplan, G.G. Evolving Epidemiology of IBD. *Curr. Gastroenterol. Rep.* **2019**, *21*, 40. [CrossRef]
57. Flynn, M.M.; Tierney, A.; Itsiopoulos, C. Is Extra Virgin Olive Oil the Critical Ingredient Driving the Health Benefits of a Mediterranean Diet? A Narrative Review. *Nutrients* **2023**, *15*, 2916. [CrossRef]
58. Alves, E.; Domingues M do, R.; Domingues, P. Chapter 4—Olive oil. In *Functional Foods and Their Implications for Health Promotion*; Zabetakis, I., Tsoupras, A., Lordan, R., Ramji, D., Eds.; Academic Press: Cambridge, MA, USA, 2023; pp. 97–129. [CrossRef]
59. Mayr, L.; Grabherr, F.; Schwärzler, J.; Reitmeier, I.; Sommer, F.; Gehmacher, T.; Niederreiter, L.; He, G.-W.; Ruder, B.; Kunz, K.T.R.; et al. Dietary lipids fuel GPX4-restricted enteritis resembling Crohn's disease. *Nat. Commun.* **2020**, *11*, 1775. [CrossRef]
60. Haskey, N.; Ye, J.; Estaki, M.; Meza, A.A.V.; Barnett, J.A.; Yousefi, M.; Birnie, B.W.; Gruenheid, S.; Ghosh, S.; Gibson, D.L. A Mediterranean-like fat blend protects against the development of severe colitis in the mucin-2 deficient murine model. *Gut Microbes* **2022**, *14*, 2055441. [CrossRef]
61. Molina-Garcia, L.; Santos, C.S.P.; Cunha, S.C.; Casal, S.; Fernandes, J.O. Comparative Fingerprint Changes of Toxic Volatiles in Low PUFA Vegetable Oils Under Deep-Frying. *JAOCS J. Am. Oil Chem. Soc.* **2017**, *94*, 271–284. [CrossRef]
62. Jimenez-Lopez, C.; Carpena, M.; Lourenço-Lopes, C.; Gallardo-Gomez, M.; Lorenzo, J.M.; Barba, F.J.; Prieto, M.A.; Simal-Gandara, J. Bioactive compounds and quality of extra virgin olive oil. *Foods* **2020**, *9*, 1014. [CrossRef]
63. Panche, A.N.; Diwan, A.D.; Chandra, S.R. Flavonoids: An overview. *J. Nutr. Sci.* **2016**, *5*, e47. [CrossRef] [PubMed]
64. Man, A.W.C.; Zhou, Y.; Xia, N.; Li, H. Involvement of gut microbiota, microbial metabolites and interaction with polyphenol in host immunometabolism. *Nutrients* **2020**, *12*, 3054. [CrossRef] [PubMed]
65. McRae, M.P. Health Benefits of Dietary Whole Grains: An Umbrella Review of Meta-analyses. *J. Chiropr. Med.* **2017**, *16*, 10–18. [CrossRef] [PubMed]
66. Seal, C.J.; Courtin, C.M.; Venema, K.; de Vries, J. Health benefits of whole grain: Effects on dietary carbohydrate quality, the gut microbiome, and consequences of processing. *Compr. Rev. Food Sci. Food Saf.* **2021**, *20*, 2742–2768. [CrossRef]
67. Fuentes-Zaragoza, E.; Sánchez-Zapata, E.; Sendra, E.; Sayas, E.; Navarro, C.; Fernández-López, J.; Pérez-Alvarez, J.A. Resistant starch as prebiotic: A review. *Starch Stärke* **2011**, *63*, 406–415. [CrossRef]
68. Haskey, N.; Gold, S.L.; Faith, J.J.; Raman, M. To Fiber or Not to Fiber: The Swinging Pendulum of Fiber Supplementation in Patients with Inflammatory Bowel Disease. *Nutrients* **2023**, *15*, 1080. [CrossRef]
69. Balakrishna, R.; Bjørnerud, T.; Bemanian, M.; Aune, D.; Fadnes, L.T. Consumption of Nuts and Seeds and Health Outcomes Including Cardiovascular Disease, Diabetes and Metabolic Disease, Cancer, and Mortality: An Umbrella Review. *Adv. Nutr.* **2022**, *13*, 2136–2148. [CrossRef]
70. Creedon, A.C.; Hung, E.S.; Berry, S.E.; Whelan, K. Nuts and their effect on gut microbiota, gut function and symptoms in adults: A systematic review and meta-analysis of randomised controlled trials. *Nutrients* **2020**, *12*, 2347. [CrossRef]
71. Preda, C.M.; Istratescu, D.; Nitescu, M.; Manuc, T.; Manuc, M.; Stroie, T.; Catrinoiu, M.; Tieranu, C.; Meianu, C.G.; Tugui, L.; et al. Impact of Dietary Patterns in Inflammatory Bowel Disease Subtypes. *Maedica* **2023**, *18*, 174. [CrossRef]
72. Tor-Roca, A.; Garcia-Aloy, M.; Mattivi, F.; Llorach, R.; Andres-Lacueva, C.; Urpi-Sarda, M. Phytochemicals in Legumes: A Qualitative Reviewed Analysis. *J. Agric. Food Chem.* **2020**, *68*, 13486–13496. [CrossRef] [PubMed]
73. Viguiliouk, E.; Blanco Mejia, S.; Kendall, C.W.C.; Sievenpiper, J.L. Can pulses play a role in improving cardiometabolic health? Evidence from systematic reviews and meta-analyses. *Ann. N. Y. Acad. Sci.* **2017**, *1392*, 43–57. [CrossRef] [PubMed]
74. Lambert, K.; Pappas, D.; Miglioretto, C.; Javadpour, A.; Reveley, H.; Frank, L.; Grimm, M.C.; Samocha-Bonet, D.; Hold, G.L. Systematic review with meta-analysis: Dietary intake in adults with inflammatory bowel disease. *Aliment. Pharmacol. Ther.* **2021**, *54*, 742–754. [CrossRef] [PubMed]
75. Nieman, K.M.; Anderson, B.D.; Cifelli, C.J. The Effects of Dairy Product and Dairy Protein Intake on Inflammation: A Systematic Review of the Literature. *J. Am. Coll. Nutr.* **2021**, *40*, 571–582. [CrossRef]
76. Kempinski, R.; Arabasz, D.; Neubauer, K. Effects of Milk and Dairy on the Risk and Course of Inflammatory Bowel Disease versus Patients' Dietary Beliefs and Practices: A Systematic Review. *Nutrients* **2024**, *16*, 2555. [CrossRef]
77. Chiba, M.; Nakane, K.; Komatsu, M. Westernized Diet is the Most Ubiquitous Environmental Factor in Inflammatory Bowel Disease. *Perm. J.* **2019**, *23*, 18–107. [CrossRef]
78. Jia, X.; Hu, C.; Wu, X.; Qi, H.; Lin, L.; Xu, M.; Xu, Y.; Wang, T.; Zhao, Z.; Chen, Y.; et al. Evaluating the Effects of Omega-3 Polyunsaturated Fatty Acids on Inflammatory Bowel Disease via Circulating Metabolites: A Mediation Mendelian Randomization Study. *Metabolites* **2023**, *13*, 1041. [CrossRef]

79. Chen, J.; Jayachandran, M.; Bai, W.; Xu, B. A critical review on the health benefits of fish consumption and its bioactive constituents. *Food Chem.* **2022**, *369*, 130874. [CrossRef]
80. Monteiro, C.A.; Cannon, G.; Moubarac, J.C.; Levy, R.B.; Louzada, M.L.C.; Jaime, P.C. The un Decade of Nutrition, the NOVA food classification and the trouble with ultra-processing. *Public Health Nutr.* **2018**, *21*, 5–17. [CrossRef]
81. Babaei, A.; Pourmotabbed, A.; Talebi, S.; Mehrabani, S.; Bagheri, R.; Ghoreishy, S.M.; Amirian, P.; Zarpoosh, M.; Mohammadi, H.; Kermani, M.A.H.; et al. The association of ultra-processed food consumption with adult inflammatory bowel disease risk: A systematic review and dose-response meta-analysis of 4035694 participants. *Nutr. Rev.* **2024**, *82*, 861–871. [CrossRef]
82. Rozich, J.J.; Holmer, A.; Singh, S. Effect of Lifestyle Factors on Outcomes in Patients with Inflammatory Bowel Diseases. *Am. J. Gastroenterol.* **2020**, *115*, 832–840. [CrossRef] [PubMed]
83. Ramos, G.P.; Kane, S. Alcohol use in patients with inflammatory bowel disease. *Gastroenterol. Hepatol.* **2021**, *17*, 211.
84. Levine, A.; Rhodes, J.M.; Lindsay, J.O.; Abreu, M.T.; Kamm, M.A.; Gibson, P.R.; Gasche, C.; Silverberg, M.S.; Mahadevan, U.; Boneh, R.S.; et al. Dietary Guidance From the International Organization for the Study of Inflammatory Bowel Diseases. *Clin. Gastroenterol. Hepatol.* **2020**, *18*, 1381–1392. [CrossRef]

nutrients

MDPI

Systematic Review

Beetroot Juice Supplementation as a Healthy Aging Strategy Through Improving Physical Performance and Cognitive Functions: A Systematic Review

Anna Nowak [1,*], Angelika Szymańska [2], Magdalena Kwaśniewska [1], Ewa Kochan [2] and Anna Lipert [1,*]

1 Department of Preventive Medicine, Medical University of Lodz, 92-213 Lodz, Poland; magdalena.kwasniewska@umed.lodz.pl

2 Department of Pharmacological Biotechnology, Medical University of Lodz, 90-152 Lodz, Poland; angelika.gabrysiak@umed.lodz.pl (A.S.); ewa.kochan@umed.lodz.pl (E.K.)

* Correspondence: anna.nowak10@stud.umed.lodz.pl (A.N.); anna.lipert@umed.lodz.pl (A.L.)

Abstract: Background: Findings show that beetroot-derived nitrates can improve endurance, oxygen efficiency, muscular power, recovery and cardiovascular function, particularly in recreationally active or moderately trained individuals. However, results are mixed in elite athletes, likely due to their already optimized nitric oxide utilization. Cognitive function is a crucial aspect of athletic performance enabling athletes to adapt to dynamic environments and execute skills effectively, but evidence for cognitive benefits of nitrate-rich beetroot supplementation is limited and inconsistent. The combination of improved physical activity and cognitive functions contribute to overall healthy aging and extending life expectancy. This highlights the synergistic role of nutrition, exercise and mental agility in promoting long-term well-being. **Methods:** The literature review was conducted to summarize and systematize existing evidence on beetroot juice supplementation on physical performance and cognitive function in both, healthy adult population and athletes. **Results:** Overall, beetroot supplementation demonstrates strong potential as a natural ergogenic aid for enhancing physical performance, but current evidence on cognitive improvement remains inconclusive. **Conclusions:** Further research, particularly involving female or elite athletes, is needed to establish clear recommendations of beetroot juice supplementation as a supportive element of exercise capacity and cognitive abilities contributing to maintaining health and thus healthy aging.

Keywords: dietary nitrates; ergogenic nutrition; endurance capacity; aging physiology; cognitive outcomes

1. Introduction

Nitrogen is a vital element for all living organisms. It's main form, dinitrogen gas (N_2), cannot be utilized by plants or animals. In order to be used by humans, it has to go through numerous processes in "the nitrogen cycle" [1,2]. The oral microbiome converts nitrates into nitrites. After ingestion, nitrate-rich saliva undergoes nonenzymatic metabolism in the stomach, producing nitric oxide (NO), which triggers various biological effects, e.g., neurotransmission, vasodilation or immunomodulation [3]. Nitrate (NO_3^-), along with nitrite (NO_2^-) were viewed as cancerogenic and adverse to the human diet [4,5]. Both NO_3^- and NO_2^- have been one of the ingredients added during the process of curing certain meat products to act as a preservative against microorganisms responsible for food poisoning [6]. With today's knowledge we can say that nitrates have a wide range of

https://doi.org/10.3390/nu17243954

positive effects on the human body, such as: lowering blood pressure, increasing flow-mediated dilation, reducing platelet–monocyte aggregates and improvement in vascular function [7].

Nitrate, nitrite and N-nitroso-compounds can be synthesized endogenously. In healthy individuals, approximately 1 mmol (62 mg) of nitrate is produced per day. This endogenous production becomes particularly significant when dietary nitrate intake is low or during gastrointestinal infections that affect the stomach pH [8]. Following a comprehensive re-evaluation of their safety, the European Food Safety Authority (EFSA) has concluded that the established safe levels for nitrites and nitrates intentionally added to meat and other food products provide adequate protection for consumers. Nitrite and nitrate salts (such as sodium and potassium salts; labelled on food products as: nitrites E 249–250 and nitrates E 251–252) are approved food additives in the EU. They are used for various reasons, for example to protect products such as: meat, fish, and cheese, from microbial growth or to preserve color and flavor. The current acceptable daily intake (ADI) is 3.7 mg/kg body mass/day for nitrates and 0.07 mg/kg body mass/day for nitrites [9,10]. For humans, the lethal oral dose for nitrate can range from 67 to 833 mg/kg body mass. When it comes to nitrite the lethal dose, it ranges from 33 up to 250 mg/kg body mass [8].

Vegetables are the primary source of nitrate, contributing to about 80–85% of the daily nitrate intake and up to 43% of nitrite intake [6,11]. Nitrates can be found in a variety of vegetables and their nitrate concentration can differ due to factors such as: weather conditions, soil quality and its pH or the plant species [12]. Greatestnitrate levels (>2500 mg/kg), according to their nitrate content, are vegetables and leafy greens like spinach, lettuce and beetroot, which is both a root and a leaf crop. Beetroot is grown for its edible storage roots and leaves (mainly young) [13]. Due to its great nitrates levels, it has gained popularity among athletes and is the most commonly used form of supplementing dietary nitrate. It can enhance exercise performance through multiple pathways, including vasodilation, improving blood circulation, improving muscle and cerebral blood flow, lowering oxygen demand in skeletal muscles or decreasing the buildup of anaerobic respiration byproducts which helps to not only boost power output and muscle force but also delay fatigue (Figure 1) [7].

The concentrations of nitrate (NO_3^-) and nitrite (NO_2^-) in beetroot supplements can vary widely due to differences in beetroot sourcing, processing methods, storage conditions and addition of other compounds. Since these compounds are sensitive to factors like heat, light, and time, their levels can degrade or fluctuate during production and shelf life. Unfortunately, not all manufacturers standardize their products for nitrate or nitrite content, leading to significant disparities between brands or even batches of the same product. As a result, the actual nitrate and nitrite content in beetroot supplements may differ from what is expected or labelled [14,15].

Studies have shown that dose-dependent increase of plasma nitrate and nitrite and a reduction in the oxygen cost of moderate-intensity cycling, were noted at the same supplemented dose being ~16.8 mmol. However, lower doses of nitrate supplements were the ones to improve the time-to-task failure during severe-intensity exercise [16]. Additionally, individuals with very great levels of aerobic conditioning, particularly elite endurance athletes (with a VO_2max above 65 $mL \cdot kg^{-1} \cdot min^{-1}$), generally do not experience significant performance gains from nitrate supplementation [17,18]. Nowadays, the protocols of nitrate supplementation in sports, recommend the dose of ~6-6 mmol (350–500 mg), taken approximately around 2–3 h before planned exercise [19].

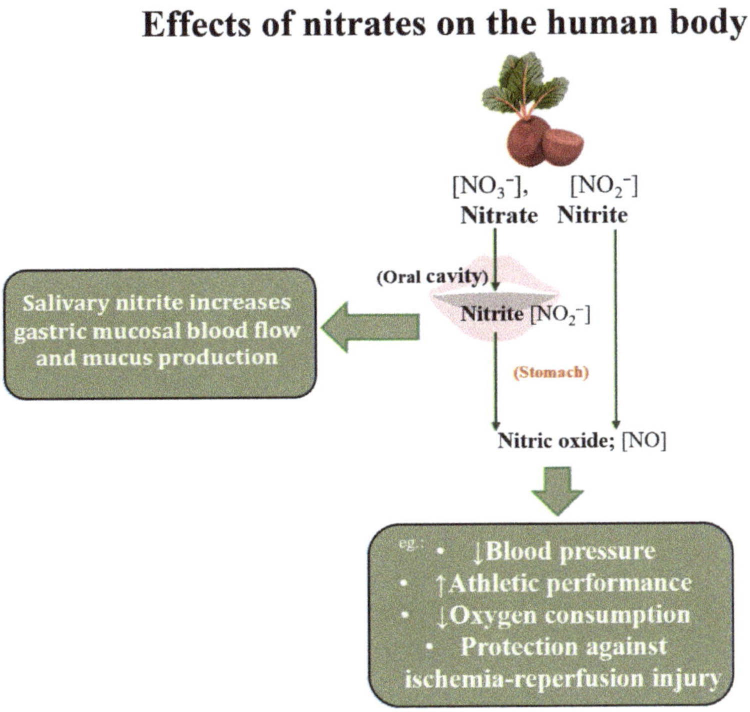

Figure 1. The effects of nitrates on the human body.

Maintaining a nutritious diet and achieving optimal nutritional balance are key strategies for supporting brain function and cognitive well-being [19]. Cognitive abilities refer to several interconnected mental operations—such as our capacity to retain and recall information (memory), the ability to concentrate and filter distractions (attention), greater level planning and self-regulation (executive functions), problem-solving, and the speed of mental processing [20]. Research suggests, that NO_3^- supplementation may positively impact these abilities. Benefits were seen in a few age-groups, including healthy young individuals, both at rest and during exercise, particularly after 5–7 days of supplementation. During intense exercise—when brain oxygen drops—cognition may suffer, and NO_3^-'s benefits appear limited. Yet, higher doses (~13 mmol) over 7 days improved decision-making during prolonged, high-intensity intermittent exercise [21].

Constantly growing evidence shows that supplements containing natural extracts, pure extracts, or juices from plants can have a positive effect and stimulate cognitive performance in humans. Peth-Nui et al. 2012, demonstrated that the use of *Bacopa monnieri* improves concentration and memory processing, as well as contributing to increased working memory, and even that the use of this plant extract may be useful in the treatment of attention deficit disorder [22]. Similar observations were related to the extracts derived from the *Panax ginseng* plant [23]. In addition, it was proved that ginseng's supplementation had a beneficial effect on cognitive impairment caused by Alzheimer's disease [23]. Other adaptogenic plant, *Rhodiola rosea* L., significantly improved reaction and choice times in healthy men in the study by Stojcheva et al. 2022 [24]. What is more, taking Ashwagandha extract resulted in improved memory and concentration, which classifies it as an effective adaptogen, improving cognitive abilities, as shown in a study by Gopukumar et al. 2021 [25]. In a similar manner, beetroot juice also deserves recognition for its cognitive benefits. Heiland E. et al. 2024, demonstrated that supplementing beetroot juice resulted in improved cognitive parameters, as study participants achieved significantly better results in serial subtraction task than those receiving a placebo [26]. Gilchrist et al. 2014, observed that two weeks of beetroot juice supplementation resulted in significant improvements in simple reaction time in individuals with type 2 diabetes [27]. In a study by Vaccaro et al. 2024, ingesting a beetroot-based supplement improved cognitive function, particularly memory capacity and frontal nerve function [28].

An increasing number of studies shows that both physical performance and endurance are strongly associated with cognitive functions. A recent umbrella review and meta-meta-analysis of 133 included studies found that physical exercise significantly improves global and executive functions. Importantly, the study highlighted that light- to moderate-intensity activities and physically interactive games (exergames) may be especially effective in enhancing mental performance [29]. Shorter reaction times and executive functions can translate into better athletic performance. Such observations were made by Trecroci et al. 2021, who demonstrated that young female volleyball players whose basic cognitive functions were better developed demonstrated better physical fitness in a given discipline than those whose cognitive functions were at a lower level [30]. Dietary nitrate supplementation, when combined with regular physical activity, can further enhance exercise efficiency by improving muscle oxygenation and endurance. Together, these effects create a synergistic benefit, promoting both cardiovascular health and extended lifespan (Figure 2). In the context of healthy aging, evaluating physical activity and cognitive function in young to middle-aged adults is crucial, as this stage represents the peak of physiological capacity and cognitive performance. Maintaining regular physical activity during adulthood supports cardiovascular, metabolic, and musculoskeletal health—fundamental components in the prevention of chronic disease and lowering mortality risk. Furthermore, improving cognitive functions reduces the risk of neurodegenerative disorders later in life [31].

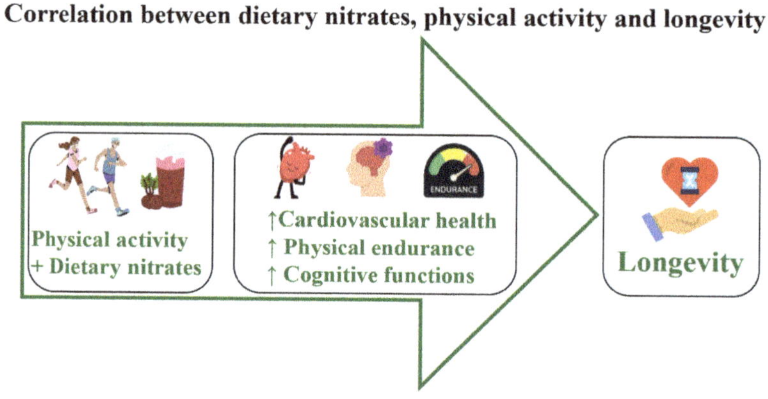

Figure 2. The correlation between dietary nitrates, physical activity and longevity.

This literature review was conducted to summarize and systematize existing evidence on beetroot juice supplementation on both physical performance and cognitive functions in healthy adult population as well as athletes. By identifying the significant variations in dosing strategies, nitrate concentrations, supplementation durations, and practical applications used across studies, we highlight how these methodological differences influence the outcomes relevant to functional capacity in older adults. This review points out the lack of a standardized beetroot juice supplementation protocol and the integration of these two areas of research. This issue currently limits the development of a clear, evidence-based guidelines for its use as a healthy aging strategy and emphasizes the need for consensus in future research. We believe that properly used supplementation with beetroot juice at a younger age, which supports exercise capacity and cognitive abilities, can contribute to maintaining health and thus healthy aging. Therefore, this paper aims to bridge this gap by examining the dual role of beetroot juice in supporting both cognitive functions and physical performance and exploring its use as a strategy for healthy aging.

2. Materials and Methods

2.1. Search Strategy

This literature review was conducted to assess the effects of beetroot juice and nitrates supplementation on cognitive function and physical performance in humans. The inclusion criteria for the review contained (a) studies conducted on humans, (b) studies conducted using beetroot and/or plants containing nitrates, (c) studies assessing cognitive functions and/or physical activity.

A literature review covering the years 2020–2025 was conducted to assess the impact of nitrate-rich beetroot supplementation on physical performance and cognitive function in healthy individuals, including both the general population and athletes aged 18–59. The search strategy was based on the use of combinations demonstrated in Table 1. The analysis included both experimental studies and review articles, allowing for the collection and critical analysis of available research findings. The aim of this study was not only to summarize existing reports and to systematize them in a way that enabled a synthetic presentation of the most current knowledge on the potential ergogenic and neurocognitive effects of beetroot supplementation in the study group, but also to indicate insufficient data for future research.

2.2. Exclusion Criteria

The first exclusion phase gathered publications on humans suffering from any chronic diseases and symptoms such as hypertension, respiratory infections, diabetes, menopause etc. Other excluded papers involved addiction and various substances use such as alcohol, drugs, smoking and others. Second exclusion phase focused on publications duplicated in both databases and, therefore, were rejected.

2.3. Search Results

This review followed the guidelines of the Preferred Reporting Items for Systematic Reviews and Meta-analyses (PRISMA). Figure 3 illustrates a PRISMA flow diagram of the study selection process for all articles. The PRISMA checklist is listed as Table S1.

All search strategies of the two databases yielded a total of 523 articles. Based on the full-text analysis, 213 records were excluded. There were 206 articles repeated in Embase and PubMed. Search terms in the electronic database Embase yielded a total of 298 matching results. A search of the electronic database PubMed yielded a total of 225 records. After subsequent comparison with the Embase database, as many as 206 results that also appeared in this database were excluded. Some articles were excluded after the screening phase because the presentation of the data did not match the inclusion criteria. In total 104 studies were selected in the present review.

Table 1. Search strategy in each database.

Database	Terms Combination
PubMed	((“Beetroot*”[Text Word] OR “beta vulgaris”[MeSH Terms] OR “beta vulgaris”[tw]) AND (“physical activit*”[Title/Abstract] OR physical[tw] OR “sport*”[Title/Abstract] OR “Athletic Performance”[MeSH Terms] OR “athletic performance*”[Title/Abstract] OR “exercise*”[Title/Abstract] OR “aerobic”[Text Word] OR “gymnastic*”[Text Word] OR “training”[Text Word]) AND “cognit*”[Text Word]) NOT (animals[mh] NOT humans[mh])
	((“Beetroot*”[Text Word] OR “beta vulgaris”[MeSH Terms] OR “beta vulgaris”[tw]) AND (“physical activit*”[Title/Abstract] OR “sport*”[Title/Abstract] OR “Athletic Performance”[MeSH Terms] OR “athletic performance*”[Title/Abstract] OR “exercise*”[Title/Abstract] OR “aerobic”[Text Word] OR “gymnastic*”[Text Word] OR “training”[Text Word])) NOT (animals[mh] NOT humans[mh])
Embase	(‘beetroot*’:ti,ab,kw,de,dn,df,mn,tn OR ‘beet’/exp OR ‘beet’ OR ‘beta vulgaris’:ti,ab,kw,de,dn,df,mn,tn) AND (‘physical activit*’:ti,ab,kw OR ‘physical’:ti,ab,kw,de,dn,df,mn,tn OR ‘sport*’:ti,ab,kw OR ‘athletic performance’/exp OR ‘athletic performance’ OR ‘athletic performance*’:ti,ab,kw OR ‘exercise*’:ti,ab,kw OR ‘aerobic’:ti,ab,kw,de,dn,df,mn,tn OR ‘gymnastic*’:ti,ab,kw,de,dn,df,mn,tn OR ‘training’:ti,ab,kw,de,dn,df,mn,tn) AND ‘cognit*’:ti,ab,kw,de,dn,df,mn,tn NOT ((‘animal’/exp OR ‘animal’) NOT (‘human’/exp OR ‘human’))
	‘beetroot*’:ti,ab,kw,de,dn,df,mn,tn OR ‘beet’/exp OR ‘beet’ OR ‘beta vulgaris’:ti,ab,kw,de,dn,df,mn,tn) AND (‘physical activit*’:ti,ab,kw OR ‘sport*’:ti,ab,kw OR ‘athletic performance’/exp OR ‘athletic performance’ OR ‘athletic performance*’:ti,ab,kw OR ‘exercise*’:ti,ab,kw OR ‘aerobic’:ti,ab,kw,de,dn,df,mn,tn OR ‘gymnastic*’:ti,ab,kw,de,dn,df,mn,tn OR ‘training’:ti,ab,kw,de,dn,df,mn,tn) NOT ((‘animal’/exp OR ‘animal’) NOT (‘human’/exp OR ‘human’))

* In database searches, the asterisk is used as a truncation symbol to substitute for zero or more characters, enabling retrieval of multiple word variants.

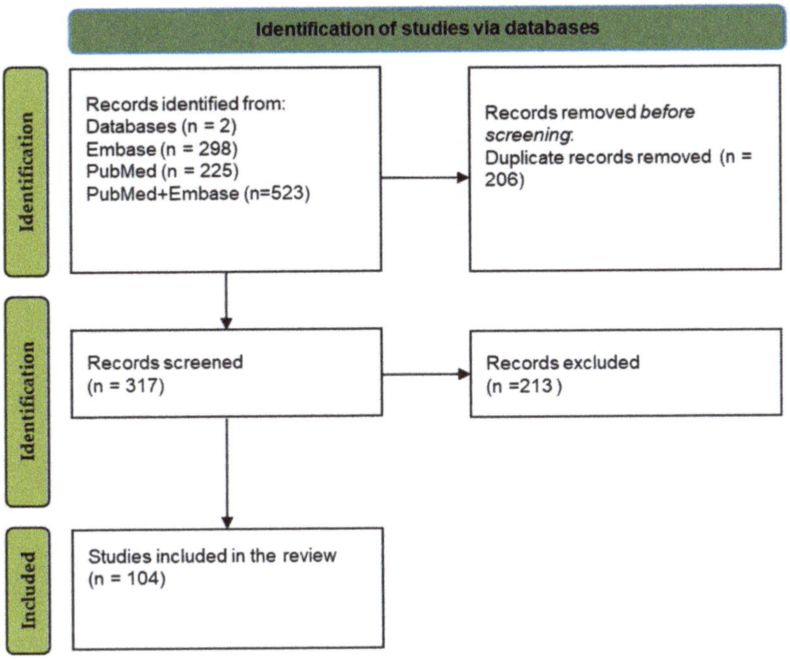

Figure 3. PRISMA flow diagram of the study selection process.

3. Results

This review analyzed data on the effects of nitrates from various forms of beetroot (juice, extracts in capsules, etc.) on physical activity and cognitive function. Tables 2–4 summarize the results based on experimental articles. Table 5 includes information from review articles and meta-analyses.

Analysis of Nitrates on Physical Activity and Cognitive Functions (Original Articles)

Studies shown in Tables 2 and 3 reported ergogenic effects of dietary nitrate (primarily sourced from beetroot) on exercise performance and cognitive functions. Endurance outcomes have improved in several studies—for example, Huang et al. observed longer time-to-exhaustion in cyclists [32], and Tirkey et al. found ~4–8% faster 10 km run times after supplementation [33]. Improvements in power and muscle strength were also noted, e.g., Rodríguez-Fernández et al. reported increased peak and mean power output during resistance exercise [34], while Jurado-Castro et al. showed greater: jump height, lifting velocity, and repetitions to failure after beetroot juice supplementation [35]. A few studies indicated enhanced recovery manifested by quicker recovery of the muscle function with less perceived soreness [36] as well as faster post-exercise cardiovascular recovery showed by Benjamim et al. [37]. In contrast, other investigations found no significant changes after nitrate supplementation (Table 4). For instance, in a study by Tan et al. no improvements in sprint, strength, or aerobic measures among female team-sport athletes were spotted. Similar observations had Burke et al.—this study reported no effect on endurance performance or exercise efficiency in elite race walkers [38]. López-Samanes et al. and Trexler et al. observed no gains in power, speed, or overall exercise performance with nitrate supplementation [39,40]. Unfortunately, only one trial showed positive visible effect of supplementing nitrates on cognitive functions. Improved cognitive performance on a Stroop-test after a moderate (400 mg of NO_3^-) nitrate dose was noted by Miraftabi et al. [41].

The analyzed studies provide overall support for the beneficial effects of beetroot supplementation on physical activity. However, inconsistencies might be due to differences in, for example: test sensitivity, participants' fitness levels or sample size.

Several trials reported improved endurance and oxygen efficiency. Beetroot supplementation has shown consistent effects in improving cardiovascular health and reducing exercise-related stress. Numerous studies reported reductions in heart rate and perceived exertion by lowering heart rate and exertion during work intervals in women or decreasing ratings of perceived exertion and muscle soreness after functional tests at altitude.

Beetroot-derived nitrates also appear to improve aerobic capacity and endurance in a variety of training situations. A growing body of literature demonstrates improved VO_2max and ventilatory efficiency in women [42] and achieving similar gains in VO_2max and rowing performance [43]. Certain studies have observed enhanced 10-km running time trial performance in both men and women, suggesting benefits across endurance modalities [33]. However, acute beetroot juice ingestion did not improve sprinting, strength, or aerobic performance in female team-sports [44], nor did it enhance tennis-specific performance in elite players [45]. Similarly, studies in trained and endurance athletes [46,47] reported no improvements, despite elevated plasma nitrate/nitrite concentrations. These mixed results may be explained by the fact that elite athletes are already very efficient at using nitric oxide, leaving little room for further improvement. As highlighted by one of the analyzed systematic reviews, the benefits of beetroot supplementation seem to be greater in individuals who are less trained [48].

Several studies highlight beetroot's potential in resistance exercise. Parameters such as increased repetitions to failure, power, and velocity, as well as improved resistance outcomes have been reported [35,49]. Higher doses of beetroot supplementation led to greater improvements in muscle torque development, while supplementation also increased resistance to fatigue during repeated knee extensions. Together, these results indicate that beetroot supplementation can enhance both the efficiency of muscle contractions and overall endurance during resistance exercise [50,51].

When considering studies used in this systematic review, most used nitrate doses between 6 mmol and 13 mmol, usually delivered in a beetroot juice or a concentrate form, consumed 2–3 h before exercise. Some of the trials tested lower doses (~4–6 mmol) and still observed some improvements in heart rate, oxygen cost, or muscular endurance [52]. Worth mentioning is the fact that higher doses (>15 mmol) did not provide clear additional benefits [50].

Table 2. Summary of the original studies examining the impact of dietary nitrates from beetroot on exercise performance—acute dosing.

	Study	Sample Size	Dose	Form	Duration	Results
	Positive Effects of Supplementation (Acute/Short-Term)					
1	Ahmadpour A. et al. [53]	10 men	PLA (<0.5 mmol NO_3^-) or BRJ 220 mL (~8.9 mmol NO_3^-) consumed 2.5 h before functional tests at 2800 m altitude.	Juice	Acute	• Beetroot juice (BRJ) improved isometric muscle endurance (wall-sit), anaerobic capacity (90 s box jump, BJ90), agility (Hex Jump), and reduced time to change directions. BRJ also lowered ratings of perceived exertion (RPE) during slalom (SL)runs and muscle soreness (MS) at 12, 24, and 48 h post-exercise.
2	Benjamim C.J.R. et al. [37]	16 men	Beetroot extract (600 mg capsule) vs. placebo, taken 120 min before exercise. The participants ingested the opposite intervention (placebo or beetroot extract) on the third and final day to guarantee the study'scross-over.	Capsules	Acute (3 days; crossover).	• Beetroot extract accelerated recovery—systolic blood pressure (SBP) and diastolic blood pressure (DBP) returned to baseline faster, heart rate (HR) recovered more quickly (elevated only 0–5 min vs. 10 min in placebo), and heart rate variability (HRV; HF index) recovered earlier.
3	Black M.I. et al. [54]	11 individuals (10 men; 1 woman)	7-day low NO_3^- diet, 3-day high NO_3^- diet, compared with a standard (control) NO_3^- diet;	Nitrates from food	Short-term dietary interventions: 7 days low NO_3^-, 3 days high NO_3^-, with controlled washout periods.	• Low NO_3^-—reduced saliva [NO_3^-] and [NO_2^-] and plasma [NO_3^-]. • High NO_3^- intake: improved sprint cycling peak power output (+4%) and mean power output (+3%), increased saliva and plasma [NO_3^-]/[NO_2^-] more when preceded by a low NO_3^- diet; BP was reduced following high NO_3^- intake when preceded by a standard diet;

Table 2. *Cont.*

	Positive Effects of Supplementation (Acute/Short-Term)					
	Study	Sample Size	Dose	Form	Duration	Results
4	Bloomer R.J. et al. [55]	10 men and 10 women	RRB1: Resync Recovery Blend, 1 serving (~7.5 g; ~4.2 g nitric oxide blend), single acute ingestion mixed with 12 fl oz water; RRB2: Resync Recovery Blend, 2 servings (~15 g; ~8.4 g nitric oxide blend), single acute ingestion mixed with 12 fl oz water; RCB1: Resync Collagen Blend, 1 serving (~21 g; ~2 g proprietary blend), single acute ingestion mixed with 12 fl oz water; PLA: Placebo, 7.5 g nitrate- and polyphenol-free powder mixed with 12 fl oz water.	Drink/juice	Acute	• Resync supplements raise plasma NO_x, especially the Recovery Blend in a dose-dependent way, without affecting heart rate or blood pressure.
5	Cocksedge S.P. et al. [56]	10 men	Nitrate-rich beetroot juice concentrate (210 mL containing ~18.6 mmol NO_3^-); 2.5 h before exercise on each testing. each trial was conducted on nine occasions over a 4–7 week timeframe, with beetroot (BR) or placebo (PL) consumed 2.5 h prior to each exercise test under normoxia, hypoxia, or hyperoxia.	Juice	Acute	• Acute BRJ (~18.6 mmol NO_3^-) increased plasma [NO_2^-] and quadriceps oxygenation during moderate-intensity cycling. During severe-intensity cycling, BR enhanced exercise tolerance in hypoxia but not in normoxia or hyperoxia, with greatest benefits observed in individuals experiencing higher skeletal muscle deoxygenation.

Table 2. *Cont.*

	Positive Effects of Supplementation (Acute/Short-Term)					
	Study	Sample Size	Dose	Form	Duration	Results
6	De Souza D.B. et al. [57]	20 men	Beetroot juice (BJ; 500 mL, 16 mmol NO_3^-); 60 min before exercise; six exercise or PLA (açaí-flavored maltodextrin, equalized the caloric content of the BJ + 20 mL of beetroot to give flavor of the PLA)	Juice	Acute	• Acute BJ supplementation significantly decreased 4-km running time in both concurrent training sessions (CT1: aerobic + resistance; CT2: resistance + aerobic) compared to placebo and control. Plasma nitric oxide concentration increased after BJ, while placebo showed no significant change.
7	Dumar A.M. et al. [58]	10 men	Single dose of 70 mL concentrated beetroot juice (~400 mg NO_3^-), consumed 2 h prior to exercise. Participants consumed the full dose within 5 min; PLA (blackcurrant juice)	Juice	Acute	• Supramaximal exercise performance (Wingate tests, 3 × 15 s) was lower in the morning with PL (AM-PL) compared to afternoon (PM) and morning BRJ (AM-BRJ). • Mean power, anaerobic capacity, and total work were all significantly higher in AM-BRJ vs. AM-PL and similar to PM. • Heart rate was lower in AM-BRJ than AM-PL. RPE—RPE was significantly lower during WAnT1 (Wingate anaerobic test) than for WAnT2 ($p = 0.002$) and WAnT3 ($p < 0.001$). • Acute BRJ ingestion mitigates the reduction in AM supramaximal exercise performance, resulting in performance comparable to PM levels, with lower HR but unchanged RPE.

Table 2. *Cont.*

	Positive Effects of Supplementation (Acute/Short-Term)					
	Study	**Sample Size**	**Dose**	**Form**	**Duration**	**Results**
8	Esen O. et al. [59]	12 men	NO_3^--rich beetroot juice (NIT, 140 mL, ~12.8 mmol NO_3^-) or NO_3^--depleted placebo (PLA, 140 mL, ~0.04 mmol NO_3^-), consumed 3 h before the Yo–Yo IR1 test.	Juice	Acute	• Acute high-dose NO_3^- supplementation with beetroot juice significantly enhanced intermittent running performance in the Yo–Yo IR1 test.
9	Forbes S. et al. [60]	14 women (including 9 using hormonal contraceptives; HC)	Nitrate-rich beetroot juice (140 mL containing ~13 mmol NO_3^-; 2,5 h before exercise or PLA (NO_3^--free blackcurrant juice)	Juice	Acute	• BRJ did not reduce VO_2 or heart rate at 50% and 70% VO_2max in the majority of participants, though 3 participants were responders showing ≥3% VO_2 reduction. • Rate of perceived exertion (RPE) was significantly reduced with BRJ compared to placebo, especially at higher intensity (70% VO_2max)
10	Garnacho-Castaño M.V. et al. [61]	10 men	BRJ—140 mL (~12.8 mmol, ~808 mg NO_3^-), consumed 3 h before the 2000-m rowing ergometer test; or PLA (made by dissolving 2 g of powdered SUPER BEETROOT (~0.01 mmol, 0.620 mg of NO_3^-) in 1 L of water))	Juice	Acute	• Possibly improved 2000-m time trial performance (mean difference 4 s) • Increased relative and absolute VO_2 max (mean difference 2.10 $mL \cdot kg^{-1} \cdot min^{-1}$ and 0.16 $L \cdot min^{-1}$).
11	Garnacho-Castaño M.V et al. [43]	11 men	Beetroot juice (BJ, 140 mL, ~12.8 mmol NO_3^-/808 mg) administered 3 h before exercise; or PLA (prepared by dissolving 2 g of powdered BJ (~ 0.01 mmol, 0.620 mg of NO_3^-)	Juice	Acute	• Plasma NOx levels after BJ: reduced pulmonary oxygen uptake (VO_2) during rest and full back squat exercise. • BJ: plasma myoglobin levels increased;

Table 2. *Cont.*

	Positive Effects of Supplementation (Acute/Short-Term)					
	Study	Sample Size	Dose	Form	Duration	Results
12	Garnacho-Castaño M.V. et al. [62]	12 men	Beetroot juice (140 mL; ~12.8 mmol NO_3^- (~808 mg)); 3 h before exercise (of each test) or PLA (prepared by dissolving 2 g of powdered BJ (~ 0.01 mmol, 0.620 mg of NO_3^-)	Juice	Acute	• Acute BJ (~12.8 mmol NO_3^-) enhanced CrossFit WOD (short and high intensity daily sessions) performance when rest periods were included between exercises, but also increased muscle fatigue, cortisol, and arterial desaturation.
13	Hemmatinafar M. et al. [63]	12 women	Beetroot juice (BRJ) vs. placebo (PLA), 50 mL per serving, 8 servings over 2 days (total 400 mL), ingested at 2, 6, 10, 14, 26, 30, 34, and 38 h post-exercise.	Juice	Acute (2-days)	• BRJ improves static muscular endurance performance (in female volleyball players) 48 h after exercise-induced muscle damage, which is also associated with reducing the perception of muscle soreness and tissue edema.
14	Jiaqi Z. et al. [52]	13 women	BJ 2.5 h before exercise; single dose 70 mL (~6.45 mmol NO_3^-) or double dose (2 × 70 mL; ~12.9 mmol NO_3^-). or PLA (BJ with extracted nitrates)	Juice	Acute	• Decreased mean heart rate (HR) and ratings of perceived exertion (RPE) during work intervals, recovery periods, and across the overall protocol in women; no additional benefits were observed with the higher 12.9 mmol dose.

Table 2. *Cont.*

	Positive Effects of Supplementation (Acute/Short-Term)					
	Study	Sample Size	Dose	Form	Duration	Results
15	Jurado-Castro J.M. et al. [64]	11 men	70 mL beetroot juice (BJ; 400 mg NO_3^-, 6.4 mmol/L or NO_3^--depleted placebo, consumed 120 min before resistance training sessions.	Juice	Acute	• BJ enhanced performance in resistance training tests, improving the number of repetitions completed. • Max HR higher in BJ compared to placebo. • Root Mean Square of the Successive Differences (RMSSD) decreased during exercise with BJ ($p = 0.023$; ES = 0.999), indicating greater parasympathetic withdrawal during activity. • RMSSD-Slope (internal load indicator) improved with BJ (BJ: 3 ± 3 vs. placebo: 0.5 ± 0.7; $p = 0.025$; ES = 1.104), suggesting lower internal load despite better performance. • Acute BJ supplementation 120 min before resistance training reduces internal load during exercise (improved RMSSD-Slope) while enhancing muscular endurance performance.
16	Jurado-Castro J.M. et al. [35]	14 women (2 on contraceptives)	70 mL NO_3^--rich beetroot juice (BRJ; 400 mg nitrate) or NO_3^--depleted placebo, consumed 2 h before exercise (during each visit—3 visits)	Juice	Acute	• Greater maximum height in countermovement jump (CMJ) after BRJ compared with PLA (+6%) • Increased mean velocity, peak velocity mean power and peak power; • Higher repetitions to failure (RTF) in back squat, leg press, and leg extension exercises; significant main effects for time, supplement, and supplement × time interaction in all exercises.

Table 2. *Cont.*

	Positive Effects of Supplementation (Acute/Short-Term)					
	Study	Sample Size	Dose	Form	Duration	Results
17	Macuh M. et al. [65]	15 men	70 mL concentrated beetroot juice (~400 mg nitrate)) or nitrate-depleted placebo (~0 mg nitrate), consumed 2 h before exercise	Juice	Acute	• Running performance (Cooper test) improved significantly with nitrate supplementation when baseline dietary nitrate intake was <300 mg/day (+0.145 km on average).
18	Miraftabi H. et al. [41]	8 men	four experimental trials: BJ-400, BJ-800, PL, CON; 2.5 h before the tests, each participant ingested either one bottle of 60 mL BJ + one bottle of 60 mL of PL or two bottles of BJ (120 mL) (=400 mg NO_3^- per bottle) or depleted dried powder NO_3^- for PL (1 g of dried powder of BJ dissolved in 1 L of water + lemon juice for taste)	Juice	Acute	• Moderate to large effect sizes on anaerobic performance and a large effect size on aerobic performance, • BJ-400 improved cognitive function (word–color and total scores).
19	Neteca J. et al. [42]	18 women	BJG- 50 mL of nitrate-rich beetroot juice concentrate (~6.2 mmol of nitrates (NO_3^-) consumed once before second exercise test; or PLA (nitrate-free beverage).	Juice	Acute	• VO_2 max increased by 4.82%, ventilation efficiency (VE/VO_2 and VE/VCO_2) improved; • Heart rate decreased, indicating enhanced cardiovascular and respiratory function and reduced fatigue during prolonged exercise.
20	Ranchal-Sanchez A. et al. [66]	12 men	Beetroot juice (70 mL containing ~400 mg NO_3^- per serving); 120 min before exercise, single acute dose, across three visits; or PLA (blackcurrant juice with depleted nitrates)	Juice	Acute	• Acute BJ (~400 mg NO_3^-) enhanced muscular endurance in back squat and overall session repetitions.

Table 2. *Cont.*

	Positive Effects of Supplementation (Acute/Short-Term)					
	Study	Sample Size	Dose	Form	Duration	Results
21	Rodríguez-Fernández A. et al. [34]	18 men	Beetroot juice (BJ), 140 mL total (2 × 70 mL concentrated shots; ~800 mg NO_3^-otal); ingested 2.5 h prior to testing or PLA (2 × 70 mL providing <0.1 mmol NO_3^-)	Juice	Acute	• Mean power (MP): BJ increased MP during both concentric (CON) and eccentric (ECC) contractions across moment inertias of 0.025, 0.050, 0.075, and 0.100 kg/m^2. • Peak power (PP): BJ increased peak power during both CON and ECC contractions across all moment inertias; • Total power output increased at all moment inertias with BJ; improvements were similar for CON and ECC contractions (15–25% improvement). • Interpretation: Acute BJ ingestion enhanced skeletal muscle contractile function and power output during half-squat exercise at multiple inertial loads.
22	Rowland S.N. et al. [67]	12 men	Beetroot juice 2 × 70 mL (~13 mmol NO_3^-) with breakfast 2.5 h before exercise at morning (08:00), afternoon (12:00), or evening (15:00). Six experimental conditions, PL and BR in the morning (started at 08:00; PL-MORN and BR-MORN), afternoon (started at 12:00; PL-AFT, BR-AFT) and evening (started at 15:00; PL-EVE and BR-EVE).	Juice	Acute	• Central systolic BP was reduced 2.5 h after BR ingestion at all timepoints. BR increased salivary and plasma [NO_3^-] and [NO_2^-] similarly across morning, afternoon, and evening.

Table 2. *Cont.*

	Study	Sample Size	Dose	Form	Duration	Results
	Positive Effects of Supplementation (Acute/Short-Term)					
23	Serra-Payá N. et al. [68]	11 men	140 mL Beet-It-Pro Elite Shot (~808 mg NO_3^- (~12.8 mmol)), 3 h prior to testing or PLA (2 g of powdered BJ (~0.01 mmol, 0.620 mg of NO_3^-, dissolved in 1 L of water + lemon juice for flavor)).	Juice	Acute	• Acute BJ intake improves FS (full squad) resistance exercise performance, ventilatory efficiency (VE/VCO_2 slope), and $PetCO_2$ when rest is provided between exercises, likely due to enhanced $NO_3^- \rightarrow NO_2^- \rightarrow$ NO conversion and pulmonary vasodilation. The effect is not observed under severe anaerobic conditions without rest.
24	Tan R. et al. [69]	14 men	2 × 70 mL doses per day of concentrated NO_3^--rich beetroot juice (BR: ~5.9 mmol of NO_3^- per 70 mL). Experimental days (day 1 and 4 of each supplementation period): 2 × 70 mL of allocated beverage 2.5 h before exercise. Days 2 and 3 of each supplementation period: 1 × 70 mL beverage twice a day; or PLA (nitrate-depleted BR)	Juice	2 × 4 days	• Acute BRJ supplementation increased upper-body muscular endurance (bench press RTF) and raised plasma [NO_3^-].

Table 2. *Cont.*

	Positive Effects of Supplementation (Acute/Short-Term)					
	Study	Sample Size	Dose	Form	Duration	Results
25	Tatlici A. et al. [70]	8 men	Second visit of the trial: 2 × 70 mL beetroot juice; Third visit of the trial: 2 × 70 mL beetroot juice, 150 min prior to testing or PLA (140 mL of cherry + lemon juice).	Juice	Acute	• Balance performance after fatigue-inducing full-squat exercise (FSE) was significantly better in the BRJ group compared to placebo. At rest, some balance parameters were also improved in the BRJ group. Static Medial-Lateral Stability Index (MLSI) improved significantly with BRJ. • Dynamic OSI (overall stability index) and APSI (anterior/posterior stability index) were improved with BRJ. Post-fatigue, BRJ supplementation improved Static OSI (ES = 1.3), APSI (ES = 1.2), Dynamic OSI (ES = 1.1), APSI (ES = 1.0), and MLSI (ES = 1.0) compared to placebo. • Acute BRJ ingestion improves balance performance both at rest and following fatigue in trained wrestlers
26	Tatlici A. et al. [71]	8 men	Beetroot juice (BJ), 2 × 70 mL shots (~140 mL), 150 min before exercise or PLA (140 mL of cherry + lemon juice).	Juice	Acute	• Acute BJ supplementation significantly increased upper-body (shoulder) strength and average lower- and upper-body strength
27	Thurston T.S. et al. [72]	11 men	Single daily dose for 2 days prior to experimental trial, plus a double dose 2 h before exercise (Nitrate-rich beetroot concentrate; 70 mL; 4.1 mmol NO_3^-) or PLA (nitrate-stripped; 0.03 mmol of NO_3^-).	Juice	Short term (3-day supplementation period; single doses for 2 days and double dose 2 h prior to exercise.)	• Acute nitrate-rich beetroot concentrate supplementation elevates plasma nitrate and nitrite, lowers mean arterial pressure (MAP) and leg blood flow during cycling.

Table 2. *Cont.*

	Positive Effects of Supplementation (Acute/Short-Term)					
	Study	Sample Size	Dose	Form	Duration	Results
28	Volino-Souza M. et al. [73]	9 women and 4 men	Beetroot juice (BJ), 140 mL containing ~8.12 ± 3.61 mmol NO_3^-; consumed 150 min before exercise or PLA (depleted nitrate beetroot juice; ~0.08 ± 0.76 mmol of nitrate).	Juice	Acute	• A single acute dose of BJ (~8.1 mmol NO_3^-) enhanced muscle reoxygenation during recovery
29	Wei C. et al. [50]	8 men and 3 women	2 bottles of NO_3^- depleted BR (placebo, PL) (~0.08 mmol NO_3^-, 2 × 70 mL); 1 bottle of NO_3^- rich BR (~6.4 mmol NO_3^-, 1 × 70 mL); 2 bottles of NO_3^- − rich BR (~12.8 mmol NO_3^-, 2 × 70 mL); 3 bottles of NO_3^- − rich BR (~19.2 mmol NO_3^-, 3 × 70 mL); 1.3 g KNO3 (~12.8 mmol NO_3^- mixed with 300 mL deionized water on separate laboratory visits.	Juice	Five visits over a period of 17–35 days	• Muscle contractile function showed dose-dependent effects: mean peak torque and torque impulse were significantly enhanced during the first 10 muscle contractions following 12.8 and 19.2 mmol NO_3^- ingestion, while mean rate of torque development (RTD) at 0–50 ms and 0–100 ms was enhanced following 6.4 mmol NO_3^-.
30	Williams T.D. et al. [49]	11 men	Beetroot juice -70 mL containing ~400 mg NO_3^-; 2 h before exercise, within 5 min or PLA (blackcurrat juice).	Juice	Acute	• Acute BRJ supplementation increased mean velocity and mean power during free-weight bench press compared to placebo. • Total repetitions across 3 sets to failure at 70% 1 RM (repetition maximum) increased. Set-to-set declines in repetitions were observed for both conditions (BRJ and PLA), but total repetitions were higher with BRJ. Overall, BRJ enhanced upper-body muscular strength, endurance and power output.

Table 2. *Cont.*

	Study	Sample Size	Dose	Form	Duration	Results
			Positive Effects of Supplementation (Acute/Short-Term)			
31	Wong T.H. et al. [74]	17 men	Two trials—2 × 285 mL of either ISO-BR (isotonic beetroot juice) or BR drink 3 h before testing Both contained 6.45 mmol, 400 mg, per 285 mL serving; 9 mg/100 mL of ascorbic acid was added into the ISO-BR drink.	Juice	Acute	• ISO-BR increased salivary NOx more than BR and improved peak power output. Rate of fatigue was higher (+7.9%) with ISO-BR. Plasma NOx increased similarly for both drinks (~4-fold), and salivary NOx strongly correlated with plasma NOx.
32	Yuschen X. et al. [75]	12 men	2.5 h before exercise- Nitrate-rich beetroot juice (NRBRJ): 70 mL shot 400 containing 400 mg NO_3^- or PLA (prune juice).	Juice	Acute	• Mean exercise load increased with NRBRJ. • Diastolic blood pressure (DBP) decreased at rest and at 5, 20, and 30 min during exercise. • Mean arterial pressure (MAP) decreased at rest and at 20 and 30 min during exercise. • Brachial–ankle pulse wave velocity (baPWV) decreased after exercise. • Flow-mediated dilation (FMD) increased before and after exercise compared to PLA.

BRJ/BJ/BR—beetroot juice; PLA/PL—placebo; CON—control condition; NRBRJ—nitrate-rich beetroot juice; ISO-BR—isotonic beetroot juice; NO_3^-—nitrate ion; NO_2^-—nitrite ion; NO—nitric oxide; NOx—combined nitrate + nitrite concentration; KNO_3—potassium nitrate; VO_2—oxygen consumption; VO_2max—maximal oxygen uptake; HR—heart rate; BP—blood pressure; DBP—diastolic blood pressure; SBP—systolic blood pressure; MAP—mean arterial pressure; baPWV—brachial–ankle pulse wave velocity; FMD—flow-mediated dilation; $PetCO_2$—end-tidal carbon dioxide pressure; VCO_2—carbon dioxide production; VE—minute ventilation; VO_2—ventilatory equivalent for oxygen; VCO_2—ventilatory equivalent for carbon dioxide; RER—respiratory exchange ratio; ΔHHb—change in deoxyhemoglobin + deoxymyoglobin; RMSSD—root mean square of successive differences; HRV—heart rate variability; RTD—rate of torque development; CMJ—countermovement jump; RTF—repetitions to failure; MP—mean power; PP—peak power; CON/ECC—concentric/eccentric muscle contractions; FS—full squat; WOD—workout of the day; WAnT—Wingate anaerobic test; IR1/Yo-Yo IR1—Yo-Yo Intermittent Recovery Test; 1RM—one-repetition maximum; TTE—time to exhaustion; RPE—rating of perceived exertion; TQR—total quality recovery; MLSI—medial–lateral stability index; OSI—overall stability index; APSI—anterior–posterior stability index; HC—hormonal contraceptives; GPS—global positioning system; CAF—caffeine; CIT—citrulline; POM—pomegranate powder; NAC—N-acetylcysteine; MAL—maltodextrin.

Table 3. Summary of the original studies examining the impact of dietary nitrates from beetroot on exercise performance—chronic dosing.

	Positive Effects of Supplementation (Chronic)					
	Study	**Sample size**	**Dose**	**Form**	**Duration**	**Results**
1	Burgos J. et al. [76]	32 men	I-placebo group (PLG); II-CIT (citrulline) group (CITG): 3 g/day (3 × 1 g) gelatin capsules III-nitrate-rich beetroot extract group (BRG); 3 gelatin capsules of 700 mg a day (5:1 beetroot extract equivalent to 3500 mg of whole dried root, standardized to contain 0.3% betanin providing 100 mg of NO_3^-) IV-CIT-BR group (CIT-BRG).	Capsules	Chronic (9 weeks)	• CIT-BRG prevented increases in cortisol and decline in testosterone/cortisol ratio (T/C) compared to PLG and showed significantly higher % change in T/C vs. PLG and CITG ($p < 0.05$). CITG and BRG alone showed decreases in testosterone levels;
2	Burgos J. et al. [77]	32 men	6 capsules/day: (I) placebo group (PLG); (II) CIT (citrulline) group (3 × 1 g CIT; CITG); (III): nitrate-rich beetroot extract group (3 × 700 mg; 100 mg of NO_3^-; BRG) and (IV) CIT-BR group (CIT-BRG)	Capsules	Chronic (9 weeks)	• Nine weeks of CIT + BR supplementation (CIT-BRG): significant improvements in aerobic power compared to PL and CIT alone. CIT-BRG also showed significant increases in maximal strength (HJUMP) and endurance-strength (1-MAT) after 9 weeks, whereas the other groups showed smaller or no improvements. Handgrip dynamometer (DYN) performance increased in all groups, but CIT-BRG displayed higher percentage improvements.
3	Daab W. et al. [36]	13 men	Beetroot juice (BET; 150 mL per serving, 250 mg NO_3^-/serving), consumed twice daily (08:00 and 18:00) for 7 consecutive days, including 3 days pre-exercise, on the trial day, and 3 days post-exercise or PLA (nonspecified)	Juice	Chronic (7-days)	• 7 days of high-nitrate BET improved recovery of muscle function and reduced perceived muscle soreness after simulated soccer match, without affecting blood markers of muscle damage.

Table 3. *Cont.*

	Positive Effects of Supplementation (Chronic)					
	Study	**Sample size**	**Dose**	**Form**	**Duration**	**Results**
4	de Oliveira G.V. et al. [78]	14 men	100 g of beetroot-based nutritional gel (BG; 12.2 ± 0.2 mmol of nitrate); On the second and third visit: a single dose of BG after measuring maximal forearm muscle isometric strength; Then 120 min before exercise, ingestion of the supplement; or PLA (nitrate-depleted BG gel).	Gel	Chronic, 8-day supplementation	• High-nitrate beetroot gel (BG) supplementation significantly attenuated the decline in handgrip strength after exercise. • A single dose of BG improved maximal forearm isometric strength recovery 20 min post-handgrip exercise.
5	Esen O. et al. [79]	14 men	2 × 70 mL/day (~12.8 mmol/day NO_3^-) for 5 days; on the experimental trial day, both shots were taken together 2.5 h before testing; or PLA (nitrate-depleted beetroot juice).	Juice	Chronic (5-day supplementation) with acute dosing on the test day	• Short-term NO_3^- supplementation reduced motor unit potential (MUP) duration during brief isometric contractions and recovery stages with and without blood flow restriction.
6	Esen O. et al. [80]	14 men	NO_3^--rich beetroot juice (BRJ; NIT: 2 × 70 mL/day, ~12.8 mmol/day NO_3^-) or NO_3^--depleted BRJ as placebo (PLA; 2 × 70 mL/day, ~0.08 mmol/day NO_3^-). For days 1–4, doses were taken morning (~9 a.m.) and evening (~9 p.m.); on day 5, both doses were taken together 2.5 h before exercise testing.		Chronic (2 × 5-days)	• Chronic NO_3^- supplementation (~12.8 mmol/day) elevated plasma NO_2^-, reduced BP at rest, and attenuated BP increases during short and sustained isometric muscle contractions.
7	Esen O. et al. [81]	10 men and 6 women	Nitrate-rich (NIT) beetroot juice 2 × 70 mL/day (~12.8 mmol/day NO_3^-) for 4 days (morning & evening), plus 2 × 70 mL 2.5 h before trial; or PLA (nitrate-depleted beetroot juice).	Juice	Chronic (short term; 2 × 5-days separated by a washout period)	• Plasma [NO_2^-] increased by ~140% in NIT vs. PLA ($p < 0.001$). • Motor unit potential (MUP) duration was significantly shorter in NIT vs. PLA during brief and sustained contractions with BFR.

Table 3. *Cont.*

	Positive Effects of Supplementation (Chronic)					
	Study	Sample size	Dose	Form	Duration	Results
8	Huang X. et al. [32]	44 men and 36 women	Concentrated beetroot juice (BRJ; 6.5 mmol NO_3^-/70 mL) or nitrate-free placebo (PL; 0.065 mmol NO_3^-/70 mL), 3 × 70 mL/day for 7 days.	Juice	Chronic (7-days)	• Running economy: Lower mean VO_2, RER, and blood lactate (BLA) during submaximal treadmill running at high speed (V3: males 13.3 km/h, females 11.6 km/h) in BRJ vs. PL. • Time-to-exhaustion (TTE) during cycling at 85% peak power output (PPO): Significantly increased in BRJ vs. PL (male: 16.50 ± 3.09 min vs. 14.42 ± 2.62 min, $p = 0.02$; female: 12.38 ± 2.23 min vs. 10.86 ± 2.21 min, $p = 0.04$). • Rating of perceived exertion (RPE): Lower with BRJ, though differences were not statistically significant. • One week of BRJ supplementation improved submaximal running economy and cycling endurance (TTE) but did not enhance cross-country skiing performance; RPE tended to decrease but not significantly.
9	Khosravi S. et al. [51]	12 men	Beetroot juice (BRJ), 2 × 70 mL/day (~12.8 mmol NO_3^- per day) for 6 days; exercise testing on day 6, 2–2.5 h after the final dose; or PLA (blackcurrant juice).	Juice	Chronic; (6 days)	• Six days of BRJ supplementation increased peak torque during bilateral isokinetic knee extensions. Improvements were observed at high angular velocities: 180 and 360°/s for the dominant leg and 360°/s for the non-dominant leg. BRJ also enhanced muscle fatigue resistance during 50 maximal knee extensions at 180°/s, with an increase in peak torque.

Table 3. *Cont.*

	Positive Effects of Supplementation (Chronic)					
	Study	Sample size	Dose	Form	Duration	Results
10	Kozłowska L. et al. [82]	10 men and 10 women	Freeze-dried beetroot juice (BRJ), 26 g/day (~200 mL juice equivalent, ~2.1 mmol NO_3^-), taken once daily with a meal 2 h before VO_2max testing; or PLA (ID-dietary recommendations without additional BRJ).	Freeze-dried juice	Chronic (4-weeks)	• VO_2max significantly increased after BRJ supplementation. Muscle damage marker LDH stabilized after BRJ supplementation. Serum creatine kinase (CK) activity was consistently higher in men than women across all stages. Oxidative stress marker malondialdehyde concentration (MDA) increased after BRJ, while antioxidant defense markers (selenium, glutathione peroxidase activity- GPx1, GPx3) increased.
11	Liubertas T. et al. [83]	13 men	Oat bar (60 g; 4 g standardized *Amaranthus hypochondriacus* concentrate; ≈400 mg NO_3^-), consumed 1 h before exercise during single-dose testing, and daily for 6 days before long-term testing; or PLA (60 g-oat bar with excluded *Amaranthus hypochondriacus*).	Oat bar	Chronic (6 days) and single-dose test performed 1 h after first ingestion	• Increase of peak power of increasing cycling exercise (ICE); Long-term use of dietary amaranth: VO_2max demonstrated a significant increase.
12	Nicholas C. et al. [84]	10 men	140 mL/day of NO_3^-–-rich (12.8 mmol·d^{-1}; BRJ + lemon juice); 2.5 h before the trial; or PLA (nitrate-depleted BRJ + lemon juice for taste).	Juice	Chronic (6 days)	• Improved heavy load carriage; • Increased heart rate, mean tidal volume, and performance during time trial with BRJ.

Table 3. *Cont.*

	Study	Sample size	Dose	Form	Duration	Results
	Positive Effects of Supplementation (Chronic)					
13	Rowland S.N. et al. [85]	9 men	Beetroot powder—NO_3^--rich (BR, 6% NO_3^-, 8 mmol NO_3^-). Participants consumed 8.4 g/day in ≥250 mL water for 6 days. On day 7, a pre-exercise dose 2 h before cycling and a top-up 8.4 g dose 1 h into the 2-h exercise.	Powder dissolved in water	Chronic (Two 7-day supplementation periods (BR or PL), cross-over, with experimental testing on day 7 including pre- and mid-exercise top-up doses)	• Short-term nitrate-rich beetroot powder supplementation increased plasma [NO_3^-] and [NO_2^-], improved end-sprint mean power output, and enhanced muscle oxygenation (deoxyhaemoglobin + deoxymyooglobin concentration [HHb] (kinetics)).
14	Tan R. et al. [86]	8 men and 4 women	Nitrate-rich beetroot juice (BR, ~6.2 mmol NO_3^- – per 70 mL, 2 × 70 mL/day) compared to NO_3^--depleted beetroot juice placebo (PL, ~0.04 mmol NO_3^- – per 70 mL) and control water (CON); (Three separate 4-day supplementation periods (2 × 70 mL/day; days 1–2 one morning + one evening, days 3–4 both in morning ~2.5 h before exercise).	Juice	Chronic	• BR supplementation significantly increased plasma [NO_3^-] and [NO_2^-] compared to PL and CON. During moderate-intensity cycling, BR reduced the O_2 cost of exercise by ~2% when ensemble-averaged over four-step exercise transitions
15	Tirkey D. et al. [33]	15 men and 15 women	Beetroot juice (BRJ) 250 mL/day in natura, providing ~5.00 mmol NO_3^- per day; or PLA (nitrate-depleted beverage).	Juice	Chronic (15 days)	• Fifteen days of daily BRJ supplementation improved 10-km running time trial performance in both male and female trained athletes. Male experimental group showed a 4.2% improvement. Female experimental group showed a 7.5% improvement.

Table 3. *Cont.*

	Positive Effects of Supplementation (Chronic)					
	Study	Sample size	Dose	Form	Duration	Results
16	Viribay A. et al. [87]	20 men	Per day: (I) 5 capsules of placebo and 6 g of maltodextrin in powder; (II) 5 capsules (500 mg) of BR and 6 g of maltodextrin in powder; (III) 5 capsules of BR (500 mg) and 6 g of CIT in powder.	Capsules	Chronic (7-days)	• 7 days of combined BR extract and CIT supplementation enhances lactate clearance after high-intensity exercise and improves peak power during aerobic testing in elite rowers, providing modest ergogenic benefits.

BRJ/BJ/BR—beetroot juice; PLA/PL—placebo; CON—control condition; NRBRJ—nitrate-rich beetroot juice; ISO-BR—isotonic beetroot juice; NO_3^-—nitrate ion; NO_2^-—nitrite ion; NO—nitric oxide; NOx—combined nitrate + nitrite concentration; KNO_3—potassium nitrate; VO_2—oxygen consumption; VO_2max—maximal oxygen uptake; HR—heart rate; BP—blood pressure; DBP—diastolic blood pressure; SBP—systolic blood pressure; MAP—mean arterial pressure; baPWV—brachial–ankle pulse wave velocity; FMD—flow-mediated dilation; $PetCO_2$—end-tidal carbon dioxide pressure; VCO_2—carbon dioxide production; VE—minute ventilation; VO_2—ventilatory equivalent for oxygen; VCO_2—ventilatory equivalent for carbon dioxide; RER—respiratory exchange ratio; ΔHHb—change in deoxyhemoglobin + deoxymyoglobin; RMSSD—root mean square of successive differences; HRV—heart rate variability; RTD—rate of torque development; CMJ—countermovement jump; RTF—repetitions to failure; MP—mean power; PP—peak power; CON/ECC—concentric/eccentric muscle contractions; FS—full squat; WOD—workout of the day; WAnT—Wingate anaerobic test; IR1/Yo-Yo IR1—Yo-Yo Intermittent Recovery Test; 1RM—one-repetition maximum; TTE—time to exhaustion; RPE—rating of perceived exertion; TQR—total quality recovery; MLSI—medial–lateral stability index; OSI—overall stability index; APSI—anterior–posterior stability index; HC—hormonal contraceptives; GPS—global positioning system; CAF—caffeine; CIT—citrulline; POM—pomegranate powder; NAC—N-acetylcysteine; MAL—maltodextrin.

Table 4. Summary of the original studies examining the impact of dietary nitrates from beetroot on exercise performance.

	Non-Significant/No Effects of Supplementation					
	Study	Sample Size	Dose	Form	Duration	Results
1	Berjisian, E. et al. [88]	16 men	One 60-mL bottle of fluid containing either 6.4 mmol (NO_3^-), 500 mg L-Arginine, and L-Ornithine or NO_3^- depleted dried powder as placebo and ingested a capsule containing 5 mg/kg body mass of caffeine (CAF) or cellulose as PL 60 min before the start of the Stroop test. Four experimental trials: BJ + CAF, CAF + PL, BJ + PL, and PL + PL.	Juice	Acute	• No significant effect of BJ, CAF, or BJ + CAF on total distance covered (YYIR1 test (intermittent running) • No significant effect of supplementation on CMJ height and power. • RPE increased over time; no supplementation effect. • No supplementation effect on cognitive performance.

Table 4. *Cont.*

	Non-Significant/No Effects of Supplementation					
	Study	**Sample Size**	**Dose**	**Form**	**Duration**	**Results**
2	Berlanga L.A. et al. [89]	10 men	150 min before testing: 70-mL dose of BJ (6.4 mmol of NO_3^-); or PLA (nitrate-depleted BJ).	Juice	Acute	• Acute ingestion of 70 mL beetroot juice (6.4 mmol NO_3^-) did not improve neuromuscular performance.
3	Burke L.M. et al. [38]	21 men	Study 1: two evenings before the experimental trial (−36, and −12 h): 70 mL shot of NO_3^--rich beetroot juice (BRJ; 6.45 mmol NO_3^-); Morning of the experimental trial: 140 mL (~12.9 mmol NO_3^-) of BRJ supplement with breakfast+ second treatment after 7 km exercise: 70 mL BRJ (6.45 mmol NO_3^-); after each treadmill 26-km protocol: 190 mL of allocated test drink Study 2: Carb Max	Juice	Acute	• Two-day preload plus pre- and mid-exercise ingestion of beetroot juice increased plasma nitrate concentrations throughout the ~2 h exercise session. • Plasma nitrite concentrations were elevated only during the first half of exercise; levels declined in the second half. • Beetroot juice did not alter oxygen uptake or the oxygen cost of exercise at race-relevant speeds. • Beetroot juice supplementation did not improve endurance performance, exercise efficiency, or oxygen utilization in elite race walkers
4	Collins S.M. et al. [90]	15 men and 9 women	Subjects performed two counterbalanced trials, once with a control and another after consuming 70 mL (~4.2 mmol NO_3^-) of beetroot concentrate nitrate supplement 2 h prior to physical activity; or PLA (strongly flavored water).	Beetroot concentrate	Acute	• Acute ingestion of 70 mL beetroot nitrate did not improve high-intensity functional training (HIFT) performance, lactate or perceived exertion.

Table 4. *Cont.*

	Non-Significant/No Effects of Supplementation					
	Study	Sample Size	Dose	Form	Duration	Results
5	Conger S.A. et al. [91]	14 men	The supplement was provided to the participant 24 to 72 h preceding the trial. One dose of red beet juice powder containing ~8 mmol (496 mg) NO_3^- mixed with 237 mL of water (this dose is considered "high" (high > 7.5 mmol); or PLA (cherry-apple-cranberry juice blend).	Juice	Acute	• Beet juice did not enhance overall power output, endurance, or performance in short-term maximal anaerobic cycling; minor reduction in fatigue was only observed in the 30-s test.
6	Esen O. et al. [92]	12 men	140 mL NO_3^--rich (BRJ; 2 × 70 mL; ~12.8 mmol NO_3^-) or NO_3^--depleted (PLA) BRJ, 3 h before two experimental trials three.	Juice	Acute	• Acute high-dose BRJ (12.8 mmol NO_3^-) increases plasma NO_3^-/NO_2^- but does not improve intermittent running performance, CMJ (counter-movement jump), or blood lactate responses in trained male rugby players.
7	Fernández-Elías V. et al. [45]	9 men	3 h prior to exercise: 70 mL of concentrated beetroot juice (6.4 mmol NO_3^-); or PLA (0.005 mmol of NO_3^-) prepared by dissolving 1 g of powdered beetroot and lemon juice in water.	Juice	Acute	• Acute ingestion of nitrate-rich beetroot juice did not increase total distance covered, running speed, or high-intensity running during a 3-set tennis match. • Serve speed before and after the match was unchanged between beetroot juice and placebo conditions. • Isometric handgrip strength before and after the match showed no differences between treatments. • RPE post-match was not affected by beetroot juice ingestion. • Beetroot juice did not improve pre-to-post match changes in tennis-specific performance measures.

Table 4. *Cont.*

	Non-Significant/No Effects of Supplementation					
	Study	Sample Size	Dose	Form	Duration	Results
8	Hennis P.J. et al. [93]	21 men and 6 women	3 days prior to exercise trials and continued throughout the exercise trials: 3 × 200 mL, daily nitrate consumption of ~0.18 [18.5 (±2.0) mmol]; or PLA (nitrate-depleted beetroot/fruit juice [1.4 (0.1) mmol]).	Juice	Chronic	• Dietary nitrate did not alter exercise efficiency, anaerobic threshold, peak work rate, heart rate, or ventilation. • Plasma nitrate, nitrite, and nitroso product concentrations were largely unchanged during exercise tests, with some post-exercise spikes in nitrite and S-nitrosothiol in a few individuals.
9	López-Samanes Á. et al. [39]	11 women	3 h before each testing session: 70 mL dose of beetroot juice (6.4 mmol of NO_3^-); or PLA (nitrate-depleted beetroot juice).	Juice	Acute	• No effects of acute beetroot juice on countermovement jump height, isometric handgrip strength, 20 m sprint, repeated sprint ability, GPS-measured match-play activity, or perceived exertion in elite female field hockey players.
10	López-Samanes Á. [94]	13 men	Two separate occasions: 3 h before testing; 70 mL of either BJ (containing 6.4 mmol of NO_3^-) or PLA; (in each trial, 50% of participants ingested PLA and 50% ingested BJ beverages) with random assignment to each supplement.	Juice	Acute	• Acute ingestion of 70 mL beetroot juice (BJ, 4.2–6.4 mmol NO_3^-) did not improve tennis-specific neuromuscular performance. • No effects were observed on serve velocity, countermovement jump height, isometric handgrip strength, 5-0-5 agility, or 10 m sprint speed. • RPE was unaffected. • Low doses of nitrate precursors do not provide ergogenic benefits for highly trained tennis players.

Table 4. *Cont.*

	Non-Significant/No Effects of Supplementation					
	Study	**Sample Size**	**Dose**	**Form**	**Duration**	**Results**
11	Moreno B. et al. [95]	6 women and 7 men	Beetroot juice (BJ, 70 mL, 6.4 mmol NO_3^-) or nitrate-depleted placebo (PLA, 70 mL), ingested 3 h before swimming test. Two sessions separated by 18-day washout.	Juice	Acute	• 100-m times showed no difference between the BJ and (possible shorter time for BJ in the last repetition); • BJ—possibly lower RPE in the first and second repetition; Total Quality Recovery scale scores likely higher in the first and third repetition (than in PLA). • No difference in blood lactate concentration between; an increase in 100-m times for both BJ and PLA after the fifth repetition. • No significant differences in performance in a 6 × 100-m repeated sprint test. Possible trend toward a better recovery and a better tolerance of fatigue after supplementing BJ.
12	Ortiz de Zevallos J. et al. [96]	12 women and 14 men	70 mL of beetroot juice (BRJ ~6.5 mmol NO_3^-) twice/day (~13 mmol total NO_3^-) for ~3 days or an identical NO_3^--depleted placebo (PL). On testing days—the last two 70 mL shots 2 h before their laboratory arrival time. Female subjects were given additional bottles and were instructed to start consuming the juice the day before the estimated day of menses to consider any changes in the start of the menstrual cycle and guarantee consumption of at least 3 days of supplementation before experimental visits.	Juice	Acute (3-days)	• Plasma NO_3^- and NO_2^- increased after supplementation. Cognitive tests showed no significant changes. Submaximal exercise economy and time-to-exhaustion improved only in males, not females. Muscular endurance, jump height and low power improved/increased only in some cases. No improvement in sprinting, high-load strength, and intermittent running. Post-exercise lactate clearance improved with some BR + CIT supplementation.

Table 4. *Cont.*

	Non-Significant/No Effects of Supplementation					
	Study	**Sample Size**	**Dose**	**Form**	**Duration**	**Results**
13	Robinson G.P. et al. [47]	8 men	3 h prior to testing: 140 mL of beetroot juice (providing ~12.4 mmol NO_3^-) daily for 7 days. On nonexperimental days (days 1–2, 4, and 6)—1 × 70 mL in the morning (~09:00) and 1 × 70 mL in the evening (~19:00); or PLA (~0.08 mmol NO_3^-).	Juice	Chronic	• Beetroot juice (BR) supplementation increased plasma NO_2^-, providing more substrate for O_2-independent nitric oxide synthesis during exercise but BR did not improve high-intensity intermittent running performance in endurance-trained males. • Effects were consistent in normoxia and low-to-moderate hypoxia (~1200–2400 m). • Overall, BR does not enhance high-intensity intermittent running performance in trained endurance athletes under these conditions.
14	Rokkedal-Lausch T. et al. [46]	12 well-trained cyclists (gender not specified)	140 mL of concentrated beetroot juice (~12.4 mmol nitrate) per day; one dose (70 mL) in the morning and one dose (70 mL) in the evening. On the days of the experimental trials: total dose 2-h before arriving at the laboratory; or PLA (nitrate-depleted BR).	Juice	Chronic (7 days)	• BR supplementation did not alter oxygen uptake (VO_2) or muscle deoxygenation (ΔHHb) kinetics during moderate-intensity cycling (~60–62% VO_2max). • BR reduced the amplitude of the VO_2 response (~2.1%), but steady-state VO_2, exercise efficiency, and steady-state ΔHHb remained unchanged. • Effects of BR were similar in normoxia and hypoxia; no supplementation-by-condition interactions were observed. • Hypoxia increased heart rate, carbon dioxide production (VCO_2), minute ventilation (VE), and respiratory exchange ratio (RER), and reduced VO_2 time delay, independently of BR supplementation.

Table 4. *Cont.*

	Non-Significant/No Effects of Supplementation					
	Study	Sample Size	Dose	Form	Duration	Results
15	Sousa A. et al. [97]	30 men	Three experimental groups: (I) HNO: high-intensity exercise training sessions in normobaric hypoxia with NO_3^- supplement; (II) HPL: high-intensity exercise training sessions in normobaric hypoxia with placebo and (III) CON: high-intensity exercise training sessions in normoxia with placebo. Supplements given 2.5–3 h prior to each session. ((NO_3^- beetroot juice; 400 mg of a powdered standardized beetroot extract (2% of NO_3^-, ~8.4 mmol))	Juice	Chronic	• NO_3^- supplementation did not enhance exercise performance at simulated altitude compared to placebo.
16	Tan R. et al. [98]	16 men	Four supplementation conditions: (1) PL with MAL (PL + MAL), (2) PL with NAC (PL + NAC), (3) BR with MAL (BR + MAL) (4) BR with NAC (BR + NAC); 2 × 70 mL doses per day of either BR (~6.2 mmol of NO_3^-per 70 mL) or PL. On day 1–5: one 70 mL beverage in the morning and one in the evening. On the experimental day: 2 × 70 mL of allocated beverage 2.5 h prior to exercise and 70 mg/kg of NAC (N-acetylcysteine; 600 mg NAC per capsule)) or maltodextrin (MAL; 600 mg per capsule) 1 h prior to exercise.	Juice	Chronic (6 days)	• Muscle excitability decline during 1 h cycling was attenuated by NAC (PL + NAC) but not by BR or BR + NAC. • Time to exhaustion (TTE) during severe-intensity cycling was not affected by BR, NAC, or their combination. • Voluntary muscle activation and neural drive were unchanged across conditions. • Co-ingestion of BR and NAC maintained plasma NO_3^- but did not enhance endurance or performance.

Table 4. *Cont.*

	Non-Significant/No Effects of Supplementation					
	Study	**Sample Size**	**Dose**	**Form**	**Duration**	**Results**
17	Tan R. et al. [99]	15 men	(1) PL; (2) NO_3^--rich beetroot juice (BR: ~12 mmol of NO_3^-) with 2 empty gelatin capsules; (3) BR with 2 capsules with pomegranate powder (POM: 1000 mg; BR + POM; On experimental: 2 × 70 mL of allocated beverage and capsules 2.5 h before exercise + on a separate visit: two capsules containing 1000 mg of POM 2.5 h prior to a blood draw	Juice + Capsules	Acute	• POM did not increase plasma [NO_3^-] and [NO_2^-] compared to PL. • BR + POM did not alter plasma [NO_3^-] and [NO_2^-] compared to BR. • BR did not affect performance in vertical CMJ, explosive push-ups, or back squats.
18	Tan R. et al. [44]	15 women	2 × 70 mL of concentrated NO_3^--depleted placebo (PL; 0.10 mmol NO_3^- total) or NO_3^--rich beetroot juice (BR; ~ 12.0 mmol NO_3^- total) with a washout-out period of at least 5 days separating the two supplementation periods.	Juice	Acute	• Acute nitrate-rich beetroot juice did not improve sprinting, strength, or aerobic performance in female team-sport players.
19	Trexler E.T. et al. [40]	27 men	2 h before exercise: (1) 70-mL beetroot juice beverage (400 mg dietary nitrate); (2) placebo (PLA); (3) 8 g of unflavored citrulline malate (CitMal)	Juice	Acute	• A single dose of beetroot juice or CitMal does not improve physical performance, endurance, or exercise efficiency in resistance performance.

Table 4. *Cont.*

	Non-Significant/No Effects of Supplementation					
	Study	**Sample Size**	**Dose**	**Form**	**Duration**	**Results**
20	Viribay A. [100]	20 men	(I) Placebo group (PLAG); (II) Beetroot extract group (BRG); and (III) BR supplemented with L-citrulline group (BR-CITG). The intervention spanned 3 consecutive weeks, with each week corresponding to a distinct supplement-intake condition. Daily dosages for 7 days: (I) five placebo capsules per, alongside 6 g of maltodextrin powder; (II) five capsules (each containing 500 mg) per day of BR accompanied by 6 g of maltodextrin powder; or (III) 5 capsules per day (each containing 500 mg) of BR alongside 6 g of L-citrulline powder.	Capsules	Chronic (7-days)	• 7 days of co-ingestion of BR extract and CIT (citrulline) did not enhance physiological or metabolic outcomes during submaximal or maximal rowing exercise.

BRJ/BJ/BR—beetroot juice; PLA/PL—placebo; CON—control condition; NRBRJ—nitrate-rich beetroot juice; ISO-BR—isotonic beetroot juice; NO_3^-—nitrate ion; NO_2^-—nitrite ion; NO—nitric oxide; NOx—combined nitrate + nitrite concentration; KNO_3—potassium nitrate; VO_2—oxygen consumption; VO_2max—maximal oxygen uptake; HR—heart rate; BP—blood pressure; DBP—diastolic blood pressure; SBP—systolic blood pressure; MAP—mean arterial pressure; baPWV—brachial–ankle pulse wave velocity; FMD—flow-mediated dilation; $PetCO_2$—end-tidal carbon dioxide pressure; VCO_2—carbon dioxide production; VE—minute ventilation; VO_2—ventilatory equivalent for oxygen; VCO_2—ventilatory equivalent for carbon dioxide; RER—respiratory exchange ratio; ΔHHb—change in deoxyhemoglobin + deoxymyoglobin; RMSSD—root mean square of successive differences; HRV—heart rate variability; RTD—rate of torque development; CMJ—countermovement jump; RTF—repetitions to failure; MP—mean power; PP—peak power; CON/ECC—concentric/eccentric muscle contractions; FS—full squat; WOD—workout of the day; WAnT—Wingate anaerobic test; IR1/Yo-Yo IR1—Yo-Yo Intermittent Recovery Test; 1RM—one-repetition maximum; TTE—time to exhaustion; RPE—rating of perceived exertion; TQR—total quality recovery; MLSI—medial–lateral stability index; OSI—overall stability index; APSI—anterior–posterior stability index; HC—hormonal contraceptives; GPS—global positioning system; CAF—caffeine; CIT—citrulline; POM—pomegranate powder; NAC—N-acetylcysteine; MAL—maltodextrin.

Table 5. Summary of the review articles and meta-analyses on the impact of dietary nitrates from beetroot on exercise performance.

	Review Articles		
	Study	Included Articles	Conclusions
1	Abreu R. et al. [101]	• 1 out of 18 included studies was about nitrate supplementation from beets; • semi-professional soccer players were given nitrate-rich beetroot juice, simulated a soccer match, and their post-exercise performance was assessed;	Performance decreased after exercise in both groups, but the reduction was smaller with beetroot juice, suggesting possible benefits during long-term recovery.
2	Alsharif N. et al. [102]	• 27 studies—24 of them were describing supplementation of nitrogen coming from beetroot juice; • Studies differed in the methods and duration of supplementation, age of participants, training levels, and sports disciplines.	It was noted that supplementation contributed to the improvement of: total distance covered, peak power, mean power output, total work done. The results from this review and meta-analysis confirm the ergogenic potential of dietary NO_3 supplementation in some aspects of high-intensity exercise capacity
3	Antonio J. et al. [103]	• 5 studies about the supplementation of beetroot juice; the duration and method of administration (varied between the studies); • examining parameters related to endurance and physical performance;	All five studies in the review reported benefits of beetroot supplementation, including increased time to exhaustion, reduced oxygen consumption, and improved training load. Beetroot juice supplementation by athletes may have a positive impact on their performance and physical endurance during training
4	Apte M. et al. [3]	• 10 studies assessing the effect of beetroot juice on physical performance; specifically time trial performance, • 4 studies assessing the effect of beetroot juice on cognitive functions	Beetroot juice supplementation consistently improved time-trial performance across studies, with some evidence of cognitive benefits in young adults (18–30 years), though results were mixed. Natural dietary nitrates appear to be an accessible and low-cost ergogenic aid.
5	Calvo J. et al. [104]	• 27 studies—23 of them used beetroot as the supplemented nitrate source; • studies varied in: duration and supplementation method, and the participants differed in their training levels and chosen sports.	Supplementation reduced VO_2, improved pain threshold, and enhanced performance in sprint interval training, but heterogeneity requires more trials.

Table 5. *Cont.*

	Review Articles		
	Study	**Included Articles**	**Conclusions**
6	Chen L. et al. [105]	• The review article discusses the health-promoting properties of beetroot, including its anti-cancer, antioxidant, kidney and liver protective properties, and its impact on physical performance.	Some studies showed gains in kayaking, resistance, and mountaineering performance, confirming the ergogenic potential of beetroot, though results remain varied.
7	Delleli S. et al. [106]	• 9 studies on athletes practicing various combat sports; (different age groups, different levels of training, supplementing beetroot in various forms, e.g., juice, capsules or gel)	In combat sports, six studies reported improved performance with beetroot supplementation, while three found no benefit or deterioration. Effectiveness may depend on training level, and further confirmation is required.
8	Domínguez R. et al. [107]	• The aim of the review was to discuss the state of knowledge about nutrition and dietary practices in tennis players in order to maximize sports performance	Beetroot juice supplementation improved agility and handgrip strength in tennis players and improved performance in endurance, high-intensity sports and resistance training.
9	d'Unienville N.M.A. et al. [48]	• meta-analysis included a total of 118 studies; • 56 studies were related to nitrates from beetroot, red spinach, Swiss chard and rhubarb.	Nitrate supplementation showed benefits only when derived from beetroot, especially in less trained individuals, while no clear effects were observed in women. Sex differences and limited data in female athletes highlight the need for more targeted research.
10	Esen O. et al. [108]	• 19 studies on beetroot juice (the chosen placebo varied across studies); • Age, athletic ability, and disciplines varied significantly among the included studies. • The duration of administration and supplementation doses were inconsistent;	Beetroot juice slightly enhanced peak and mean power and time to peak power but showed no effect on isometric strength. Wide variability among studies limits practical interpretation.
11	Gamonales J.M. et al. [109]	• 15 studies; 14 of them administered nitrates in the form of beetroot juice; • these studies were characterized by significant heterogeneity in terms of dosing regimen, participant characteristics, and the parameters studied;	Some studies reported benefits in jump performance, pain threshold, and VO_2 recovery, while five found no differences. Effects appear small, inconsistent, and require further exploration. Over 60% indicated positive effects on regeneration, but evidence remains heterogeneous.

Table 5. *Cont.*

	Review Articles		
	Study	**Included Articles**	**Conclusions**
12	Gilsanz L. et al. [110]	• 6 studies in which subjects of various stages of advancement and different ages were given beetroot juice, caffeine, their combination or placebo; • sportsmen practiced various sport disciplines (e.g., cycling, triathlon, soccer)	No studies demonstrated improvements in physical performance parameters with beetroot juice compared to placebo.
13	Harlow J. et al. [111]	• one study was included in the review; • assessment of the effects of beetroot juice supplementation (by soldiers) on exercise capacity and high-altitude acclimatization;	Beetroot juice improved exercise performance compared with placebo and promoted faster post-exercise heart rate recovery. Beetroot juice may have a positive effect on performance during high-intensity, moderate-duration workouts.
14	Hogwood A. et al. [112]	• 11 studies, only 8 of them were conducted on healthy people	A small, non-significant trend toward improved VO_2peak was observed, but overall effects were inconsistent. Adding beetroot juice to training did not enhance outcomes beyond exercise alone.
15	Jones L. et al. [113]	• 9 studies—8 of which administered nitrates in the form of beetroot juice; 6 of these studies were included in the meta-analysis; • Included studies differed in protocols and supplementation regimens; • Participants varied in age and athletic ability; • no professional athletes were included;	Beetroot juice improved recovery of isometric strength and jumping ability but had no effect on oxidative stress markers. Benefits may depend on training modality.
16	Kiani A. et al. [114]	• This review discusses various positive aspects associated with supplementation that increases blood nitrogen levels. Two studies were included that examined the effect of supplementation on improving physical performance in athletes.	Beetroot supplementation significantly improved completion time, average power output, and time to exhaustion in cycle ergometer time trials compared with placebo. These findings suggest benefits for high-intensity endurance exercise, though further studies are needed to define optimal supplementation strategies.

Table 5. *Cont.*

	Review Articles	
Study	**Included Articles**	**Conclusions**
17 Kim J. et al. [115]	• The review included studies that examined the effects of supplementation with caffeine, beta-alanine, sodium bicarbonate, β-hydroxy-β-methylbutyric acid, and beetroot juice. The latter included two studies in which well-trained rowers were given beetroot juice at varying doses and with different supplementation schedules.	Rowing studies demonstrated improved repetitions and 2000-m performance, particularly in moderately trained athletes, alongside rises in plasma nitrite levels.
18 Lago-Rodríguez Á. et al. [116]	• 5 studies—all involving 60 participants; • 4 of these studies involved healthy individuals and both sexes from different age groups; • The supplementation model differed in the administered dose of nitrates from beetroot juice.	Studies on healthy individuals found no effect on isokinetic torque but suggested potential benefits in less trained or short-term contexts. Evidence remains limited.
19 López-Laval I. et al. [117]	• 19 studies, two of which concerned beetroot supplementation in gel form, and the remaining studies concerned other nutrients. The volunteers studied varied in their discipline, age, supplementation regimen, and the parameters examined	Supplementation improved muscle oxygen saturation, recovery of strength, and reduced exercise-induced strength loss, though variability limits firm conclusions.
20 López-Torres O. et al. [118]	• 6 studies in which women were given beetroot juice and their athletic performance was assessed; • In other 5 studies, women were given beetroot juice; various sports and different fitness levels;	Results were mixed in women and elite athletes, with no benefits reported in some groups, while kayakers and runners showed significant improvements. More research in women is particularly needed.
21 Mohd Daud S.M. et al. [119]	• 26 studies, 5 of which administered beetroot juice; • different supplementation protocols and examined parameters between the studies	Supplementation improved muscle recovery in volunteers and also reduces post-exercise muscle pain. Fruit juices may be the best natural-based dietary supplements, replacing other supplement products in supporting muscle recovery and improving athletic performance in trained athletes. Future research, focusing on optimal dose, timing, and frequency of consumption, is needed.

Table 5. *Cont.*

	Review Articles		
	Study	**Included Articles**	**Conclusions**
22	O'Connor E. et al. [120]	• 5 studies that assessed the effect of this supplementation on post-exercise recovery. • The athletes' disciplines, their training levels, and the parameters studied and supplementation parameters varied between studies.	Supplementation reduced post-exercise muscle soreness in soccer players and sprinters, but not in endurance athletes. Blood markers of damage, oxidative stress, and inflammation were unaffected.
23	Poulios A. et al. [121]	• one paper on long-term supplementation with beetroot juice in semi-professional football player; • study examined vertical jump, speed and strength, as well as reduction of post-exercise muscle pain	Supplementation enhanced jump height, strength, speed, and reduced muscle soreness, but did not alter biochemical markers of muscle damage.
24	Rojano-Ortega D. et al. [122]	• 9 studies; • Volunteers: were of different age groups, participated in a big of sports, and the supplementation regimen varied between the studies; • The protocols for the parameters studied were also uniform	Four of these studies demonstrated improvement in these variables, four studies also demonstrated improvement in muscle soreness, and only one study demonstrated a significant difference in creatine kinase levels after beetroot supplementation versus placebo. However, no effect of supplementation on inflammatory markers was demonstrated.
25	San Juan A. et al. [123]	• 4 studies involving 49 men exercising at least twice a week; • The studies differed in: duration, supplementation method, and the examined parameters. • In 3 of the 4 included studies, volunteers were given nitrogen coming from beets.	All included studies showed gains in resistance training outcomes like repetitions, bench press power, and VO_2 reduction. Beetroot may benefit both racquet sports and weightlifting, though mechanisms remain unclear.
26	Silva K. et al. [124]	• Non-disclosed number of studies; only information about the number of participants; • 168 participants, from included studies, received nitrates in the form of beetroot juice and 9 in the form of beetroot gel;	A meta-analysis concluded that beetroot juice is more effective than other nitrate sources, particularly for exercise lasting 2–10 min.

Table 5. *Cont.*

	Review Articles		
	Study	**Included Articles**	**Conclusions**
27	Tan R. et al. [125]	• 6 studies on cyclists performing sprints; • Examining: average power, peak power, time to peak power and minimum power during 30-s sprints;	Supplementation positively influenced time to peak power during short sprints, but had no effect on average or peak power. Findings are promising but limited, requiring further research.
28	Tan R. et al. [126]	• 6 studies about nitrate-rich beetroot juice supplementation; • the model and methods of supplementation in these studies were different, as were the methods of testing performance; • studies were not standardized;	Supplementation improved repetitions to failure, average power, and velocity in resistance exercise. However, study heterogeneity limits the strength of conclusions.
29	Tan R. et al. [127]	• 18 studies—in 17 of them, the chosen form of supplement was beetroot juice; • Training levels, age, methods of supplementation, tested parameters and sports disciplines, as well as the testing methods differed between the studies;	Positive effects were observed in squat, knee strength, and bench press velocity, but further standardized studies are needed to confirm findings.
30	Tanabe Y. et al. [128]	• 8 studies on beetroot juice supplementation; • Different physical activities across the studies (including the disciplines and level of advancement) • The study and supplementation protocols varied;	Some studies reported improvements in creatine kinase and faster recovery in strength and VO_2, but no reductions in blood markers of muscle damage.
31	Vicente-Salar N. et al. [129]	• 6 studies on supplementing nitrates from beetroot in the form of juice, extract, or gel; • The volunteers varied in terms of their sport, skill level, and age; • The supplementation regimen and the parameters examined were also not identical in each study;	In combat sports, several studies found improved physical performance and reduced soreness, though no effects were seen on inflammation markers (only one study demonstrated a significant difference in creatine kinase levels). A supplement such as beetroot juice needs further research to strengthen the evidence of its positive effect in improving performance in combat sports and other disciplines.
32	Vicente-Salar N. et al. [130]	• 21 studies; only one study involved beetroot juice supplementation.	In elite tennis players, supplementation did not improve explosive movements or perceptual effort. Further research is needed to assess strength-related outcomes.

Table 5. *Cont.*

	Review Articles		
	Study	**Included Articles**	**Conclusions**
33	Wong T.H. et al. [131]	• 17 studies on supplementing nitrates in the form of beetroot; • age, training level, method of supplementation and tested parameters differed between the studies;	Evidence was mixed: some studies showed improvements in power and performance whereas others showed no change or declines. Supplementation may help alleviate muscle soreness, but variability remains high.
34	Wong T.H. et al. [132]	• 24 studies—20 of them were about supplementing nitrogen coming from beets; • studies differed in terms of protocol and method of supplementation, age and training levels of participants and practiced disciplines.	Time trial performance improved in cycling trials (4–5 km), with slightly faster completion after beetroot versus placebo.
35	Zamani H. et al. [133]	• The impact of a single dose and the length of supplementation was assessed for men and women with different fitness levels.	A single dose improved blood flow, sprint and interval performance, time to exhaustion, and post-exercise recovery, particularly in less trained athletes.
36	Zoughaib W.S. et al. [134]	• 5 studies on nitrates derived from salt or beetroot juice; • The study groups were of different ages and fitness level; • 4 of the included studies involved healthy individuals;	Beetroot improved distance, power, and work done, and may be more effective than nitrate salts, though study numbers are small.

4. Discussion

Beetroot (*Beta vulgaris rubra*) has been a part of the human diet for centuries, originally valued for its pigments, fiber, vitamins, and minerals [135]. More recently, however, attention has shifted toward its high dietary nitrate (NO_3^-)content. Although the biological effects of nitrates have been recognized since antiquity—early records describe the use of potassium nitrate (KNO_3) in ancient China to treat heart problems [136]—beetroot has only begun to be systematically examined as a natural source of nitrate in the past two decades, particularly after discoveries that dietary nitrate could lower blood pressure and improve vascular function in humans. Modern research began around 2007, when controlled trials showed that nitrate supplementation reduced the oxygen cost of submaximal exercise [137]. This has sparked widespread interest in beetroot as both a cardiovascular and performance-enhancing nutritional aid.

This systematic review examined studies published between 2020 and 2025 on beetroot supplementation and its effect on physical activity and cognitive functions.

In the late 1980s, researchers discovered that blood vessels release a substance called endothelium-derived relaxing factor (EDRF), which turned out to be nitric oxide (NO). They demonstrated that NO is made from an amino acid called L-arginine, and that drugs, such as nitroglycerin, exert their effects by releasing this "newly" identified molecule. This finding changed the view of nitrates and nitrites—from being seen only as chemicals or pollutants to being seen as important natural molecules that help regulate blood flow and vascular function [138].

For many years, dietary nitrate (NO_3^-) and nitrite (NO_2^-) were believed to play no significant physiological role in the body and were mainly associated with potential toxicity. It is now clear that both can act as alternative sources of nitric oxide (NO), especially when oxygen levels are low [139]. The physiological effects ofnitrates begin with the so called "enterosalivary mechanism". Nitrates (NO_3^-) consumed with food are absorbed in the intestines and then secreted to saliva, where they are reduced to nitrite (NO_2^-). The final step is the conversion of nitrite to nitric oxide (NO), which occurs under conditions of hypoxia and low pH found in working muscles. This phenomenon is often observed during intense physical exercise [140,141].

The most important effect of nitric oxide, in terms of physical exercise, is the activation of guanylate cyclase in vascular muscles, which leads to an increase in cGMP concentration and, consequently, vasodilation. This increases the blood flow to the muscles, which allows a more efficient delivery of oxygen and energy substrates, and faster removal of exercise-related metabolites [142]. Another important mechanism involves the effects of NO and its derivatives on mitochondrial function. Research shows that nitrates increase the efficiency of oxidative phosphorylation and improve the ATP-to-oxygen ratio. This results in a lower oxygen cost, observed as a decrease in oxygen consumption under the same mechanical load [143].

Researchers have also shown that NO influences the muscle contractile apparatus. Its effect on calcium channels and proteins regulating Ca^{2+} release in the sarcoplasmic reticulum promotes more efficient energy utilization during contraction. Studies suggest that this effect is most pronounced in fast-twitch muscles, documenting improved performance during very high-intensity exercise with a predominance of anaerobic metabolism [144].

The effects of beetroot-derived nitrates on cognitive function remain unclear. Unlike in physical performance, where moderate doses show consistent benefits, there is no consensus regarding the nitrate dose or concentration most effective for improving executive function, attention, or memory. Further research using standardized cognitive tests is needed to determine whether moderate or prolonged supplementation can enhance brain function. Given the limited number of trials, systematic investigations are crucial to clarify how nitrates from beetroot juice affect cognition and to establish effective dosing strategies.

In recent years, inorganic (dietary) nitrates have been increasingly recognized as potential ergogenic agents due to their role in enhancing nitric oxide's bioavailability. NO is a signaling molecule that relaxes blood vessels, allowing better blood flow and oxygen delivery to working muscles and reduces pulmonary vascular resistance, improving ventilation, perfusion and oxygen uptake. It also improves mitochondrial efficiency and reduces the oxygen cost of exercise, supporting endurance and recovery [18,143]. The multidirectional mechanisms of the physiological effects of nitrates on the human body discussed above suggest that they may result in an increased physical performance. Such effects have been observed in studies indicating a positive impact of beetroot supplementation on physical performance (Tables 2 and 3).

Dietary nitrates in the most part (around 80% of dietary nitrate) come from vegetables. Vegetables with the greatest nitrate content (>1000 mg/kg) include are arugula, spinach, beetroot, lettuce, and celery. Nitrate levels are typically greater in leaves than in stems or roots. Vegetables with medium nitrate levels (100–1000 mg/kg) include cabbage, turnip, and green beans, while those with low levels (<100 mg/kg) include onions and tomatoes [137]. In the studies included in this paper, beetroot juice (BRJ) was the most commonly used form of nitrate supplementation. This vegetable has more practical advantages over other mentioned leafy greens, such as: it is easier to consume in effective amounts, is supported by a stronger research and provides other bioactive compounds (e.g., betalains, polyphenols). This supplement contains high concentrations of inorganic nitrates, and its liquid form facilitates precise dose determination and manipulation under controlled conditions [14,21]. An additional advantage of using juice supplementation is the possibility of concentrating it, which allows for the preparation of smaller, more convenient portions. The combination of elements such as rapid absorption, predictable pharmacokinetics, and extensive experimental control makes beetroot juice preferred in studies over powders, gels, or capsules.

Despite the large number of studies on this topic, findings on beetroot supplementation remain inconsistent. Several trials reported positive outcomes, such as improved muscular power and endurance time, reduced fatigue, better recovery, and in some cases enhanced VO_2max or cardiovascular efficiency. The results of this re- view also show that there are studies on the basis of which it cannot be stated that supplementation with beetroot juice has a positive effect on the increasing body performance (Table 4). Ambiguous research outcomes may result, for instance, from different supplementation durations or varying experimental conditions. Mixed findings have also been reported for other nitrate-rich foods that may influence physical performance. Vegetables such as spinach, arugula, swiss chard and amaranth, have also been examined, though to a much smaller extent. Consistent with the findings from this review, one systematic review reported that, in randomized trials, red spinach extract improved several performance parameters, such as time, average power, relative power and average speed [145]. One study also tried to assess the effect of red spinach extract on cognitive functions, after a 7-day supplementation period. However, compared to placebo, the results were similar to studies included in this review, meaning red spinach extract supplementation had no significant effect on cognitive performance, nor subjective feelings of focus, energy, and fatigue [146].

Researchers have not only been investigating vegetables (also mentioned in this review), but also herbs have been given a closer look. One of the compounds with positive effects on exercise performance is caffeine. This plant-derived alkaloid has been proven to have positive ergogenic and cognitive effects. A study by Kovacs et al. showed that enhancement of endurance and anaerobic performance, similar to beetroot, can be achieved with doses between 2–9 mg/kg ~1 h pre-exercise [147]. Alongside positively affecting strength and endurance, based on reviewed articles, beetroot can lower blood pressure. Lowering blood pressure is also one of the effects that a plant called *Tribulus Terrestris* has on the human body [148]. However, this plant and beetroot share another similarity. Both have mixed results when it comes to such as: maximal strength or muscular endurance in resistance-trained men [149]. While nitrate appears to have ergogenic benefits, beetroot may show additional effects due to containing compounds such as betalains and polyphenols.

The present review identified only one study that examined the effects of nitrates on both physical performance and cognitive function [41]. As was previously revealed, these two elements are not only interconnected but also highly interdependent. Previous studies suggest that nitrates may affect both cognitive function and physical performance. Therefore, further studies should be conducted to examine the effects of nitrates on both parameters, so that clear conclusions can be drawn from a larger sample size and a variety of supplementation regimens, allowing creating optimal supplementation protocols.

Another limitation in drawing concrete conclusions and presenting the most favorable conditions for supplementation—its duration, administration schedule, and form—is the significant heterogeneity of the studies included in the review, with these parameters differing significantly. The studies often included individuals of varying ages, with significantly varying levels of training, and those practicing various sports. The studies lacked protocol consistency [106,108,110]. This problem, however, turns out to be quite common, as similar conclusions regarding the significant heterogeneity of studies documenting the effect of supplementation on physical performance were observed [150,151].

The above conclusions suggest that such research is necessary, as identifying the weaknesses of existing studies may support the development of more consistent future investigations which may lead to the discovery of new, interesting evidence on the benefits of supplementation to improve physical efficacy.

5. Summary and Conclusions

This literature review attempted to analyze existing evidence of the effects of nitrates, mostly derived from beetroot, on physical activity and cognitive functions and their influence on healthy aging. Evaluating physical activity and cognitive function in young to middle-aged adults is crucial, as this period represents the peak of physiological and cognitive performance as well as reproductive health and productivity. Sustaining regular physical activity during adulthood supports cardiovascular and metabolic health alongside musculoskeletal strength—key determinants of long-term health and disease prevention. What is more, preserving cognitive function enhances decision-making, and mental health, reducing the risk of neurodegenerative diseases later in life. Monitoring these factors promotes healthy aging and contributes to extending life expectancy. Research shows consistent improvements in cardiovascular health, endurance, and resistance exercise, especially in less trained individuals, usually supplementing beetroot juice in moderate doses of 6–12 mmol. However, findings in elite athletes remain inconsistent. Overall, beetroot supplementation shows strong potential as a natural ergogenic aid for physical performance. Evidence regarding cognitive improvement is still limited and inconclusive, proving the need for creating standardized protocols, larger trials, and detailed dose–response investigations. This gap in knowledge creates an opportunity for future researchers to examine the relationship between beetroot-derived nitrates and cognitive functions.

Supplementary Materials: The following supporting information can be downloaded at: https://www.mdpi.com/article/10.3390/nu17243954/s1, Table S1: PRISMA checklist.

Author Contributions: Conceptualization, A.N. and A.L.; methodology, A.N. and A.L.; software, A.N. and A.S.; validation, E.K., A.L. and M.K.; formal analysis, A.N. and A.S.; investigation, A.N. and A.S.; resources, A.N. and A.S.; data curation, A.N. and A.S.; writing—original draft preparation, A.N. and A.S.; writing—review and editing, E.K. and A.L.; visualization, A.N. and A.S.; supervision, A.L. and M.K.; project administration, A.L.; funding acquisition, M.K. and E.K. All authors have read and agreed to the published version of the manuscript.

Funding: This research received no external funding.

Institutional Review Board Statement: Not applicable.

Informed Consent Statement: Not applicable.

Data Availability Statement: Data sharing is not applicable (only appropriate if no new data is generated or the article describes entirely theoretical research).

Acknowledgments: The authors have reviewed and edited the output and take full responsibility for the content of this publication.

Conflicts of Interest: The authors declare no conflicts of interest.

References

1. Stein, L.Y.; Klotz, M.G. The Nitrogen Cycle. *Curr. Biol.* **2016**, *26*, R94–R98. [CrossRef] [PubMed]
2. Lundberg, J.O.; Weitzberg, E. Biology of Nitrogen Oxides in the Gastrointestinal Tract. *Gut* **2013**, *62*, 616–629. [CrossRef] [PubMed]
3. Apte, M.; Nadavade, N.; Sheikh, S.S. A Review on Nitrates' Health Benefits and Disease Prevention. *Nitric Oxide* **2024**, *142*, 1–15. [CrossRef] [PubMed]
4. Lundberg, J.O.; Weitzberg, E.; Gladwin, M.T. The Nitrate-Nitrite-Nitric Oxide Pathway in Physiology and Therapeutics. *Nat. Rev. Drug Discov.* **2008**, *7*, 156–167. [CrossRef]
5. Ma, L.; Hu, L.; Feng, X.; Wang, S. Nitrate and Nitrite in Health and Disease. *Aging Dis.* **2018**, *9*, 938. [CrossRef]
6. Chou, S.-S.; Chung, J.-C.; Hwang, D.-F.; Chou, S.-S.; Chung, J.-C.; Hwang, D.-F. A High Performance Liquid Chromatography Method for Determining Nitrate and Nitrite Levels in Vegetables. *Available J. Food Drug Anal.* **2003**, *11*, 11. [CrossRef]
7. Rossi, I.; Mignogna, C.; Del Rio, D.; Mena, P. Health Effects of 100% Fruit and Vegetable Juices: Evidence from Human Subject Intervention Studies. *Nutr. Res. Rev.* **2024**, *37*, 194–238. [CrossRef]
8. WHO. *Nitrate and Nitrite in Drinking-Water Background Document for Development of WHO Guidelines for Drinking-Water Quality*; WHO: Geneva, Switzerland, 2003.
9. EFSA. *Confirms Safe Levels for Nitrites and Nitrates Added to Food*; EFSA: Parma, Italy, 2025. Available online: https://www.efsa.europa.eu/en/press/news/170615 (accessed on 31 August 2025).
10. Regulation–EU–2023/2108–EN–EUR-Lex. Available online: https://eur-lex.europa.eu/eli/reg/2023/2108/oj/eng (accessed on 31 August 2025).
11. Bryan, N.S.; van Grinsven, H. The Role of Nitrate in Human Health. *Adv. Agron.* **2013**, *119*, 153–182. [CrossRef]
12. Salehzadeh, H.; Maleki, A.; Rezaee, R.; Shahmoradi, B.; Ponnet, K. The Nitrate Content of Fresh and Cooked Vegetables and Their Health-Related Risks. *PLoS ONE* **2020**, *15*, e0227551. [CrossRef]
13. Moreno, B.C.; Soto, K.O.; González, D.R.; Gonzalez Reinoso, D. El Consumo de Nitrato y Su Potencial Efecto Benéfi Co Sobre La Salud Cardiovascular Nitrate Consumption and Potential Benefi Cial Effect on Cardiovascular Health. *Rev. Chil. Nutr.* **2015**, *42*, 199–205. [CrossRef]
14. Gallardo, E.J.; Coggan, A.R. What Is in Your Beet Juice? Nitrate and Nitrite Content of Beet Juice Products Marketed to Athletes. *Int. J. Sport Nutr. Exerc. Metab.* **2019**, *29*, 345–349. [CrossRef] [PubMed]
15. Bescos, R.; Rollason, M.L.; Davies, T.S.; Casas-Agustench, P. Content of Nitrate and Nitrite in Commercial and Self-made Beetroot Juices and the Effect of Storage Temperature. *Food Sci. Nutr.* **2023**, *11*, 6376. [CrossRef] [PubMed]
16. Wylie, L.J.; Kelly, J.; Bailey, S.J.; Blackwell, J.R.; Skiba, P.F.; Winyard, P.G.; Jeukendrup, A.E.; Vanhatalo, A.; Jones, A.M. Beetroot Juice and Exercise: Pharmacodynamic and Dose-Response Relationships. *J. Appl. Physiol.* **2013**, *115*, 325–336. [CrossRef] [PubMed]
17. Dietary Nitrate/Beetroot Juice | Australian Sports Commission. Available online: https://www.ausport.gov.au/ais/nutrition/supplements/group_a/performance-supplements2/beetroot-juicenitrate (accessed on 2 September 2025).
18. Senefeld, J.W.; Wiggins, C.C.; Regimbal, R.J.; Dominelli, P.B.; Baker, S.E.; Joyner, M.J. Ergogenic Effect of Nitrate Supplementation: A Systematic Review and Meta-Analysis. *Med. Sci. Sports Exerc.* **2020**, *52*, 2250. [CrossRef]
19. Siervo, M.; Babateen, A.; Alharbi, M.; Stephan, B.; Shannon, O. Dietary Nitrate and Brain Health. Too Much Ado about Nothing or a Solution for Dementia Prevention? *Br. J. Nutr.* **2022**, *128*, 1130–1136. [CrossRef]
20. Gareau, M.G. Cognitive Function and the Microbiome. *Int. Rev. Neurobiol.* **2016**, *131*, 227–246. [CrossRef]

21. Jones, A.M.; Thompson, C.; Wylie, L.J.; Vanhatalo, A. Dietary Nitrate and Physical Performance. *Annu. Rev. Nutr.* **2018**, *38*, 303–328. [CrossRef]
22. Peth-Nui, T.; Wattanathorn, J.; Muchimapura, S.; Tong-Un, T.; Piyavhatkul, N.; Rangseekajee, P.; Ingkaninan, K.; Vittaya-Areekul, S. Effects of 12-Week Bacopa Monnieri Consumption on Attention, Cognitive Processing, Working Memory, and Functions of Both Cholinergic and Monoaminergic Systems in Healthy Elderly Volunteers. *Evid. Based Complement. Altern. Med.* **2012**, *2012*, 606424. [CrossRef]
23. Lee, B.C.; Choe, Y.M.; Suh, G.H.; Choi, I.G.; Kim, H.S.; Hwang, J.; Yi, D.; Jhoo, J.H.; Kim, J.W. Ginseng Intake and Alzheimer Disease-Specific Cognition in Older Adults According to Apolipoprotein E4 Allele Status. *Front. Aging Neurosci.* **2023**, *15*, 1152626. [CrossRef]
24. Stojcheva, E.I.; Quintela, J.C. The Effectiveness of Rhodiola Rosea L. Preparations in Alleviating Various Aspects of Life-Stress Symptoms and Stress-Induced Conditions—Encouraging Clinical Evidence. *Molecules* **2022**, *27*, 3902. [CrossRef]
25. Gopukumar, K.; Thanawala, S.; Somepalli, V.; Rao, T.S.S.; Thamatam, V.B.; Chauhan, S. Efficacy and Safety of Ashwagandha Root Extract on Cognitive Functions in Healthy, Stressed Adults: A Randomized, Double-Blind, Placebo-Controlled Study. *Evid. Based Complement. Altern. Med.* **2021**, *2021*, 8254344. [CrossRef]
26. Heiland, E.G.; Lindh, F.; Regan, C.; Ekblom, Ö.; Kjellenberg, K.; Larsen, F.J.; Fernström, M.; Nyberg, G.; Ekblom, M.M.; Helgadóttir, B. A Randomised Crossover Trial of Nitrate and Breakfast on Prefrontal Cognitive and Haemodynamic Response Functions. *npj Sci. Food* **2024**, *8*, 64. [CrossRef] [PubMed]
27. Gilchrist, M.; Winyard, P.G.; Fulford, J.; Anning, C.; Shore, A.C.; Benjamin, N. Dietary Nitrate Supplementation Improves Reaction Time in Type 2 Diabetes: Development and Application of a Novel Nitrate-Depleted Beetroot Juice Placebo. *Nitric Oxide* **2014**, *40*, 67–74. [CrossRef] [PubMed]
28. Vaccaro, M.G.; Innocenti, B.; Cione, E.; Gallelli, L.; De Sarro, G.; Bonilla, D.A.; Cannataro, R. Acute Effects of a Chewable Beetroot-Based Supplement on Cognitive Performance: A Double-Blind Randomized Placebo-Controlled Crossover Clinical Trial. *Eur. J. Nutr.* **2024**, *63*, 303–321. [CrossRef] [PubMed]
29. Singh, B.; Bennett, H.; Miatke, A.; Dumuid, D.; Curtis, R.; Ferguson, T.; Brinsley, J.; Szeto, K.; Petersen, J.M.; Gough, C.; et al. Effectiveness of Exercise for Improving Cognition, Memory and Executive Function: A Systematic Umbrella Review and Meta-Meta-Analysis. *Br. J. Sports Med.* **2025**, *59*, e108589. [CrossRef]
30. Trecroci, A.; Duca, M.; Cavaggioni, L.; Rossi, A.; Scurati, R.; Longo, S.; Merati, G.; Alberti, G.; Formenti, D. Relationship between Cognitive Functions and Sport-Specific Physical Performance in Youth Volleyball Players. *Brain Sci.* **2021**, *11*, 227. [CrossRef]
31. Brooks-Wilson, A.R. Genetics of Healthy Aging and Longevity. *Hum. Genet.* **2013**, *132*, 1323. [CrossRef]
32. Huang, X.; Zhang, Z.; Wang, X.; Wang, G.; Wang, Y.; Tang, K.; Gao, B. Influence of Chronic Nitrate-Rich Beetroot Juice Supplementation on the Endurance Performance of Active Winter Triathletes: A Randomized Controlled Trial. *J. Am. Nutr. Assoc.* **2023**, *42*, 195–206. [CrossRef]
33. Tirkey, D.; Anant, S.K.; Venugopal, R. Effect of Beetroot Supplementation on 10 Km Time Trial Performance of Distance Runners. *Res. J. Pharm. Technol.* **2021**, *14*, 6423–6429. [CrossRef]
34. Rodríguez-Fernández, A.; Castillo, D.; Raya-González, J.; Domínguez, R.; Bailey, S.J. Beetroot Juice Supplementation Increases Concentric and Eccentric Muscle Power Output. Original Investigation. *J. Sci. Med. Sport* **2021**, *24*, 80–84. [CrossRef]
35. Jurado-Castro, J.M.; Campos-Perez, J.; Ranchal-Sanchez, A.; Durán-López, N.; Domínguez, R. Acute Effects of Beetroot Juice Supplements on Lower-Body Strength in Female Athletes: Double-Blind Crossover Randomized Trial. *Sports Health* **2022**, *14*, 812. [CrossRef]
36. Daab, W.; Bouzid, M.A.; Lajri, M.; Bouchiba, M.; Saafi, M.A.; Rebai, H. Chronic Beetroot Juice Supplementation Accelerates Recovery Kinetics Following Simulated Match Play in Soccer Players. *J. Am. Coll. Nutr.* **2021**, *40*, 61–69. [CrossRef] [PubMed]
37. Benjamim, C.J.R.; de Sousa Júnior, F.W.; Porto, A.A.; Andrade, C.V.G.; de Figueiredo, M.Í.L.S.; Benjamim, C.J.R.; da Silva Rodrigues, G.; Rocha, E.M.B.; Cavalcante, T.F.; Garner, D.M.; et al. Negligible Effects of Nutraceuticals from Beetroot Extract on Cardiovascular and Autonomic Recovery Response Following Submaximal Aerobic Exercise in Physically Active Healthy Males: A Randomized Trial. *Int. J. Environ. Res. Public Health* **2023**, *20*, 4019. [CrossRef] [PubMed]
38. Burke, L.M.; Hall, R.; Heikura, I.A.; Ross, M.L.; Tee, N.; Kent, G.L.; Whitfield, J.; Forbes, S.F.; Sharma, A.P.; Jones, A.M.; et al. Neither Beetroot Juice Supplementation nor Increased Carbohydrate Oxidation Enhance Economy of Prolonged Exercise in Elite Race Walkers. *Nutrients* **2021**, *13*, 2767. [CrossRef] [PubMed]
39. López-Samanes, Á.; Pérez-Lopez, A.; Morencos, E.; Muñoz, A.; Kühn, A.; Sánchez-Migallón, V.; Moreno-Pérez, V.; González-Frutos, P.; Bach-Faig, A.; Roberts, J.; et al. Beetroot Juice Ingestion Does Not Improve Neuromuscular Performance and Match-Play Demands in Elite Female Hockey Players: A Randomized, Double-Blind, Placebo-Controlled Study. *Eur. J. Nutr.* **2023**, *62*, 1123–1130. [CrossRef]
40. Trexler, E.T.; Keith, D.S.; Lucero, A.A.; Stoner, L.; Schwartz, T.A.; Persky, A.M.; Ryan, E.D.; Smith-Ryan, A.E. Effects of Citrulline Malate and Beetroot Juice Supplementation on Energy Metabolism and Blood Flow During Submaximal Resistance Exercise. *J. Diet. Suppl.* **2020**, *17*, 698–717. [CrossRef]

41. Miraftabi, H.; Avazpoor, Z.; Berjisian, E.; Sarshin, A.; Rezaei, S.; Domínguez, R.; Reale, R.; Franchini, E.; Samanipour, M.H.; Koozehchian, M.S.; et al. Effects of Beetroot Juice Supplementation on Cognitive Function, Aerobic and Anaerobic Performances of Trained Male Taekwondo Athletes: A Pilot Study. *Int. J. Environ. Res. Public Health* **2021**, *18*, 10202. [CrossRef]
42. Neteca, J.; Veseta, U.; Liepina, I.; Volgemute, K.; Dzintare, M.; Babarykin, D. Effect of Beetroot Juice Supplementation on Aerobic Capacity in Female Athletes: A Randomized Controlled Study. *Nutrients* **2024**, *17*, 63. [CrossRef]
43. Garnacho-Castaño, M.V.; Sánchez-Nuño, S.; Molina-Raya, L.; Carbonell, T.; Maté-Muñoz, J.L.; Pleguezuelos-Cobo, E.; Serra-Payá, N. Circulating Nitrate-Nitrite Reduces Oxygen Uptake for Improving Resistance Exercise Performance after Rest Time in Well-Trained CrossFit Athletes. *Sci. Rep.* **2022**, *12*, 9671. [CrossRef]
44. Tan, R.; Merrill, C.; Riley, C.F.; Hammer, M.A.; Kenney, R.T.; Riley, A.A.; Li, J.; Zink, A.C.; Karl, S.T.; Price, K.M.; et al. Acute Inorganic Nitrate Ingestion Does Not Impact Oral Microbial Composition, Cognitive Function, or High-Intensity Exercise Performance in Female Team-Sport Athletes. *Eur. J. Appl. Physiol.* **2024**, *124*, 3511–3525. [CrossRef]
45. Fernandez-Elias, V.; Courel-Ibanez, J.; Perez-Lopez, A.; Jodra, P.; Moreno-Perez, V.; Coso, J.D.; Lopez-Samanes, A. Acute Beetroot Juice Supplementation Does Not Improve Match-Play Activity in Professional Tennis Players. *J. Am. Nutr. Assoc.* **2022**, *41*, 30–37. [CrossRef] [PubMed]
46. Rokkedal-Lausch, T.; Franch, J.; Poulsen, M.K.; Thomsen, L.P.; Weitzberg, E.; Kamavuako, E.N.; Karbing, D.S.; Larsen, R.G. Multiple-Day High-Dose Beetroot Juice Supplementation Does Not Improve Pulmonary or Muscle Deoxygenation Kinetics of Well-Trained Cyclists in Normoxia and Hypoxia. *Nitric Oxide* **2021**, *111–112*, 37–44. [CrossRef] [PubMed]
47. Robinson, G.P.; Killer, S.C.; Stoyanov, Z.; Stephens, H.; Read, L.; James, L.J.; Bailey, S.J. Influence of Dietary Nitrate Supplementation on High-Intensity Intermittent Running Performance at Different Doses of Normobaric Hypoxia in Endurance-Trained Males. *Int. J. Sport Nutr. Exerc. Metab.* **2020**, *31*, 1–8. [CrossRef] [PubMed]
48. d'Unienville, N.M.A.; Blake, H.T.; Coates, A.M.; Hill, A.M.; Nelson, M.J.; Buckley, J.D. Effect of Food Sources of Nitrate, Polyphenols, L-Arginine and L-Citrulline on Endurance Exercise Performance: A Systematic Review and Meta-Analysis of Randomised Controlled Trials. *J. Int. Soc. Sports Nutr.* **2021**, *18*, 76. [CrossRef]
49. Williams, T.D.; Martin, M.P.; Mintz, J.A.; Rogers, R.R.; Ballmann, C.G. Effect of Acute Beetroot Juice Supplementation on Bench Press Power, Velocity, and Repetition Volume. *J. Strength. Cond. Res.* **2020**, *34*, 924–928. [CrossRef]
50. Wei, C.; Vanhatalo, A.; Black, M.I.; Rajaram, R.; Massey, G.; Jones, A.M. Dose-Response Relationship between Dietary Nitrate Intake and Nitric Oxide Congeners in Various Blood Compartments and Skeletal Muscle: Differential Effects on Skeletal Muscle Torque and Velocity. *Free Radic. Biol. Med.* **2025**, *229*, 520–533. [CrossRef]
51. Khosravi, S.; Ahmadizad, S.; Yekaninejad, M.S.; Karami, M.R.; Djafarian, K. The Effect of Beetroot Juice Supplementation on Muscle Performance during Isokinetic Knee Extensions in Male Taekwondo Athletes. *Sci. Sports* **2021**, *36*, 483.e1–483.e7. [CrossRef]
52. Jiaqi, Z.; Zihan, D.; Wong, S.H.-S.; Chen, Z.; Poon, E.T.-C. Acute Effects of Various Doses of Nitrate-Rich Beetroot Juice on High-Intensity Interval Exercise Responses in Women: A Randomized, Double-Blinded, Placebo-Controlled, Crossover Trial. *J. Int. Soc. Sports Nutr.* **2024**, *21*, 2334680. [CrossRef]
53. Ahmadpour, A.; Fashi, M.; Hemmatinafar, M. Consuming Beetroot Juice Improves Slalom Performance and Reduces Muscle Soreness in Alpine Skiers under Hypoxic Conditions. *Curr. Dev. Nutr.* **2024**, *8*, 104408. [CrossRef]
54. Black, M.I.; Wylie, L.J.; Kadach, S.; Piknova, B.; Park, J.W.; Stoyanov, Z.; L'Heureux, J.E.; Schechter, A.N.; Vanhatalo, A.; Jones, A.M. Effects of Low and High Dietary Nitrate Intake on Human Saliva, Plasma and Skeletal Muscle Nitrate and Nitrite Concentrations and Their Functional Consequences. *Free Radic. Biol. Med.* **2024**, *225*, 881–893. [CrossRef]
55. Bloomer, R.J.; Butawan, M.; Pigg, B.; Martin, K.R. Acute Ingestion of a Novel Nitrate-Rich Dietary Supplement Significantly Increases Plasma Nitrate/Nitrite in Physically Active Men and Women. *Nutrients* **2020**, *12*, 1176. [CrossRef] [PubMed]
56. Cocksedge, S.P.; Breese, B.C.; Morgan, P.T.; Nogueira, L.; Thompson, C.; Wylie, L.J.; Jones, A.M.; Bailey, S.J. Influence of Muscle Oxygenation and Nitrate-Rich Beetroot Juice Supplementation on O_2 Uptake Kinetics and Exercise Tolerance. *Nitric Oxide* **2020**, *99*, 25–33. [CrossRef]
57. DE SOUZA, D.B.; Ribeiro, J.N.; Simão, A.N.C.; Aguilar-Navarro, M.; Polito, M.D. The Acute Effect of In Natura Beetroot Juice Intake on Intra-Session Exercise Sequences During Concurrent Training. *Int. J. Exerc. Sci.* **2022**, *15*, 1075. [CrossRef] [PubMed]
58. Dumar, A.M.; Huntington, A.F.; Rogers, R.R.; Kopec, T.J.; Ballmann, C.G. Acute Beetroot Juice Supplementation Attenuates Morning-Associated Decrements in Supramaximal Exercise Performance in Trained Sprinters. *Int. J. Environ. Res. Public Health* **2021**, *18*, 412. [CrossRef] [PubMed]
59. Esen, O.; Domínguez, R.; Karayigit, R. Acute Beetroot Juice Supplementation Enhances Intermittent Running Performance but Does Not Reduce Oxygen Cost of Exercise among Recreational Adults. *Nutrients* **2022**, *14*, 2839. [CrossRef]
60. Forbes, S.P.A.; Spriet, L.L. Potential Effect of Beetroot Juice Supplementation on Exercise Economy in Well-Trained Females. *Appl. Physiol. Nutr. Metab.* **2022**, *47*, 106–109. [CrossRef]

61. Garnacho-Castaño, M.V.; Pleguezuelos-Cobo, E.; Berbel, M.; Irurtia, A.; Carrasco-Marginet, M.; Castizo-Olier, J.; Veiga-Herreros, P.; Faundez-Zanuy, M.; Serra-Payá, N. Effects of Acute Beetroot Juice Intake on Performance, Maximal Oxygen Uptake, and Ventilatory Efficiency in Well-Trained Master Rowers: A Randomized, Double-Blinded Crossover Study. *J. Int. Soc. Sports Nutr.* **2024**, *21*, 2373170. [CrossRef]
62. Garnacho-Castaño, M.V.; Palau-Salvà, G.; Serra-Payá, N.; Ruiz-Hermosel, M.; Berbell, M.; Viñals, X.; Bataller, M.G.; Carbonell, T.; Vilches-Saez, S.; Cobo, E.P.; et al. Understanding the Effects of Beetroot Juice Intake on CrossFit Performance by Assessing Hormonal, Metabolic and Mechanical Response: A Randomized, Double-Blind, Crossover Design. *J. Int. Soc. Sports Nutr.* **2020**, *17*, 56. [CrossRef]
63. Hemmatinafar, M.; Zaremoayedi, L.; Koushkie Jahromi, M.; Alvarez-Alvarado, S.; Wong, A.; Niknam, A.; Suzuki, K.; Imanian, B.; Bagheri, R. Effect of Beetroot Juice Supplementation on Muscle Soreness and Performance Recovery after Exercise-Induced Muscle Damage in Female Volleyball Players. *Nutrients* **2023**, *15*, 3763. [CrossRef]
64. Jurado-Castro, J.M.; Casanova-Rodriguez, D.; Campos-Perez, J.; Llorente-Cantarero, F.J.; De La Florida-Villagran, C.A.; Diaz-Bernier, V.M.; Ranchal-Sanchez, A. Beetroot Juice Produces Changes in Heart Rate Variability and Reduces Internal Load during Resistance Training in Men: A Randomized Double-Blind Crossover. *Nutrients* **2022**, *14*, 5119. [CrossRef]
65. Macuh, M.; Kojić, N.; Knap, B. The Effects of Nitrate Supplementation on Performance as a Function of Habitual Dietary Intake of Nitrates: A Randomized Controlled Trial of Elite Football Players. *Nutrients* **2023**, *15*, 3721. [CrossRef] [PubMed]
66. Ranchal-Sanchez, A.; Diaz-Bernier, V.M.; De La Florida-Villagran, C.A.; Llorente-Cantarero, F.J.; Campos-Perez, J.; Jurado-Castro, J.M. Acute Effects of Beetroot Juice Supplements on Resistance Training: A Randomized Double-Blind Crossover. *Nutrients* **2020**, *12*, 1912. [CrossRef] [PubMed]
67. Rowland, S.N.; James, L.J.; O'Donnell, E.; Bailey, S.J. Influence of Acute Dietary Nitrate Supplementation Timing on Nitrate Metabolism, Central and Peripheral Blood Pressure and Exercise Tolerance in Young Men. *Eur. J. Appl. Physiol.* **2023**, *124*, 1381. [CrossRef] [PubMed]
68. Serra-Payá, N.; Garnacho-Castaño, M.V.; Sánchez-Nuño, S.; Albesa-Albiol, L.; Girabent-Farrés, M.; Arcone, L.M.; Fernández, A.P.; García-Fresneda, A.; Castizo-Olier, J.; Viñals, X.; et al. The Relationship between Resistance Exercise Performance and Ventilatory Efficiency after Beetroot Juice Intake in Well-Trained Athletes. *Nutrients* **2021**, *13*, 1094. [CrossRef]
69. Tan, R.; Pennell, A.; Price, K.M.; Karl, S.T.; Seekamp-Hicks, N.G.; Paniagua, K.K.; Weiderman, G.D.; Powell, J.P.; Sharabidze, L.K.; Lincoln, I.G.; et al. Effects of Dietary Nitrate Supplementation on Performance and Muscle Oxygenation during Resistance Exercise in Men. *Nutrients* **2022**, *14*, 3703. [CrossRef]
70. Tatlici, A.; Lima, Y.; Yilmaz, S.; Ekin, A.; Okut, S.; Ceviz, E. The Effects of Beetroot Juice Supplementation on Balance Performance of Wrestlers. *Arch. Razi Inst.* **2021**, *15*, pjmhs211572234. [CrossRef]
71. Tatlici, A. The Effects of Acute Beetroot Juice Supplementation on Lower and Upper Body Isokinetic Strength of the Wrestlers. *J. Mens. Health* **2021**, *17*, 249–254. [CrossRef]
72. Thurston, T.S.; Weavil, J.C.; Hureau, T.J.; Gifford, J.R.; Georgescu, V.P.; Wan, H.Y.; la Salle, D.T.; Richardson, R.S.; Amann, M. On the Implication of Dietary Nitrate Supplementation for the Hemodynamic and Fatigue Response to Cycling Exercise. *J. Appl. Physiol.* **2021**, *131*, 1691–1700. [CrossRef]
73. Volino-Souza, M.; de Oliveira, G.V.; Barros-Santos, E.; Conte-Junior, C.A.; Alvares, T.S. The Impact of Beetroot Juice Intake on Muscle Oxygenation and Performance during Rhythmic Handgrip Exercise. *PharmaNutrition* **2020**, *14*, 100215. [CrossRef]
74. Wong, T.H.; Sim, R.; Sim, A.; Burns, S.F. Effects of an Isotonic Beetroot Drink on Power Output During Sprint Exercise and Jump Performance in Physically Active Individuals: A Randomized Crossover Trial. *J. Diet. Suppl.* **2024**, *21*, 808–824. [CrossRef]
75. Yuschen, X.; Choi, J.H.; Seo, J.; Sun, Y.; Lee, E.; Kim, S.W.; Park, H.Y. Effects of Acute Beetroot Juice Supplementation and Exercise on Cardiovascular Function in Healthy Men in Preliminary Study: A Randomized, Double-Blinded, Placebo-Controlled, and Crossover Trial. *Healthcare* **2024**, *12*, 1240. [CrossRef] [PubMed]
76. Burgos, J.; Viribay, A.; Calleja-gonzález, J.; Fernández-lázaro, D.; Olasagasti-ibargoien, J.; Seco-calvo, J.; Mielgo-ayuso, J. Long-Term Combined Effects of Citrulline and Nitrate-Rich Beetroot Extract Supplementation on Recovery Status in Trained Male Triathletes: A Randomized, Double-Blind, Placebo-Controlled Trial. *Biology* **2022**, *11*, 75. [CrossRef]
77. Burgos, J.; Viribay, A.; Fernández-Lázaro, D.; Calleja-González, J.; González-Santos, J.; Mielgo-Ayuso, J. Combined Effects of Citrulline Plus Nitrate-Rich Beetroot Extract Co-Supplementation on Maximal and Endurance-Strength and Aerobic Power in Trained Male Triathletes: A Randomized Double-Blind, Placebo-Controlled Trial. *Nutrients* **2021**, *14*, 40. [CrossRef] [PubMed]
78. De Oliveira, G.V.; Do Nascimento, L.A.D.; Volino-Souza, M.; Do Couto Vellozo, O.; Alvares, T.S. A Single Oral Dose of Beetroot-Based Gel Does Not Improve Muscle Oxygenation Parameters, but Speeds up Handgrip Isometric Strength Recovery in Recreational Combat Sports Athletes. *Biol. Sport* **2020**, *37*, 93. [CrossRef] [PubMed]
79. Esen, O.; Bailey, S.J.; Stashuk, D.W.; Howatson, G.; Goodall, S. Influence of Nitrate Supplementation on Motor Unit Activity during Recovery Following a Sustained Ischemic Contraction in Recreationally Active Young Males. *Eur. J. Nutr.* **2024**, *63*, 2379–2387. [CrossRef]

80. Esen, O.; Cepicka, L.; Gabrys, T.; Karayigit, R. High-Dose Nitrate Supplementation Attenuates the Increased Blood Pressure Responses to Isometric Blood Flow Restriction Exercise in Healthy Males. *Nutrients* **2022**, *14*, 3645. [CrossRef]
81. Esen, O.; Faisal, A.; Zambolin, F.; Bailey, S.J.; Callaghan, M.J. Effect of Nitrate Supplementation on Skeletal Muscle Motor Unit Activity during Isometric Blood Flow Restriction Exercise. *Eur. J. Appl. Physiol.* **2022**, *122*, 1683. [CrossRef]
82. Kozłowska, L.; Mizera, O.; Gromadzińska, J.; Janasik, B.; Mikołajewska, K.; Mróz, A.; Wąsowicz, W. Changes in Oxidative Stress, Inflammation, and Muscle Damage Markers Following Diet and Beetroot Juice Supplementation in Elite Fencers. *Antioxidants* **2020**, *9*, 571. [CrossRef]
83. Liubertas, T.; Kairaitis, R.; Stasiule, L.; Capkauskiene, S.; Stasiulis, A.; Viskelis, P.; Viškelis, J.; Urbonaviciene, D. The Influence of Amaranth (*Amaranthus Hypochondriacus*) Dietary Nitrates on the Aerobic Capacity of Physically Active Young Persons. *J. Int. Soc. Sports Nutr.* **2020**, *17*, 37. [CrossRef]
84. Bordonie, N.C.; Saunders, M.J.; de Zevallos, J.O.; Kurti, S.P.; Luden, N.D.; Crance, J.H.; Baur, D.A. Dietary Nitrate Supplementation Enhances Heavy Load Carriage Performance in Military Cadets. *Eur. J. Appl. Physiol.* **2023**, *123*, 91–102. [CrossRef]
85. Rowland, S.N.; Da Boit, M.; Tan, R.; Robinson, G.P.; O'Donnell, E.; James, L.J.; Bailey, S.J. Dietary Nitrate Supplementation Enhances Performance and Speeds Muscle Deoxyhaemoglobin Kinetics during an End-Sprint after Prolonged Moderate-Intensity Exercise. *Antioxidants* **2022**, *12*, 25. [CrossRef] [PubMed]
86. Tan, R.; Wylie, L.J.; Wilkerson, D.P.; Vanhatalo, A.; Jones, A.M. Effects of Dietary Nitrate on the O_2 Cost of Submaximal Exercise: Accounting for "Noise" in Pulmonary Gas Exchange Measurements. *J. Sports Sci.* **2022**, *40*, 1149–1157. [CrossRef] [PubMed]
87. Viribay, A.; Alcantara, J.M.A.; López, I.; Mielgo-Ayuso, J.; Castañeda-Babarro, A. Impact of a Short-Term Nitrate and Citrulline Co-Supplementation on Sport Performance in Elite Rowers: A Randomized, Double-Blind, Placebo-Controlled Crossover Trial. *Eur. J. Appl. Physiol.* **2024**, *124*, 1911. [CrossRef]
88. Berjisian, E.; McGawley, K.; Saunders, B.; Domínguez, R.; Koozehchian, M.S.; de Oliveira, C.V.C.; Rafiei, R.; Miraftabi, H.; Sarshin, A.; Naderi, A. Acute Effects of Beetroot Juice and Caffeine Co-Ingestion during a Team-Sport-Specific Intermittent Exercise Test in Semi-Professional Soccer Players: A Randomized, Double-Blind, Placebo-Controlled Study. *BMC Sports Sci. Med. Rehabil.* **2022**, *14*, 52. [CrossRef] [PubMed]
89. Berlanga, L.A.; Lopez-Samanes, A.; Martin-Lopez, J.; de la Cruz, R.M.; Garces-Rimon, M.; Roberts, J.; Bertotti, G. Dietary Nitrate Ingestion Does Not Improve Neuromuscular Performance in Male Sport Climbers. *J. Hum. Kinet.* **2023**, *87*, 47. [CrossRef]
90. Collins, S.M.; Kearns, D. The Effect of Beetroot Supplementation on High-Intensity Functional Training Performance. *Int. J. Exerc. Sci.* **2020**, *13*, 667. [CrossRef]
91. Conger, S.A.; Zamzow, C.M.; Darnell, M.E. Acute Beet Juice Supplementation Does Not Improve 30- or 60-Second Maximal Intensity Performance in Anaerobically Trained Athletes. *Int. J. Exerc. Sci.* **2021**, *14*, 60. [CrossRef]
92. Esen, O.; Karayigit, R.; Peart, D.J. Acute Beetroot Juice Supplementation Did Not Enhance Intermittent Running Performance in Trained Rugby Players. *Eur. J. Sport. Sci.* **2023**, *23*, 2321–2328. [CrossRef]
93. Hennis, P.J.; Cumpstey, A.F.; O'Doherty, A.F.; Fernandez, B.O.; Gilbert-Kawai, E.T.; Mitchell, K.; Moyses, H.; Cobb, A.; Meale, P.; Pöhnl, H.; et al. Dietary Nitrate Supplementation Does Not Alter Exercise Efficiency at High Altitude–Further Results From the Xtreme Alps Study. *Front. Physiol.* **2022**, *13*, 827235. [CrossRef]
94. López-Samanes, Á.; Pérez-López, A.; Moreno-Pérez, V.; Nakamura, F.Y.; Acebes-Sánchez, J.; Quintana-Milla, I.; Sánchez-Oliver, A.J.; Moreno-Pérez, D.; Fernández-Elías, V.E.; Domínguez, R. Effects of Beetroot Juice Ingestion on Physical Performance in Highly Competitive Tennis Players. *Nutrients* **2020**, *12*, 584. [CrossRef]
95. Moreno, B.; Morencos, E.; Vicente-Campos, D.; Muñoz, A.; González-García, J.; Veiga, S. Effects of Beetroot Juice Intake on Repeated Performance of Competitive Swimmers. *Front. Physiol.* **2023**, *13*, 1076295. [CrossRef]
96. de Zevallos, J.O.; Hogwood, A.C.; Kruse, K.; De Guzman, J.; Buckley, M.; Weltman, A.L.; Allen, J.D. Sex Differences in the Effects of Inorganic Nitrate Supplementation on Exercise Economy and Endurance Capacity in Healthy Young Adults. *J. Appl. Physiol.* **2023**, *135*, 1157–1166. [CrossRef] [PubMed]
97. Sousa, A.; Viana, J.L.; Milheiro, J.; Reis, V.M.; Millet, G.P. Dietary Nitrate Supplementation Is Not Helpful for Endurance Performance at Simulated Altitude Even When Combined With Intermittent Normobaric Hypoxic Training. *Front. Physiol.* **2022**, *13*, 839996. [CrossRef] [PubMed]
98. Tan, R.; Black, M.; Home, J.; Blackwell, J.; Clark, I.; Wylie, L.; Vanhatalo, A.; Jones, A.M. Physiological and Performance Effects of Dietary Nitrate and N-Acetylcysteine Supplementation during Prolonged Heavy-Intensity Cycling. *J. Sports Sci.* **2023**, *40*, 2585–2594. [CrossRef]
99. Tan, R.; Price, K.M.; Wideen, L.E.; Lincoln, I.G.; Karl, S.T.; Seals, J.P.; Paniagua, K.K.; Hagen, D.W.; Tchaprazian, I.; Bailey, S.J.; et al. Dietary Nitrate Ingested with and without Pomegranate Supplementation Does Not Improve Resistance Exercise Performance. *Front. Nutr.* **2023**, *10*, 1217192. [CrossRef] [PubMed]
100. Viribay, A.; Alcantara, J.M.A.; López, I.; Mielgo-Ayuso, J.; Castañeda-Babarro, A. No Evidence of Improvements in Energy Metabolism after 1 Week of Nitrate and Citrulline Co-Supplementation in Elite Rowers. *Eur. J. Appl. Physiol.* **2025**, *125*, 715–728. [CrossRef]

101. Abreu, R.; Oliveira, C.B.; Costa, J.A.; Brito, J.; Teixeira, V.H. Effects of Dietary Supplements on Athletic Performance in Elite Soccer Players: A Systematic Review. *J. Int. Soc. Sports Nutr.* **2023**, *20*, 2236060. [CrossRef]
102. Alsharif, N.S.; Clifford, T.; Alhebshi, A.; Rowland, S.N.; Bailey, S.J. Effects of Dietary Nitrate Supplementation on Performance during Single and Repeated Bouts of Short-Duration High-Intensity Exercise: A Systematic Review and Meta-Analysis of Randomised Controlled Trials. *Antioxidants* **2023**, *12*, 1194. [CrossRef]
103. Antonio, J.; Pereira, F.; Curtis, J.; Rojas, J.; Evans, C. The Top 5 Can't-Miss Sport Supplements. *Nutrients* **2024**, *16*, 3247. [CrossRef]
104. Calvo, J.L.; Alorda-Capo, F.; Pareja-Galeano, H.; Jiménez, S.L. Influence of Nitrate Supplementation on Endurance Cyclic Sports Performance: A Systematic Review. *Nutrients* **2020**, *12*, 1796. [CrossRef]
105. Chen, L.; Zhu, Y.; Hu, Z.; Wu, S.; Jin, C. Beetroot as a Functional Food with Huge Health Benefits: Antioxidant, Antitumor, Physical Function, and Chronic Metabolomics Activity. *Food Sci. Nutr.* **2021**, *9*, 6406–6420. [CrossRef] [PubMed]
106. Delleli, S.; Ouergui, I.; Messaoudi, H.; Trabelsi, K.; Glenn, J.M.; Ammar, A.; Chtourou, H. Does Beetroot Supplementation Improve Performance in Combat Sports Athletes? A Systematic Review of Randomized Controlled Trials. *Nutrients* **2023**, *15*, 398. [CrossRef] [PubMed]
107. Domínguez, R.; Oliver, A.J.S.; Da Silva, S.F.; López-Samanes, A.; Martínez-Sanz, J.M.; Mata, F. Dietary-Nutritional Needs in Tennis: A Narrative Review Necesidades Dietético-Nutricionales En El Tenis: Una Revisión Narrativa. *Rev. Esp. Nutr. Humana Diet.* **2021**, *25*, e1029. [CrossRef]
108. Esen, O.; Dobbin, N.; Callaghan, M.J. The Effect of Dietary Nitrate on the Contractile Properties of Human Skeletal Muscle: A Systematic Review and Meta-Analysis. *J. Am. Nutr. Assoc.* **2023**, *42*, 327–338. [CrossRef]
109. Gamonales, J.M.; Rojas-Valverde, D.; Muñoz-Jiménez, J.; Serrano-Moreno, W.; Ibáñez, S.J. Effectiveness of Nitrate Intake on Recovery from Exercise-Related Fatigue: A Systematic Review. *Int. J. Environ. Res. Public Health* **2022**, *19*, 12021. [CrossRef]
110. Gilsanz, L.; Del Coso, J.; Jiménez-Saiz, S.L.; Pareja-Galeano, H. Effect of Caffeine and Nitrates Combination on Exercise Performance, Heart Rate and Oxygen Uptake: A Systematic Review and Meta-Analysis. *Nutrients* **2024**, *16*, 3352. [CrossRef]
111. Harlow, J.; Blodgett, K.; Stedman, J.; Pojednic, R. Dietary Supplementation on Physical Performance and Recovery in Active-Duty Military Personnel: A Systematic Review of Randomized and Quasi-Experimental Controlled Trials. *Nutrients* **2024**, *16*, 2746. [CrossRef]
112. Hogwood, A.C.; Anderson, K.C.; Ortiz de Zevallos, J.; Paterson, C.; Weltman, A.; Allen, J.D. Limited Effects of Inorganic Nitrate Supplementation on Exercise Training Responses: A Systematic Review and Meta-Analysis. *Sports Med. Open* **2023**, *9*, 84. [CrossRef]
113. Jones, L.; Bailey, S.J.; Rowland, S.N.; Alsharif, N.; Shannon, O.M.; Clifford, T. The Effect of Nitrate-Rich Beetroot Juice on Markers of Exercise-Induced Muscle Damage: A Systematic Review and Meta-Analysis of Human Intervention Trials. *J. Diet. Suppl.* **2022**, *19*, 749–771. [CrossRef]
114. Kiani, A.K.; Bonetti, G.; Medori, M.C.; Caruso, P.; Manganotti, P.; Fioretti, F.; Nodari, S.; Connelly, S.T.; Bertelli, M. Dietary Supplements for Improving Nitric-Oxide Synthesis. *J. Prev. Med. Hyg.* **2022**, *63*, E239–E245. [CrossRef]
115. Kim, J.; Kim, E.K. Nutritional Strategies to Optimize Performance and Recovery in Rowing Athletes. *Nutrients* **2020**, *12*, 1685. [CrossRef] [PubMed]
116. Lago-Rodríguez, Á.; Domínguez, R.; Ramos-álvarez, J.J.; Tobal, F.M.; Jodra, P.; Tan, R.; Bailey, S.J. The Effect of Dietary Nitrate Supplementation on Isokinetic Torque in Adults: A Systematic Review and Meta-Analysis. *Nutrients* **2020**, *12*, 3022. [CrossRef] [PubMed]
117. López-Laval, I.; Mielgo-Ayuso, J.; Terrados, N.; Calleja-González, J. Evidence-Based Post Exercise Recovery in Combat Sports: A Narrative Review. *J. Sports Med. Phys. Fit.* **2021**, *61*, 386–400. [CrossRef] [PubMed]
118. López-Torres, O.; Rodríguez-Longobardo, C.; Capel-Escoriza, R.; Fernández-Elías, V.E. Ergogenic Aids to Improve Physical Performance in Female Athletes: A Systematic Review with Meta-Analysis. *Nutrients* **2022**, *15*, 81. [CrossRef]
119. Daud, S.M.M.; Sukri, N.M.; Johari, M.H.; Gnanou, J.; Manaf, F.A. Pure Juice Supplementation: Its Effect on Muscle Recovery and Sports Performance. *Malays. J. Med. Sci.* **2023**, *30*, 31–48. [CrossRef]
120. O'Connor, E.; Mündel, T.; Barnes, M.J. Nutritional Compounds to Improve Post-Exercise Recovery. *Nutrients* **2022**, *14*, 5069. [CrossRef]
121. Poulios, A.; Papanikolaou, K.; Draganidis, D.; Tsimeas, P.; Chatzinikolaou, A.; Tsiokanos, A.; Jamurtas, A.Z.; Fatouros, I.G. The Effects of Antioxidant Supplementation on Soccer Performance and Recovery: A Critical Review of the Available Evidence. *Nutrients* **2024**, *16*, 3803. [CrossRef]
122. Rojano-Ortega, D.; Peña Amaro, J.; Berral-Aguilar, A.J.; Berral-de la Rosa, F.J. Effects of Beetroot Supplementation on Recovery After Exercise-Induced Muscle Damage: A Systematic Review. *Sports Health* **2022**, *14*, 556–565. [CrossRef]
123. San Juan, A.F.; Dominguez, R.; Lago-Rodríguez, Á.; Montoya, J.J.; Tan, R.; Bailey, S.J. Effects of Dietary Nitrate Supplementation on Weightlifting Exercise Performance in Healthy Adults: A Systematic Review. *Nutrients* **2020**, *12*, 2227. [CrossRef]

124. Silva, K.V.C.; Costa, B.D.; Gomes, A.C.; Saunders, B.; Mota, J.F. Factors That Moderate the Effect of Nitrate Ingestion on Exercise Performance in Adults: A Systematic Review with Meta-Analyses and Meta-Regressions. *Adv. Nutr.* **2022**, *13*, 1866–1881. [CrossRef]
125. Tan, R.; Cass, J.K.; Lincoln, I.G.; Wideen, L.E.; Nicholl, M.J.; Molnar, T.J.; Gough, L.A.; Bailey, S.J.; Pennell, A. Effects of Dietary Nitrate Supplementation on High-Intensity Cycling Sprint Performance in Recreationally Active Adults: A Systematic Review and Meta-Analysis. *Nutrients* **2024**, *16*, 2764. [CrossRef] [PubMed]
126. Tan, R.; Pennell, A.; Karl, S.T.; Cass, J.K.; Go, K.; Clifford, T.; Bailey, S.J.; Perkins Storm, C. Effects of Dietary Nitrate Supplementation on Back Squat and Bench Press Performance: A Systematic Review and Meta-Analysis. *Nutrients* **2023**, *15*, 2493. [CrossRef] [PubMed]
127. Tan, R.; Cano, L.; Lago-Rodríguez, Á.; Domínguez, R. The Effects of Dietary Nitrate Supplementation on Explosive Exercise Performance: A Systematic Review. *Int. J. Environ. Res. Public Health* **2022**, *19*, 762. [CrossRef] [PubMed]
128. Tanabe, Y.; Fujii, N.; Suzuki, K. Dietary Supplementation for Attenuating Exercise-Induced Muscle Damage and Delayed-Onset Muscle Soreness in Humans. *Nutrients* **2021**, *14*, 70. [CrossRef]
129. Vicente-Salar, N.; Fuster-Muñoz, E.; Martínez-Rodríguez, A. Nutritional Ergogenic Aids in Combat Sports: A Systematic Review and Meta-Analysis. *Nutrients* **2022**, *14*, 2588. [CrossRef]
130. Vicente-Salar, N.; Santos-Sánchez, G.; Roche, E. Nutritional Ergogenic Aids in Racquet Sports: A Systematic Review. *Nutrients* **2020**, *12*, 2842. [CrossRef]
131. Wong, T.H.; Sim, A.; Burns, S.F. The Effect of Beetroot Ingestion on High-Intensity Interval Training: A Systematic Review and Meta-Analysis. *Nutrients* **2021**, *13*, 3674. [CrossRef]
132. Wong, T.H.; Sim, A.; Burns, S.F. The Effects of Nitrate Ingestion on High-Intensity Endurance Time-Trial Performance: A Systematic Review and Meta-Analysis. *J. Exerc. Sci. Fit.* **2022**, *20*, 305–316. [CrossRef]
133. Zamani, H.; de Joode, M.E.J.R.; Hossein, I.J.; Henckens, N.F.T.; Guggeis, M.A.; Berends, J.E.; de Kok, T.M.C.M.; van Breda, S.G.J. The Benefits and Risks of Beetroot Juice Consumption: A Systematic Review. *Crit. Rev. Food Sci. Nutr.* **2021**, *61*, 788–804. [CrossRef]
134. Zoughaib, W.S.; Fry, M.J.; Singhal, A.; Coggan, A.R. Beetroot Juice Supplementation and Exercise Performance: Is There More to the Story than Just Nitrate? *Front. Nutr.* **2024**, *11*, 1347242. [CrossRef]
135. Neelwarne, B.; Halagur, S.B. Red Beet: An Overview. *Red. Beet Biotechnol. Food Pharm. Appl.* **2013**, *11*, 1347242. [CrossRef]
136. Butler, A.; Moffett, J. Saltpetre in Early and Medieval Chinese Medicine. *Asian Med.* **2009**, *5*, 173–185. [CrossRef]
137. Larsen, F.J.; Weitzberg, E.; Lundberg, J.O.; Ekblom, B. Effects of Dietary Nitrate on Oxygen Cost during Exercise. *Acta Physiol.* **2007**, *191*, 59–66. [CrossRef] [PubMed]
138. Moncada, S.; Palmer, R.M.J.; Higgs, E.A. The Discovery of Nitric Oxide as the Endogenous Nitrovasodilator. *Hypertension* **1988**, *12*, 365–372. [CrossRef]
139. Lidder, S.; Webb, A.J. Vascular Effects of Dietary Nitrate (as Found in Green Leafy Vegetables and Beetroot) via the Nitrate-nitrite-nitric Oxide Pathway. *Br. J. Clin. Pharmacol.* **2013**, *75*, 677. [CrossRef]
140. Kapil, V.; Khambata, R.S.; Jones, D.A.; Rathod, K.; Primus, C.; Massimo, G.; Fukuto, J.M.; Ahluwalia, A. The Noncanonical Pathway for in Vivo Nitric Oxide Generation: The Nitrate-Nitrite-Nitric Oxide Pathway. *Pharmacol. Rev.* **2020**, *72*, 692–766. [CrossRef]
141. Jones, A.M. Dietary Nitrate Supplementation and Exercise Performance. *Sports Med.* **2014**, *44*, 35. [CrossRef]
142. Joyner, M.J.; Casey, D.P. Regulation of Increased Blood Flow (Hyperemia) to Muscles during Exercise: A Hierarchy of Competing Physiological Needs. *Physiol. Rev.* **2015**, *95*, 549–601. [CrossRef]
143. Larsen, F.J.; Schiffer, T.A.; Borniquel, S.; Sahlin, K.; rn Ekblom, B.; Lundberg, J.O.; Weitzberg, E. Dietary Inorganic Nitrate Improves Mitochondrial Efficiency in Humans. *Cell Metab.* **2011**, *13*, 149–159. [CrossRef]
144. Kumar, R.; Coggan, A.R.; Ferreira, L.F. Nitric Oxide and Skeletal Muscle Contractile Function. *Nitric Oxide* **2022**, *122–123*, 54–61. [CrossRef]
145. Wen, J.; Syed, B.; Abed, I.; Manguerra, D.; Shehabat, M.; Razick, D.I.; Nadora, D.; Nadora, D.; Akhtar, M.; Pai, D. Improved Effect of Spinach Extract on Physical Performance: A Systematic Review of Randomized Controlled Trials. *Cureus* **2025**, *17*, e77840. [CrossRef]
146. Haynes, J.T.; Townsend, J.R.; Aziz, M.A.; Jones, M.D.; Littlefield, L.A.; Ruiz, M.D.; Johnson, K.D.; Gonzalez, A.M. Impact of Red Spinach Extract Supplementation on Bench Press Performance, Muscle Oxygenation, and Cognitive Function in Resistance-Trained Males. *Sports* **2021**, *9*, 77. [CrossRef] [PubMed]
147. Kovacs, E.M.R.; Stegen, J.H.C.H.; Brouns, F. Effect of Caffeinated Drinks on Substrate Metabolism, Caffeine Excretion, and Performance. *J. Appl. Physiol.* **1998**, *85*, 709–715. [CrossRef] [PubMed]
148. Williams, M. Dietary Supplements and Sports Performance: Herbals. *J. Int. Soc. Sports Nutr.* **2006**, *3*, 1. [CrossRef] [PubMed]
149. Sellami, M.; Slimeni, O.; Pokrywka, A.; Kuvačić, G.; Hayes, L.D.; Milic, M.; Padulo, J. Herbal Medicine for Sports: A Review. *J. Int. Soc. Sports Nutr.* **2018**, *15*, 14. [CrossRef]

150. Szymańska, A.; Nowak, A.; Lipert, A.; Kochan, E. Effect of Ginseng Supplementation on Exercise Endurance as a Support for Cardiovascular Disease Management: A Systematic Review and Meta-Analysis. *Antioxidants* **2025**, *14*, 32. [CrossRef]
151. Bonilla, D.A.; Moreno, Y.; Gho, C.; Petro, J.L.; Odriozola-Martínez, A.; Kreider, R.B. Effects of Ashwagandha (*Withania somnifera*) on Physical Performance: Systematic Review and Bayesian Meta-Analysis. *J. Funct. Morphol. Kinesiol.* **2021**, *6*, 20. [CrossRef]

MDPI AG
Grosspeteranlage 5
4052 Basel
Switzerland
Tel.: +41 61 683 77 34

Nutrients Editorial Office
E-mail: nutrients@mdpi.com
www.mdpi.com/journal/nutrients

www.ingramcontent.com/pod-product-compliance
Lightning Source LLC
Chambersburg PA
CBHW061603210926
51850CB00009B/2194